REHABILITATION MANAGEMENT OF AMPUTEES

This volume is one of the series,
Rehabilitation Medicine Library,
Edited by John V. Basmajian,

New books and new editions published, in press or in preparation for this series:

BANERJEE: Rehabilitation Management of Amputees
BASMAJIAN: Therapeutic Exercise, third edition*
BISHOP: Behavioral Problems and the Disabled: Assessment and Management
BROWNE, KIRLIN AND WATT: Rehabilitation Services and the Social Work Role: Challenge for Change
CHYATTE: Rehabilitation in Chronic Renal Failure
EHRLICH: Rehabilitation Management of Rheumatic Conditions
FISHER AND HELM: Rehabilitation of the Burn Patient
HAAS ET AL: Pulmonary Therapy and Rehabilitation: Principles and Practice
INCE: Behavioral Psychology in Rehabilitation Medicine: Clinical Applications
JOHNSON: Practical Electromyography
LEHMANN: Therapeutic Heat and Cold, third edition*
LONG: Prevention and Rehabilitation in Ischemic Heart Disease
REDFORD: Orthotics Etcetera, second edition*
ROGOFF: Manipulation, Traction and Massage, second edition*
ROY AND TUNKS: Chronic Pain: Psychosocial Factors in Rehabilitation
SHA'KED: Human Sexuality in Rehabilitation Medicine
STILLWELL: Therapeutic Electricity and Ultraviolet Radiation, third edition

* Originally published as part of the Physical Medicine Library, edited by Sidney Licht.

REHABILITATION MANAGEMENT OF AMPUTEES

Edited by

Sikhar Nath Banerjee,

M.B.B.S., F.R.C.P. (C)

Associate Professor, Department of Medicine, McMaster University

Director, Amputee Programme, Chedoke-McMaster Hospitals, Hamilton, Ontario, Canada

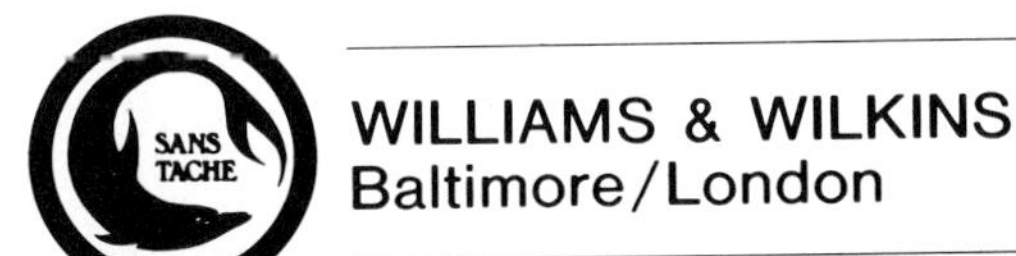

WILLIAMS & WILKINS
Baltimore/London

428 E. Preston Street
Baltimore, Md. 21202, U.S.A.

Made in the United States of America

Library of Congress Cataloging in Publication Data

Main entry under title:

Rehabilitation management of amputees.

(Rehabilitation medicine library)
Includes index.
1. Amputees—Rehabilitation. 2. Prosthesis.
I. Banerjee, Sikhar Nath. II. Series. [DNLM:
1. Amputation—Rehabilitation. 2. Amputees. WE 172 R345]
RD553.R34 362.4′38 81-16295
ISBN 0-683-00470-0 AACR2

Composed and printed at the
Waverly Press, Inc.
Mt. Royal and Guilford Aves.
Baltimore, Md. 21202, U.S.A.

Dedicated to the Memory of
Terry Fox (1958 to 1981)
Who Dreamt the Impossible Dream
and Made It Come True

Series Editor's Foreword

Rehabilitation Management of Amputees is a book that has been needed for several decades. While surgical considerations have been the subject of a considerable number of books and articles in orthopaedics, this is the first comprehensive and thorough book on the broad rehabilitation aspects. The editor and his authors have brought together here all the significant problems and solutions beginning with prevention, *i.e.* the hygienic care of the limbs to make amputation unnecessary, through all the theoretical and practical approaches to achieve the best known results.

The authors include rehabilitation physicians, surgeons, physical and occupational therapists, social workers, and a representative of a large organization of war amputees. These writers have a wide experience and a profound interest in amputation of the limbs and especially the human beings who have lost a precious part of their physical structure. The psychosocial consequences are no less important in rehabilitation and are given prominence in more than just the excellent chapter devoted to them.

The editor, Dr. Banerjee, is my close associate at the Chedoke-McMaster Rehabilitation Centre where I have followed the progress of his special rehabilitation program for amputees. Increasingly, he and his multidisciplinary team of professionals have elaborated better and better techniques for optimizing recovery. Ideally, this must begin with early consultations between the surgeon and those who must accept the responsibility even before the operation is over nowadays. Modern progress in surgery requires at least commensurate progress in rehabilitation. This ideal is far from achieved, but this volume should make a major contribution to achieving it.

The Rehabilitation Medicine Library consists of a burgeoning number of books that are planned to interest a wide spectrum of rehabilitation professionals. This book exemplifies the attempt to interest everyone in rehabilitation while also becoming the touchstone for the narrower band of specialists with a very intense interest in the topic of the book's title.

JOHN V. BASMAJIAN, M.D.

Preface

Our understanding of problems faced by an amputee and available solutions for these problems have undergone radical changes in the last 3 or 4 decades. Health professionals responsible for the care of amputees today, need to understand many aspects of amputee management, even though they may be responsible only for one aspect of patient care relevant to their own expertise. Several books and monographs dealing with part of the total patient management have been available in recent years. It was believed that there exists a need for a book encompassing all aspects of amputee care, taking into account physical, psychosocial, environmental and vocational problems faced by an amputee. This book was designed to meet that need.

This volume has been organized in the same sequential fashion as a prospective amputee might be expected to go through the different phases of his/her treatment, beginning with preoperative assessment and ending with reintegration into family and society. The chapter authors for this book were selected not only on the basis of their academic excellence and many years of experience in amputee rehabilitation, but also because of their lifelong dedication toward improvement of the quality of life for all amputees.

It is hoped that this book will be a resource for current information regarding the basic principles of rehabilitation management of amputees and, also, provide solutions for specific patient problems a health professional might encounter in his/her day-to-day care of patients.

Dr. J. V. Basmajian, the Series Editor, and James L. Sangston, Senior Editor at Williams & Wilkins Company, deserve special thanks for their patience and confidence in the editor and chapter authors. I am personally indebted to my secretary, Catherine Rushton, for typing and retyping many parts of this book and spending many evenings in front of the typewriter far beyond the call of her duties. Roger Young, Ralph Heather and Peter Foulds, of the Audiovisual Department of the Chedoke-McMaster Hospitals, were extremely helpful in preparing several illustrations in this book and my special thanks go to them for responding to my last minute requests. On behalf of all health professionals involved in the care of amputees, I want to express our indebtedness to our patients who have taught us so much and will continue to inspire us to perform better in the future.

Sikhar Nath Banerjee

Contributors

Sikhar Nath Banerjee, M.B.B.S., F.R.C.P.(C)
Associate Professor, Department of Medicine, McMaster University. Director Amputee Programme, Chedoke-McMaster Hospitals, Hamilton, Ontario, Canada

John V. Basmajian, M.D., F.A.C.A., F.R.C.P.(C)
Director, Rehabilitation Programmes, McMaster University School of Medicine Rehabilitation Centre, Chedoke-McMaster Hospitals, Hamilton, Ontario, Canada

Pat Bolton, O.T.(C)
formerly of Community Occupational Therapy Association, Toronto, Ontario, Canada

Ernest M. Burgess, M.D.
Principal Investigator of Prosthetics Research Study, Seattle, Washington

Hugh C. Chadderton, CM, CAE
National Secretary, The War Amputations of Canada, Ottawa, Ontario, Canada

Patricia Ellis, Dip. P. & O.T., M.C.P.A.
Assistant Chief Physical Therapist, Henderson General Hospital, Hamilton, Ontario, Canada

James Foort
Department of Surgery, Faculty of Medicine, University of British Columbia, Vancouver, B.C., Canada

Donald A. Gibson, M.D., F.R.C.S.(C)
Medical Director, Ontario Crippled Children's Centre, Toronto, Ontario, Associate Professor, Department of Surgery and Rehabilitation Medicine, University of Toronto, Ontario, Canada

Hanna Heger, O.T.(C)
Workmen's Compensation Board Hospital and Rehabilitation Centre, Downsview, Ontario, Canada

Dianne Kindon, B.A., M.S.W.
Formerly of Department of Social Work, Chedoke-McMaster Hospitals, Hamilton, Ontario, Canada

V. Nanda Kumar, M.D.
Clinical Assistant Professor in Rehabilitation Medicine, University of Kansas City, Kansas

Gertrude Mensch, M.C.P.A.
Chief Physical Therapist, Henderson General Hospital, Hamilton, Ontario, Canada

Terry Pearce, B.A., B.Ed., M.S.W.
Department of Social Work, Chedoke-McMaster Hospitals, Hamilton, Ontario, Canada

John B. Redford, M.D.
Professor and Chairman, Department of Rehabilitation Medicine, University of Kansas Medical Center, Kansas City, Kansas

George Varghese, M.D.
Assistant Professor, Department of Rehabilitation Medicine, University of Kansas Medical Center, Kansas City, Kansas

A. Bennett Wilson, Jr., B.Sc. (Mech. Eng.)
Formerly of Division of Orthopaedics, Southwestern Medical School, The University of Texas Health Science Center at Dallas, Dallas, Texas

Contents

1

Limb Amputation—Incidence, Causes, and Prevention

S. N. BANERJEE, B.SC., M.B.B.S., F.R.C.P.(C)

Amputation of any part of the human body is the most destructive and mutilating procedure that a human being may endure during his life. The scar left by the procedure is much more devastating than one sees by looking at the residual part.

Moreover, amputation of an extremity is quite frequently a symptomatic treatment and rarely cures the underlying cause, and the procedure may have to be repeated for another extremity affected by the same underlying disease. Therefore, rehabilitation management of the amputee requires understanding of the nature of multidimensional effects of amputation on the affected person and his environment, as well as expertise in each area in order to facilitate full functional restoration. This understanding helped establish multidisciplinary amputee clinic teams after the Second World War when the civilized world was suddenly faced with thousands of young amputees who had survived the ordeal, unlike their forefathers during previous wars.

Historical Perspective

Archeological evidence suggests that Neanderthal man may have survived amputation of the limbs, and Rig Veda mentions artificial limbs, but whether these amputations were done for disease conditions still remain unclear (18). As with any other facets of medicine, Hippocrates is credited as being the first in describing amputation as a planned surgical procedure for saving life. William Clowes (1588) apparently carried out the first above-knee amputation, though, Paré (1515) illustrated an above-knee prosthesis (18).

The current practice of amputation surgery and prosthetics owes a great deal to the research and developments during and after the First and Second World Wars. Before the Second World War, the residual limb use to be considered as a passive structure and surgeons tried to design a conical stump by allowing the muscles to retract. It was not until after the Second World War that myoplasty became a standard procedure for amputations at all levels and the residual limb became a dynamic structure providing power and proprioception to the amputee for successful use of the prosthesis. Berlemont *et al.* (2) presented their pioneering work on immediate postoperative fitting, and later Weiss (19) and Burgess *et al.* (3) modified this technique for dysvascular amputees. Inman, Eberhart and Radcliffe at the Biomechanics Laboratory at the Univesity of California in Berkeley carried out a detailed study of human locomotion and, as a continuation of this work, designed a quadrilateral suction socket for above-knee (1955) (11a) and patellar tendon bearing (PTB) socket for below-knee amputation (1958) (11b). The Canadian Department of Veterans Affairs (20) designed the Canadian hip disarticulation socket (1954) and Syme prosthesis (1955). These four basic socket types for lower extremity amputation still remain the most commonly used sockets although there have been various modifications of these sockets in order to satisfy individual needs of patients. When one reviews the developments in upper extremity prosthetics it becomes quite apparent that apart from externally powered prostheses there have been no revolutionary changes in upper extremity prostheses. The hook remains the most universally used terminal device as it has been for several centuries. The electronic hand does not provide any more additional function to the amputee apart from three-jaw chuck grip which is not much different from the old mechanical hand. Possibly for these reasons, the rejection rate of a prosthesis by unilateral arm amputees still remains rather high.

Incidence of Amputation

The incidence and causes of amputation varies widely throughout the world. Accurate statistical data on the incidence of amputation in the world is difficult if not impossible to obtain. According to the Committee on Prosthetics Research and Development of the National Academy of Sciences, there were 311,000 persons in the United States in 1971 with major extremity amputation (10). Annual incidence of major extremity amputation in the United States during this period was 43,000. In 1970 there were 6528 amputations of extremities done in Canada as reported by *Statistics Canada* (14). Of these, 2593 were major amputations excluding minor amputations of toes and fingers. Corresponding figures for 1975 were 7081 and 3294, respectively (15). This modest increase can be accounted for by the increase in the population. Between 1970 and 1975 there has been no significant change in the incidence of amputation in Canada when one considers the rate per 100,000 populatioon. In 1970 the amputation rate in Canada was 30.5, as opposed to 30/100,000 population in 1975.

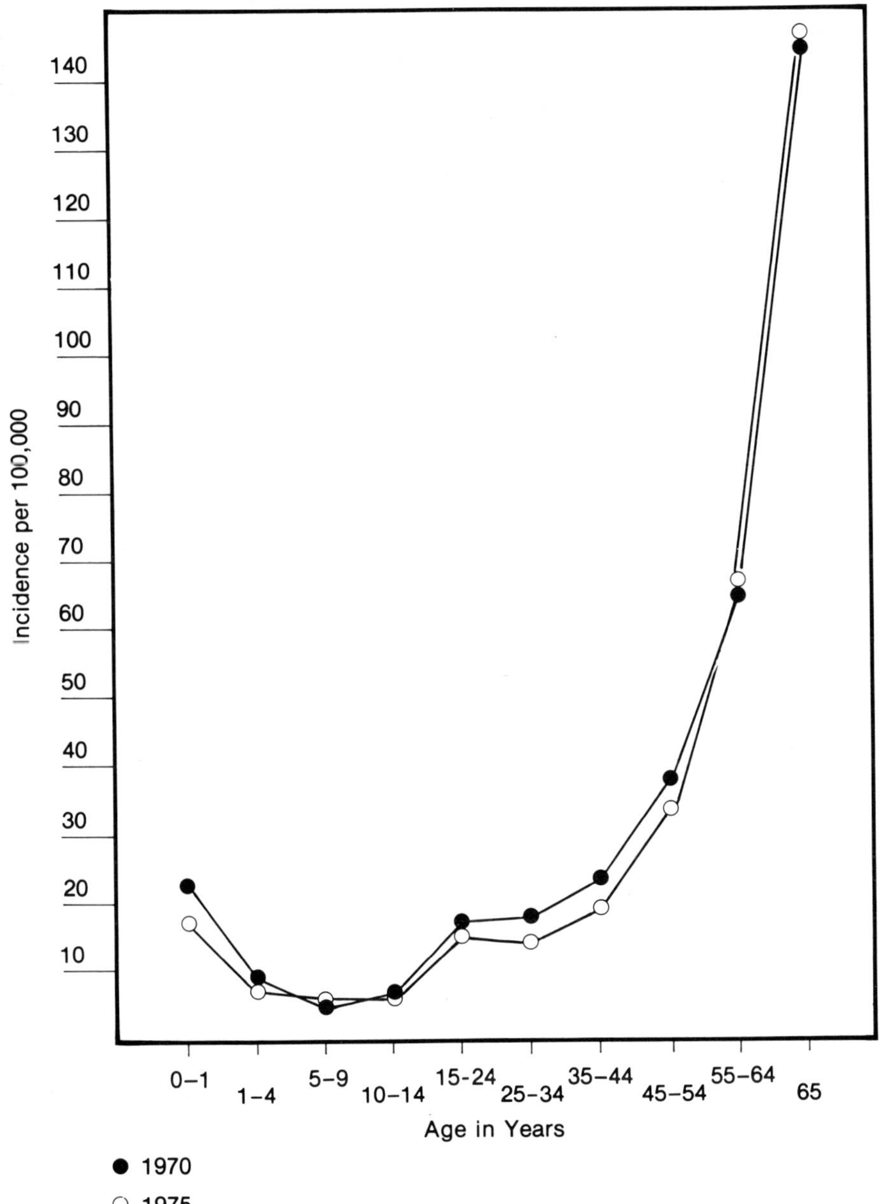

Fig. 1.1. Incidence of amputation per 100,000 population in different age groups in Canada.

The distribution of amputation done in different age groups shows a characteristic pattern (Fig. 1.1). The incidence in the 1st year of life is higher and this can be accounted for on the basis of congenital limb deficiencies. From the age of 1–15 years, the incidence remains fairly constant and there is a gradual rise up to the age of 54 related to increased exposure to trauma at work and highway traffic. From age 55 and upwards there is a sharp increase in the incidence indicating a larger number of patients with peripheral vascular disease. Hansson (7) in his study of incidence of leg amputation in Göteborg, Sweden, reported a similar rise in the amputation rate among men over 60 years of age. He also noted that the incidence of leg amputations due to peripheral vascular disease has risen sharply between the periods of 1926 and 1955. In 1926 only 2% of patients fitted with lower limb prostheses had amputations due to peripheral vascular disease and in 1955 this figure had risen to 57%. Both Canadian and Göteborg statistical data indicate distinct preponderance of males in all age groups. The male/female ratio in the Göteborg series (7) was 1.4:1 and in the 1975 Canadian data (15) the ratio was 2.2:1. In the Göteborg series, the male preponderance is more marked among amputees under 60 years old (4.1:1) than in amputees over 60 years old (1.2:1).

Levels of Amputation

It is common knowledge that in clinics one sees more lower extremity amputees than upper extremity amputees. However, when one takes into account all amputations including toes and fingers this disparity of numbers is not so evident. In 1975 the ratio of lower and upper extremity amputations in Canada was 2.4:1 (15). If, however, one excludes the minor toe and finger amputations, then the preponderance of lower extremity amputations become more evident. In fact the ratio between lower and upper exremities climbs to 16:1. Glattly (6) reported a 3-year survey (1961–1963) by the National Academy of Sciences which showed that 85% of all amputees surveyed had major lower extremity amputations. Vitali (18) reported a similar ratio between lower and upper extremity amputees in a survey of several thousand amputees between 1959 and 1973.

The distribution of various levels of amputation in the amputee population varies widely depending on the availability of advance techniques for level determination, quality of surgical care, and the socioeconomic status of the population. However, there are some similarities between amputee populations when one compares the various levels of amputation. Table 1.1 shows two populations where data was collected at two different stages. The Glattly data (6) was collected from 1961–1963 through prosthetic shops in various parts of the United States and, as such, excludes patients who did not attend prosthetic facilities. The Statistics Canada data (15) were compiled from hospital records of the year 1975 and specific percentage figures for various levels have been calculated by the author on the basis of raw data.

As pointed out earlier, the specific level of amputation is influenced, among other factors, by the philosophy with regard to amputee care at the institution. This is particularly true when dealing with an elderly person facing an amputation for peripheral vascular disease. Sarmiento *et al.* (12)

TABLE 1.1

Levels of amputation	Glattly (1964) (6)	Statistics Canada (1975) (15)
	%	%
Shoulder disarticulation	1.1	0.07
Elbow disarticulation and above-elbow	4	2.3
Wrist disarticulation and below-elbow	9.4	2.4
Hip disarticulation	1.8	1.2
Knee disarticulation and above-knee	45.2	45
Below-knee	36.8	38
Syme	1.7	10 (includes foot)

TABLE 1.2

Levels of amputation	Initial	Final
Knee disarticulation and above-knee	31	43
Below-knee	157	145
Syme	2	2

in reviewing lower extremity amputations at the University of Miami during the period 1960 through 1968, found a complete reversal of ratio between amputations performed at above-knee and below-knee levels. During the period 1960–1963, out of a total of 297 cases 69.3% had an above-knee amputation and 28% had a below-knee amputation. However, during the next 4 years (1964–1968), out of a total of 328 cases, 17% had above-knee and 68% had below-knee amputations. The reamputations from below-knee to above-knee level were 47.6% in the earlier series and only 7.5% in the later cases. This trend of making every effort to save the knee, especially when dealing with an elderly patient with peripheral vascular disease, has been noted in various other centers. Burgess *et al.* (4) in 1971 reported results of amputations performed in 177 patients with peripheral vascular disease. In total, 190 amputations were performed using the rigid dressing immediate postsurgical prosthetic regimen developed at the Seattle Prosthetic Research Study Center. Table 1.2 is a breakdown of levels of amputation.

Again in this series (4), 78% of amputations at below-knee level healed and only 22% required above-knee or knee disarticulation. Only 6% of patients required above-knee amputation who had below-knee amputations initially. The author attributed this failure to an incorrect level selection by the surgeon.

In spite of this overwhelming evidence, one still sees too many above-knee amputations being performed in elderly dysvascular patients. It is high time that rehabilitation teams looking after amputees send a plea to the surgeon—"Surgeon spare that knee," as suggested by Newton McCollough III (10).

Causes of Amputation

"For the management of the problem of prevention of amputation and rehabilitation of amputees a reasonable knowledge of incidence and causation is indispensable."

The above remark by Dr. Knud Jansen (8) is still valid today when one considers the importance of prevention of unnecessary limb loss. The cause of amputations and their frequency among a population varies considerably between developing nations of the east and the industrialized nations of the west. In eastern developing countries, trauma, infection and Buerger's disease are three leading causes of amputation, and amputation due to atherosclerosis is a rather uncommon occurrence. On the other hand, in the Western industrialized world, atherosclerosis including diabetes is the leading cause for amputation except during periods of war when one sees large numbers of young traumatic amputees. Nonetheless, atherosclerosis is the major cause of amputation today. Hansson (7) in his detailed review of leg amputations in Göteborg pointed out that the increased number of amputations due to atherosclerosis is a comparatively recent phenomenon. In 1926 only 2% of amputees fitted with lower limb prosthesis had amputation due to vascular disease, whereas in 1955 the corresponding figure was 55%. In spite of rapid industrialization and extensive use of automobiles during this period, incidence of traumatic amputation in Göteborg remained rather low at around 5–8/100,000 population. In contrast, the incidence of amputation due to vascular disease rose sharply to over 30/100,000 population. It is difficult to pinpoint the reasons behind this sharp rise in the number of dysvascular amputees but the increasing number of elderly people in society as well as the affluence of western society during the post-World War II period may be contributory factors to this change.

The published report on causes of amputation shows wide variation depending upon the size of population surveyed, the method and location of survey, as well as time and place of survey. Many surveys were done by reviewing the amputees attending prosthetic shops, which tend to show a much larger proportion of traumatic amputees who are usually younger and in better health than the dysvascular amputee, many of whom may not be a user of a prosthesis. Glattly's 1961–1963 survey (6) of 7625 amputees through prosthetic shops showed the following breakdown of causes.

Traumatic	2573	(33.3%)
Disease	4491	(58%)
Tumour	257	(3.3%)
Congenital	304	(4%)

Glattly (5) reported that 85% of all amputations done in Massachusetts General Hospital during the period 1962–1964 were due to peripheral vascular disease. Similarly Hierton and James (1973) (7a) reviewed lower extremity amputations in Uppsala County, Sweden, between 1967–1969;

peripheral vascular disease accounted for 93% of all lower extremity amputation. It is apparent that an accurate estmate of incidence and cause of amputation only can be made through review of hospital records serving a large population and, when feasible, on a nationwide basis. Detailed information and analysis regarding incidence, level and causes will be essential in launching any program directed towards every possible prevention of amputation.

Prevention of Amputation

It is apparent from the limited information that is available about cause of amputations that peripheral vascular disease is the single most important causal factor for amputation of an extremity in the western world. Ideally, if one is able to prevent or cure peripheral vascular disease, then amputation of extremities will be a thing of the past. However, in reality, the exact cause and mechanism of production of atherosclerosis is unknown, although our knowledge about this ubiquitous diseae has increased significantly in the last 3 or 4 decades.

Elimination of Risk Factors

Several risk factors were identified in Framingham study (9) as contributory factors for production of coronary artery disease. These were elevated serum cholesterol (>240 mgm/dl) elevated systolic blood pressure (>160 mm Hg) and smoking more than 20 cigarettes daily. One may conclude that elimination of these risk factors may be helpful in prevention of atherosclerosis disease of the lower extremities. It appears that in addition to the measurement of simple serum cholesterol, electrophoretic separation of different fractions of serum lipoprotiens also may be helpful in identifying and treating different types of lipoproteinemia. In recent years there has been considerable excitement regarding the role of high density lipoprotein (HDL) in protecting against atherosclerotic diseases (17). There is a strong inverse relation between plasma HDL and mortality from cardiovascular disease. The level of HDL in serum can be raised by replacing saturated animal fat with unsaturated vegetable fat. Also, increased fiber content of the diet tends to increase the HDL level in serum. There is increasing evidence that lack of physical exercise is another risk factor in the production of atherosclerotic disease. There is now strong evidence that regular continuous physical exercise not only improves cardiac and pulmonary efficiency but it has a favorable effect on hormonal regulation and metabolism of cholesterol and lipids (13).

The relation between identifiable risk factors and atherosclerosis is a statistical one and other factors like heredity, environment, occupation, etc., may be equally important in production of atherosclerosis and cannot be eliminated. However, based on current knowledge, the following measures may reduce the early onset and progression of atherosclerosis.

1. Early treatment and control of hypertension
2. Stoppage of tobacco smoking
3. Restriction of animal fat and increased fiber content diet
4. Regular continuous level of physical activity
5. Maintenance of appropriate body weight

Preventive Measures for Patients Suffering from Atherosclerosis of Lower Extremities

Once the patient has developed symptoms of atherosclerosis of lower extremities, such as claudication pain, elimination of risk factors may still have beneficial effect but, equally important, is the care of the affected extremity. It appears that many amputations can be delayed for some time if not totally prevented, provided the patient is aware of the disease and knowledgeable in the care of the ischemic extremity. Elderly people may not experience claudication pain in the early stages of the disease because of lack of vigorous exercise, and the disease may remain undiagnosed for years. So it is vitally important to examine the peripheral circulation especially when examining an elderly person for routine office visit. It is not unusual to detect bruits over the major arteries or absence of a peripheral pulse even though the patient may not complain of any specific symptoms. For these patients, following simple measures will go a long way towards prevention of unnecessary early amputation of a leg, thus:

1. *Avoid trauma to the affected extremities.* A simple injury to the skin while cutting toe-nails may get infected and require amputation. Elderly people with poor vision should be advised to seek help for cutting nails and over-enthusiastic chiropody should be avoided. Ill-fitting shoes can cause blisters, so soft shoes with a wide toe box are recommended. The patient should avoid exposure of the extremity to extremes of temperature because ischemic extremity is more prone to thermal burn. Similarly, application of harsh chemicals should be avoided. The patient and family should be advised to seek medical help immediately if they notice any skin breakdown of the extremity.
2. The patient should be advised about the constricting effects of elastics in socks and stockings which will reduce blood flow further.
3. Proper hygiene of the affected extremities is crucially important. Daily washing with soap and lukewarm water followed by pat drying with a towel may prevent skin lesions produced by poor hygiene.
4. The patient should be advised on a simple daily exercise program. Most patients with claudication pain will improve their claudication distance on a daily program of brisk walking (1). Prompt attention to any systemic illness which may cause sudden drop in systolic blood pressure (myocardial infarction, gastrointestinal bleeding, sepsis, etc.) cannot be overemphasized. When treating an elderly patient

with hypotensive drugs for hypertension, one must be extra careful about an excessive fall of systolic blood pressure causing further ischemia.

Prevention of Traumatic Amputation

The causes of traumatic amputation varies widely in different parts of the world. Vitali (18) in his study of amputees referred to the limb-fitting service of England, Wales and Northern Ireland during a period of 1959–1975 noted that the causes of traumatic amputation remained fairly constant. Of all traumatic amputations, 40% were industrial and 40% were due to traffic accidents. The remaining 20% were accounted for by house accidents, armed forces and recreation activities. With the inceasing use of farm machinery in modern agriculture, one might expect a large number of amputations in the farming industry. In Ontario, Canada, there were only 35 major amputations in 1980 in accidents related to farming (16) compared to an average of 1400 major amputations (11) done in the province in a given year for other causes.

It is obvious that many traumatic amputations can be avoided by adopting proper safety measures in operating industrial and farm machineries. Also, increased emphasis on the manufacture of safe automobiles and reduction of speed limits on highways have resulted in a considerable decrease in unnecessary loss of life and limbs on our highways. It is unfortunate that similar emphasis has not been placed on manufacture and operation of safe farm machines. Too often, little children become victims of these monstrous machines, causing unnecessary loss of limbs. In 1980 in Ontario, children aged 15 and under formed 2.1% of all victims of farm accidents and people between ages of 16–25 formed the largest percentage (42.3%) among all age groups (16). One may conclude that lack of knowledge and experience in safety methods may be contributing to these accidents.

Conclusion

In order to make effective planning for amputee care, either on a regional or national basis, it is essential to have data regarding the exact incidence and causes of amputation. At present, detailed data regarding incidence and regional or national variation in incidence is not available. Similarly, there are significant differences in causes of amputation and their distribution in a given amputee population. There is a definite need for collection of these data on a national and international basis for adequate planning of amputee care facilities, as well as prevention of amputation of extremities when feasible.

REFERENCES

1. ALPERT, J. S., LARSEN, O. A., AND LASSEN, N. A. Exercise and Intermittent Claudication Blood Flow in Calf Muscle During Walking studied by the Xenon 133 Clearance Method. *Circulation, 39:* 353–359, 1969.

2. Berlemont, M., Weber, R., and Willot, J. P.Ten Years of Experience with the Immediate Application of Prosthetic Devices to Amputees of the Lower Extemities on the Operating Table. *Prosthet. Int., 3:* 8–18, 1969.
3. Burgess, E. M., Romano, R. L., and Zettl, J. H. Amputation Management Utilizing Immediate Postsurgical Prosthetic Fitting. *Prosthet. Int., 3:* 28–37, 1969.
4. Burgess, E. M., Romano, R. L., Zettl, J. H., and Schrock, R. D. Amputations of the Leg For Peripheral Vascular Insufficiency. J. Bone Jt. Surg., *53A:* 874–890, 1971.
5. Glattly, H. W. Aging and Amputation. *Artif. Limbs, 10:* 1–4, 1966.
6. Glattly, H. W. A Preliminary Report on the Amputee Census Selected Articles from Artificial Limbs, pp. 319–324. R. E. Krieger, New York, 1970.
7. Hansson, J. The Leg Amputee: A Clinical Follow-up Study. *Acta Orthop. Scand. Suppl. 69,* 1964.
7a.Hierton, T., and James, U. Lower extremity amputation in upsala county 1947–1969. Incidence and prosthetic rehabilitation. *Acta Orthop. Scand. 44:* 573–582, 1973.
8. Jansen, K. Amputation: Frequency and Causes—Prosthetics International. *Proceedings of the Second International Prosthetics Course,* Copenhagen, 1960.
9. Kagan, A., Kannel, W. B., and Dawber, T. R., *et al.* The Coronary Profile. *Ann. NY Acad. Sci., 97:* 883, 1962.
10. McCollough, N. C., III, Shea, J. D., Warren, W. D., and Sarmiento, A. The Dysvascular Amputee: Surgery and Rehabilitation. *Curr. Probl. Surg.,* P.5, 1971.
11. Ministry of Health, Province of Ontario Information Systems Division Publications, Ontario, 1978.
11a.Radcliffe, C. W. Functional considerations in fitting of above-knee prosthesis. *Artif. Limbs 2:* 35–60, 1955.
11b.Radcliffe, C. W., and Foort, J. *The Patellar Tendon Bearing Below-Knee Prosthesis.* Biomechanics Laboratory University of California, Berkeley and San Francisco, 1961.
12. Sarmiento, A., May, B. J., Sinclair, W. F., McCollough, N. C., III, and Williams, E. M. Lower Extremity Amputation, *Clin. Orthop. Relat. Res., 00:* 22–31, 1970.
13. Simko, V. Physical Exercise and the Prevention of Atherosclerosis and Cholesterol Gall Stones: *Postgrad. Med. J., 54:* 270–277, 1978.
14. Surgical Procedures and Treatments. *Statistics Canada.* Ministry, Trade and Commerce, Ottowa, Canada, 1970.
15. Surgical Procedures and Treatments. *Statistics Canada.* Ministry, Trade and Commerce, Ottowa, Canada, 1975.
16. Survey of Agricultural Lost Time Injuries for the Year 1980. Farm Safety Association Inc., Ontario, April 1981.
17. Tall, A.-R., and Small, D. M. Current Concepts: Plasma High-Density Lipoproteins. *N. Engl. J. Med., 299:* 1232–1236, 1978.
18. Vitali, M., Robinson, K. P., Andrews, B. G., and Harris, E. E. *Amputations and Prostheses,* pp. 2–12. Bailliere Tindall 1978.
19. Weiss, M. Physiologic Amputation—Immediate Prosthesis and Early Ambulation. *Prosthet. Int., 3:* 38–44, 1969.
20. Wilson, A. B., Jr. Limb prosthetics today. *Artif. Limbs 7:* 1–42, 1963.

2

Preoperative Assessment and Management of Amputees

GEORGE VARGHESE, M.D.
JOHN B. REDFORD, M.D.

Many people regard amputation of a limb as a catastrophic disability; one which produces a profound emotional response due to its effect on body image as well as a serious loss of functional ability. Therefore, it is crucial to managing prospective amputees that wise counseling be given prior to amputation on the possibilities of functional restoration and outlook for the future. Although great strides have been made in recent years in the surgical management of peripheral vascular disease and saving limbs with primary tumors and through reimplantation, the incidence of amputations, particularly for peripheral vascular disease, remains high. Amputation, unfortunately, is considered by many physicians primarily as a failure of medical or surgical treatment of arteriosclerosis or other disease processes. It really should be considered as another option in restoration of functional use of the extremity. In fact, in spite of all the publicity surrounding limb reimplantation, amputation actually might be better for the patient in many instances (1). With appropriate rehabilitation, it is quite possible for most amputees to return to a normal, productive life even with multiple limb deficiencies.

Ideally, the surgeon who does the amputation should have a thorough knowledge of the functional implications of various levels of amputation and types of prostheses available for these levels. Unfortunately, all too often this is not the case. If the surgeon does not have the time or knowledge to discuss the postamputation rehabilitation, he should consult another physician who specializes in the amputee rehabilitation. This phase of patient care is too important simply to be assigned to a nonphysician. The physician consultant should evaluate the patient and prescribe physical therapy and occupational therapy if needed and make necessary suggestions as to prosthetic possibilities and thus help prepare the patient emotionally for the amputation.

Preoperative Counseling

The emotional impact of a decision to amputate is tremendous, both on the patient and on his family. Few persons can face the mutilation of a body part and the associated functional loss with equanimity. Nevertheless, all too often, the patient goes to the operating room without any idea of what is going to happen to his limb or what kind of functional restoration he can anticipate following the amputation. He may have no idea what an artificial limb looks like; perhaps all he knows is hearsay about peg legs for lower limbs or hooks for upper limbs. Some authority must explain to him that even though the artificial limb cannot totally replace all previous function, it can replace much of it, at least in lower limb amputations. In some instances of severe deformities, the prosthesis may actually supply better function than the pathological limb. For example, the patient that has suffered for years from osteomyelitis with numerous operations, hospitalizations and braces, may have his/her life style completely changed by a successful prosthetic restoration. In addition, the prospective amputee should understand the postoperative care complications like phantom sensation and pain, the rehabilitation program and the functional possibilities. A patient who is emotionally prepared for amputation obviously will have a more positive attitude towards rehabilitation (3, 5). In spite of this, it is not always possible to prepare the patient emotionally; the amputation may be done on an emergency basis or the patient may be too toxic to understand the seriousness of the surgery. Whenever possible, in such cases, the patient's family should be counseled.

Surgeons usually explain to the patient and his family the necessity for, and the proposed level of, amputation. However, if the surgeon is not the physician who will prescribe the prosthesis, then the consulting physician and those involved in postoperative rehabilitation should evaluate and counsel the patient preoperatively as well as postoperatively. They should tell the patient how much functional loss he/she can anticipate, outline the training program and timing of the phases of prosthetic fitting and discuss possible postoperative complications that may delay rehabilitation. Special emphasis must be made on the phantom limb phenomenon. Patients should be reassured that phantom sensation occurs as a natural reaction and so they should not consider that they are crazy or are hallucinating when they still feel their absent limb with perhaps some persistent pain.

In those patients considered for immediate postoperative prosthetic fitting, it is particularly important to have the program explained in detail.

Actual demonstration of a prosthesis or illustrations presented to the patient preoperatively will be helpful in many cases. Finally, if it seems warranted in a particularly anxious patient, a successful prosthetic wearer might be introduced preoperatively to discuss his personal experiences with rehabilitation.

Assessment of Medical Problems

Many prospective amputees are elderly. The ravages of age, particularly on the cardiovascular and musculoskeletal systems and on the patient's functional status must be evaluated. In an elderly person, if a wheelchair is the only possible form of future ambulation, this could be helpful in deciding the amputation level. In cases where other extremities are already amputated, the functional restoration following previous amputations must be reviewed. If the patient did not learn prosthetic ambulation after the first lower limb amputation, predictably he/she will not ambulate with the second amputation. However, before definitely rejecting the patient for postoperative fitting with a prosthesis, it must be established whether his previous problems were some irreversible medical complications rather than a result of poor prosthetic fitting and training.

It is particularly important to assess the patient's cardiovascular and pulmonary status. Obviously a patient with Class IV cardiac decompensation or with a serious obstructive pulmonary disease is not likely to walk with a prosthesis. Even in young persons with the very best fitted artificial lower limb, prosthetic wear inevitably increases the demands on the cardiovascular system above normal (9). Under certain circumstances, even though the patient may not be able to walk, a limb might still be considered feasible as he/she will need it for transfer from the wheelchair.

Other bodily systems requiring particular medical attention are the neurologic and musculoskeletal systems. Persons with serious neurologic deficits such as paralysis or sensory loss present problems for a successful rehabilitation (8). It should be noted, however, that even blindness may not be a contraindication to prosthetic fitting. Each neurologic deficit must be evaluated in relation to function. The patient also must be evaluated preoperatively for contractures in the limbs. These possibly may respond to treatment prior to amputaton. Finally, manual muscle tests should be conducted as part of the preoperative evaluation so that, if necessary, strengthening programs for muscles weakened by disuse can commence (2).

Patients with arthritis may present special problems in preoperative assessment. Control of active inflammation by drugs, physical therapy measures to relieve pain and exercises to increase range of motion all may be required in the preoperative phase.

Level of Amputation

As mentioned earlier, amputation should not merely be considered as a last desperate effort to save life, but rather as a step in functional restoration, particularly in the patient with peripheral vascular disease. Therefore, the criteria for selection of amputation level should not be restricted to the extent of pathology or certainty of primary wound healing. Wound healing is a prime consideration but surgeons also should consider functional goals when faced with the decision of where to amputate in peripheral vascular disease. If the patient has flexion contractures of the hip or knee, for example, this will pose serious problems in prosthetic fitting. Any hip flexion contracture of more than 30° and a long stump in an above-knee amputee will make fitting very difficult. In such cases, rather than leave a long stump, the surgeon should select a more proximal level as fitting may then be somewhat easier (6). A similar problem may be anticipated with a knee flexion contracture of more than 15° (6); in such cases, a long below-knee stump must be avoided. Saving a knee in an elderly person will increase the odds for successful walking with a prosthesis by 50%. As a below-knee prosthesis requires much less energy to walk than an above knee one, the cardiovascular system is spared considerable stress. Therefore, it is universally accepted that the surgeon should try to save the knee whenever possible in patients with peripheral vascular disease. However, some exceptions from this rule may have to be made. After a thorough assessment, some patients may be considered most unlikely to ambulate after the amputation. A patient who is totally wheelchair dependent prior to amputation or one who has severe cardiac or pulmonary problems would fall into this category. In such cases, saving the knee does not have any advantage in rehabilitation. If the patient is to sit in a wheelchair, he will develop flexion contractures in the knee. A flexion contracture makes dressing very difficult and also increases the possibility of pressure sores developing at the end of the stump (4). An above-knee amputation in such cases not only avoids these complications but may reduce hospital stay because of faster wound healing.

Although, generally, the rule for the lower extremity is to select the level that is compatible with best healing, in the upper extremity functional considerations are of even more importance. In any upper limb amputation, the rule should be to save the greatest possible length. Even an extremely short below-elbow amputation is preferable to an above-elbow one.

Selection of Patients for Immediate Postoperative Fitting

There is overwhelming evidence that a rigid dressing immediately after amputation will reduce stump edema and thus facilitate early prosthetic fitting and combat the effects of prolonged immobilization of the amputee. The disadvantage of the technique has been the difficulty in checking the stump for wound infection and other problems in the immediate postoperative phase as the stump is covered with a rigid plaster dressing. Thus, the surgeon must rely on subjective reports of the patient or laboratory data to assess wound healing. If the patient can not report any increase in pain or other odd sensations during the wound healing period, it will be impossible to determine whether infection has developed. Obviously, therefore, the patient should be alert and oriented if he/she is to be considered for an immediate postoperative rigid dresssing. Sensory loss in the extremity also will make it difficult to tell whether healing has occurred. Another factor to be considered for the immediate postoperative fitting technique in lower limb amputees is the presence of contractures either in the affected limb or in the opposite lower extremity. Any deformities or significant impairments affecting the opposite side make early ambulation difficult in the immediate postoperative period. If the patient already has had an amputation on the other side, one must be certain that he/she was ambulating successfully with that prosthesis prior to planning immediate postoperative fitting of the contemplated amputation.

Another possible contraindication for the technique would be the presence of an unresolved medical condition such as an acute myocardial infarction and heart failure. Finally, a patient with a florid infection on the diseased side is not a good candidate for immediate postoperative fitting.

Even if ambulation in the immediate postoperative period is not a consideration, rigid dressings do reduce edema of the stump. Therefore, whenever possible, rigid dressings are recommended even if the patient is unlikely to be walking with a prosthesis.

Although much less has been written about the postoperative rigid dressings in the upper extremities, they also should be considered in some cases (7). The old rule about waiting 6 weeks before fitting any patient with a prosthesis must be discarded. Rigid dressings make it possible to fit patients with permanent prostheses as early as 3 weeks in an uncomplicated case. However, this is possible only with adequate resources for full follow-up by a prosthetic rehabilitation team.

Further Preoperative Considerations

It is not unusual for many potential amputees to spend weeks or months in hospitals undergoing treatment for medical complications during their surgical treatment for peripheral vascular disease. These immobilized patients are subject to potential threats of general deconditioning, disuse atrophy, thrombophlebitis, pulmonary embolism, decubitus ulcers and joint contractures. Exercise in the preoperative period definitely will help avoid many of these complications. Ideally, all patients admitted with a diagnosis of peripheral vascular disease should be evaluated for appropriate exercise program. This program should include strengthening of the trunk and both upper limbs as well as the uninvolved lower limb. Range of motion in the affected limb and careful attention to posture in bed or in a wheelchair will prevent contracture formation. The patient also should be instructed in a daily breathing exercise program and where possible, repetitive type conditioning exercises. A patient, so prepared, will be assured of much better success in early prosthetic restoration as he will not require strengthening and reconditioning of the remaining limbs.

Although the physical and occupational therapist have a major role in preparing the patient for ambulation, services provided by a hospital social worker should not be overlooked. Through interviews with the patient's family members and others in the patient's social environment, the patient's psychosocial functioning can be assessed prior to the surgery. Thus, problems with housing, finances, social isolation, and family relationships can be anticipated and perhaps dealt with more effectively than waiting until after the amputation has occurred. Ultimately, psychosocial factors often prove more important than the surgical pathology in determining successful rehabilitation.

Conclusion

Preoperative assessment and management of potential amputees is an important but unfortunately overlooked part of the overall rehabilitation process in such patients. If the surgeon is too preoccupied with other activities, he should call on the rehabilitation consultant who will set up a preoperativee program assisted by other members of the rehabilitation team. Such a procedure will insure a smooth transition for the anxious, depressed patient faced with the devastating prospect of losing a limb. We suspect that considerable emotional turmoil could be avoided if all potential amputees were thoroughly assessed prior to their amputation.

REFERENCES

1. Friedmann, L. W. Amputation or Re-Implantation: Which is Better for the Patient? *Nassau County Med. Center Proc., Autumn:* 171–173, 1979.
2. Friedmann, L. W. The Rehabilitation of the Amputee, *Lex Et Scientia 7:* 129–135, 1971.
3. Mital, M., and Pierce, D. Impact of Amputation on the Patient and Society. *Amputee and Prosthesis*, Little Brown, Boston, 1971.
4. Mooney, V., Wagner, F., Waddell, J., and Ackerson, T. The Below-the-Knee Amputation for Vascular Disease. *J. Bone Jt. Surg., 58A:* 365–368, 1976.
5. Murdoch, G. Amputation Surgery in the Lower Extremity. *Prosthet. Orthot. Int., 1:* 72–83, 1977.
6. Murdoch, G. Levels of Amputation and Limiting Factors. *Ann. R. Coll. Surg. Engl., 40:* 206–216, 1967.
7. Romano, R., and Burgess, E. The Immediate Postsurgical Prosthetic Fitting Technique Applied to Child Amputees. *Inter-Clinic Information Bulletin, 9:* June, 1970.
8. Varghese, G., Hinterbuchner, C., Mondall, P., and Sakuma, J. Rehabilitation Outcome of Patients with Dual Disability of Hemiplegia and Amputation. *Arch. Phys. Med. Rehabil., 59:* 121–123, 1978.
9. Waters, R. L., Perry, J., Antonelli, D., and Hislap, H. Energy Cost of Walking of Amputees: The Influence of Level of Amputation. *J. Bone Jt. Surg., 58A:* 42–45, 1976.

3

Amputation Surgery and Postoperative Care

ERNEST M. BURGESS, M.D.

Few conditions leave the body more disfigured than major amputation. Successful prosthetic substitution can restore function and appearance yet each day upon removal of the substitute limb the amputee is faced with the stark reality of the missing part. The surgeon performing the amputation or revision is, by the nature of his responsibility, the primary source of confidence and communication. His sensitivity and positive approach will initiate successful rehabilitation.

Amputation presents the surgeon with two directives. He must first remove the diseased or damaged part. This, the amputation, is a completely destructive surgical exercise. The second directive is exactly the opposite. The surgeon now constructs a physiological end organ, the residual limb. He is committed to restore as completely as he can, a residual limb that will provide the amputee, through the limb substitute, the best available functional contact with the environment. When viewed in this true context, amputation surgery is, in fact, plastic and reconstructive. It presents a surgical challenge certainly equivalent to peripheral vascular reconstruction or to joint reconstructive surgery.

Amputation surgery and prosthetic rehabilitation have improved remarkably during the past decade. This progress is accelerating. Traditionally, interest in amputations has been high during major wars then lagged behind other surgical achievements in peacetime. The interest in amputation surgery generated by World War II has continued on to the present. Rapidly increasing numbers of amputations required for peripheral vascular disease largely account for this circumstance. Great technical advances in areas related to prosthetics, (*i.e.* electronics; materials, especially synthetic composites; biological design engineering; and evaluation devices) all are adding rapidly to prosthetic improvements, thereby enhancing restoration. In amputation surgery as with prosthetics and other areas of amputee rehabilitation, technical advancement is outstripping knowledge dissemination. This information lag needs to be promptly bridged.

Surgical Principles

The goal of amputation surgery is to provide a physiological residual limb. A great wealth of biomechanical information exists to inform the surgeon of arm and leg function. Guided by these principles, that portion of the limb remaining after amputation should be designed surgically to retain the maximum degree of painless sensory and motor capability (Fig. 3.1).

Amputation Levels

Sites of election of amputation are listed in most surgical texts. The so-called desirable levels are based on the cross-sectional anatomy of the tissues at the level selected and on the availability of appropriate prosthetic substitutes. These long accepted conventional elective sites are now obsolete. Modern surgical techniques and currently available prostheses permit, with few exceptions, maximum conservation of limb length. Unrestrained by the dogma of elective site selection, the surgeon is free to innovate and individualize case by case. This is the basic principle of physiological amputation surgery. There still are, however, a few amputation levels best avoided. All other levels are "sites of election" when the anatomical and surgical circumstances indicate their use.

In the lower limb, amputations of the toes and through the foot are acceptable up to the level of talonavicular joint. A knowledge of foot function is necessary when planning this surgery. For example, leaving an isolated one or two toes, particularly the great toe, can result in secondary deformity which makes shoe and partial foot prosthetic substitution difficult.

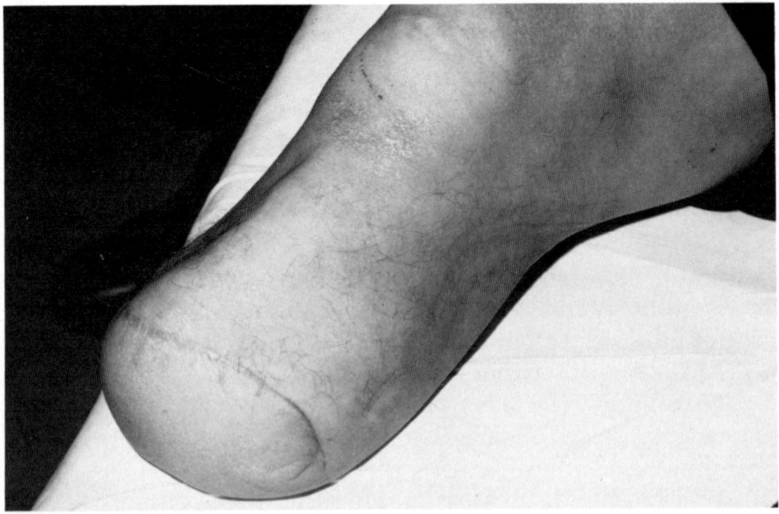

Fig. 3.1. Psysiological below-knee amputation with muscle stabilization. A degree of comfortable end bearing is achieved.

That portion of the foot remaining after amputation must be plantigrade with good weight-bearing skin. Modifications of surgical techniques at these levels require attention to remaining dynamic forces particularly muscle imbalance with resulting secondary ankle equinus, valgus or varus. After years of disrepute, forefoot and midfoot amputations are now gaining popularity. Modern prosthetic and orthotic substitutes have increased the latitude of successful amputation at these midfoot levels. Retention of the heel and talus only is rarely indicated except in certain congenital deficits. In most cases of this type, the Syme level is preferred.

The lower fourth of the leg proximal to the Syme amputation remains an unsatisfactory amputation level. The entire remaining lower leg up to the tibial tubercle is acceptable.

The very short below-knee amputation, especially in the presence of fixed knee deformity and with compromise of active extension, does not provide a satisfactory stump. The knee disarticulation level is more effective.

Throughout the thigh, all length is saved to the level of the lesser trochanter. Hip disarticulation is preferred to the very high above-knee amputation in patients where the remaining short femoral fragment is held in fixed flexion and abduction.

Level selection for amputation through the upper extremity is based on the principle of conservation. Surgery is carried out at the most distal level consistant with wound healing. The surgery is focused on the preparation of a suitable residual limb maintaining maximum length.

Lower Limb Amputations

Human bipedal gait allows us to stand upright effectively in our environment. We move about against the force of gravity adopting vast numbers of body positions, to some degree unique to each individual. During stationary and moving body attitudes, the lower limbs provide motion and stability. Both are necessary, but stability supercedes mobility in functional priority. The remarkable degree of stable body movement which can be achieved is demonstrated by the ballet dancer, the aerial high wire artist, the ice skater.

Following amputation, stable support is directly related to the length, strength and sensibility of the residual limb, the function of remaining superimposed joints and the efficiency of the prosthesis. Conservation of residual limb length, muscle strength, and the presence of proximal freely moveable, painless joints without contractures enhance rehabilitation.

The obvious role of the musculoskeletal structures as motor units should not diminish the equally important need for sensation, particularly proprioception in the residual limb. Since the mechanical properties of support, stability and motion are so evident in lower limb function, it is easy to overlook the completely correlative and necessary role of sensory input. Aware of these requirements, and with a knowledge of the functional anatomy, kinesiology and biomechanics, the surgeon proceeds to reconstruct the physiological residual limb.

TOE AND PARTIAL FOOT AMPUTATIONS

Absence of one or all of the lesser toes causes little disability. After amputation, the remaining portions of toes or metatarsal heads should be covered with pliable, nonadherent skin. Interphalangeal and metatarsal-phalangeal disarticulations are the levels of choice. Deformed stiff toes, or portions of toes, are best removed.

Loss of the first toe is appreciably disabling. Not only is the platform surface of the foot reduced but also a power lever arm has been removed resulting in some loss of strength and balance. Gait is affected, especially when running.

Forefoot amputations proximal to the toes require conservation of all length consistent with soft tissue management. Innervated plantar skin should cover the weight-bearing surfaces. Transmetatarsal levels and partial or complete ray resections are particularly useful in trauma and congenital and acquired deformities. When strict preoperative criteria are followed, they have a useful although less important place in the treatment of peripheral vascular disease (Fig. 3.2).

Amputation at all levels from the toes to the midfoot are functional and easily fit with partial foot prostheses. The prostheses will fit into a stock shoe. Skin on the plantar surface of the foot including the toes is uniquely designed to bear weight. When possible it should cover weight-bearing and pressure sensitive areas. The foot is a preimminently important sensory organ. Maximum painless skin sensation is always retained.

Midfoot and hind foot amputations in general have been considered undesirable. Today due to modern, improved, lightweight partial foot pros-

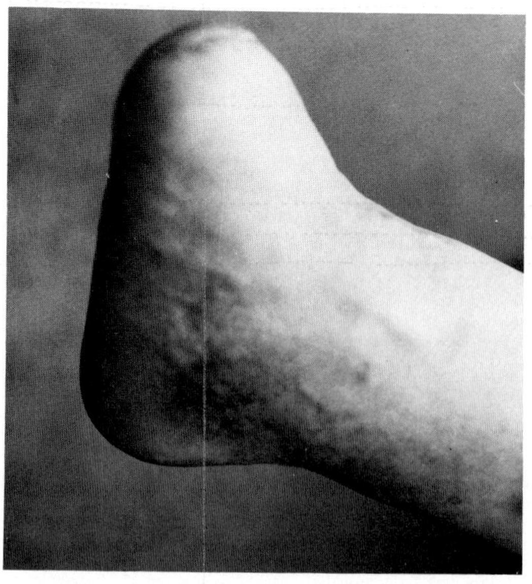

Fig. 3.2. Tarsometatarsal amputation. The foot is plantigrade. Its weight-bearing area is covered with pressure tolerant skin.

theses many of these amputations are valuable. Use of the appropriate forefoot substitute allows functional salvage of many midfoot amputations, especially in trauma, congenital deformities, and infections when good local blood supply is retained. The remaining foot segment must function in an acceptable plantigrade attitude without pain. An inclined platform surface, as with a midfoot amputation in equinus, is obviously less effective than in neutral weight-bearing position. Resulting high areas of distal pressure concentration even on good plantar skin will cause pain, skin breakdown and difficult prosthetic fit. Conservation of length alone in the midfoot area is not justified unless the attributes of stability, absence of pain, pressure tolerant skin and a useful range of ankle and tarsal movement are achieved. Occasionally appropriate tendon lengthening and soft tissue release with tendon transfer rebalancing in the foot will provide the two-fold benefit of motor control and prevention of contractures. Intertarsal or ankle arthrodesis which would be used to place the foot in a neutral weight-bearing attitude eliminates accommodating and compensatory joint movement, thus diminishing the value of joint fusion at these more distal amputation levels.

SYME AMPUTATION

The Scottish surgeon, James Syme, first performed amputation at the ankle in 1842. Surgery was then carried out without anesthesia or knowledge of antisepsis. Syme designed the surgery to permit full weight bearing on the retained plantar heel skin firmly fixed and centered over the distal tibia and fibula at ankle level. The surgery was, in concept and practice, so effective that the Syme amputation remains today little changed (Fig. 3.3).

The classical one-stage Syme amputation is indicated when it is the most distal level that can be expected to heal without complication. It is especially effective in trauma, deformities, tumors of the foot, and certain congenital anomalies. Healthy, well vascularized, plantar heel skin is necessary for its effective use. Harris of Toronto has written a lucid description of the classical one-stage Syme amputation. No deviation is recommended other than minor skin flap modifications as dictated by the pathology present.

Peripheral vascular disease and infection generally have been considered contraindications to the Syme amputation. Wagner (28) has made a critical study of this amputation for these conditions. His excellent contribution of a two-stage technique has revived the Syme level when ischemia and infection are present yet the plantar heel skin is viable and of good quality. This two-stage operation is gaining acceptance on the basis of his experience and that of others, including ourselves. Careful selection of cases and precise technique are required. The two-stage technique as practiced by Wagner is not an initial open amputation later converted by wound closure. The heel flap is placed and the wound closed primarily over irrigation drainage and without removal of the malleoli. At the second stage, the healed amputation is revised and recontoured by removal of the malleoli through two small incisions which are closed primarily.

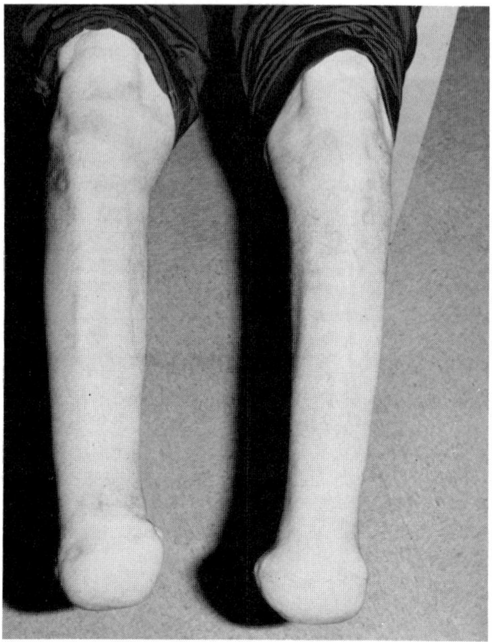

Fig. 3.3. Bilateral Syme amputations.

A major criticism of the Syme level amputation has been the unsightly prosthesis required. Its use in women has been avoided for this reason. The combination of carefully performed surgery with some reduction of the bony bulbous ankle contour, then fitting with now available cosmetically acceptable prosthesis, extends the usefulness of the Syme amputation in many circumstances to women as well as men. Its durability, strength, end bearing capacity and length commend it as the lowest major level of leg amputation to be considered.

BELOW-KNEE AMPUTATION

The successful use of amputation through the lower leg for peripheral vascular disease makes it the most frequently performed and important level for major limb ablation in peacetime. In many medical centers this amputation is performed more often than all other major levels combined. Retention of the knee joint is critical to lower limb function. The knee is the keystone for rehabilitation of below-knee amputees. This fact applies to young and old, athletic or sedentary, the weak and multiply disabled, as well as the vigorous. The importance of knee function is foremost in the surgeon's mind when the level of leg amputation is being determined (Fig. 3.4).

There is no specific site of election for below-knee amputation. Only the lower one-fourth of the leg is avoided. The tibia and fibula are subcutaneous or surrounded by tendons and fascia in this area. Here, total contact prosthetic socket fitting is difficult and attractive cosmesis is compromised. The suspension and end-bearing advantages of the Syme amputation are not available and scars tend to be adherent and painful. Thus, the surgical and prosthetic problems presented at this level outweigh the possible advantages of the slightly longer below-knee lever arm.

Excluding the area described, the surgeon may individualize the level of below-knee amputation for each patient. All length should be saved consistent with the pathology present. Length is translated directly to function by a longer lever arm, greater strength, increased proprioception and a larger total below-knee area for weight transfer. Scar placement is irrelevant as long as plastic principles are practiced and the scar is nontender, nonadherent and pliable. There is no major amputation allowing greater opportunity to use plastic and reconstructive techniques. Scar placement, muscle stabilization, bone contouring, end-bearing capacity, conservation of length and, on occasions, tibiofibular synostosis, all challenge the ingenuity of the surgeon to design a below-knee residual limb capable of nearly normal function through prosthetic rehabilitation.

Standard below-knee scar placement includes the long posterior flap, sagittal skin flaps and equidistant anterior and posterior flaps. Many modifications of these classical incisions are acceptable especially in trauma.

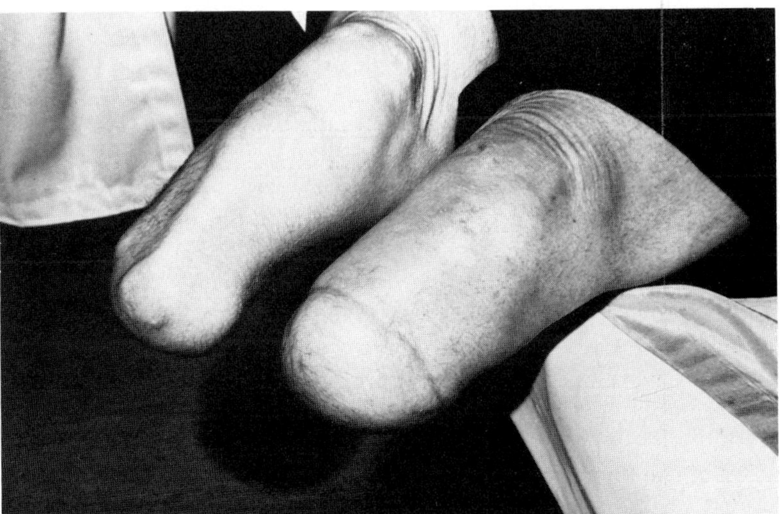

Fig. 3.4. Bilateral below-knee amputations for peripheral vascular disease. The *right* residual limb reflects older nonphysiological amputation technique. The skin closure is posterior. No muscle stabilization has been carried out. The limb is atrophying and difficult to fit with a prosthesis. The below-knee amputation on the *left* conforms to modern techniques.

Limb viability and skin blood flow research, together with clinical experience in thousands of cases, have established the long posterior skin flap technique as most appropriate when amputating for ischemia.

A normal knee with strong active extension is essential to good below-knee amputee performance. Knee contractures, instability, malalignment and thigh muscle weakness influence below-knee amputee performance in a manner quite similar to persons with an intact limb. Prosthetic accommodation can compensate for some degree of lost knee function, however, fixed-knee flexion of more than 40° is severely disabling. When the amputation is very short and the knee is in more than 40° flexion, either conversion to knee disarticulation or the use of a bent-knee prosthesis may be indicated. Occasionally persisting knee flexion deformity can be corrected successfully by posterior release, or by osteotomy. Knee ligament instability and thigh muscle weakness can more easily be overcome by prosthetic modifications.

The below-knee amputation has become one of the most challenging and rewarding of operations. Its wide application in trauma and disease, particularly peripheral vascular disease, place it high in importance in reconstructive surgery of the lower limb. A patient coming to below-knee amputation will be best served by an experienced, technically competent surgeon familiar with the anatomy and physiology of the area, the biomechanics, the kinesiology, the nature of wound healing and the prosthetic substitutes available. This is not surgery to be placed at the end of the schedule and delegated to an unsupervised, junior surgical registrar.

KNEE DISARTICULATION

Knee disarticulation is an excellent level of amputation. It provides a long strong stump with good end-bearing quality. Distal bone contours aid in prosthetic suspension and socket control. Sectioned thigh muscle tendons are easily stabilized. A number of skin incisions are acceptable including sagittal flaps. Disadvantages of through-knee amputation have related to the prosthesis. External hinges, the bulky distal prosthetic socket and the discrepancy of thigh-to-knee length when compared to the opposite, intact, limb have discouraged its use.

Surgical shaping of the femoral condyles and prosthetic improvements have largely eliminated these objections (Fig. 3.5).

The patella has been dealt with in a number of ways which include the well known Gritti-Stokes technique and more recently the Burgess (11) osteoplasty. The Burgess osteoplasty incorporates patellectomy with muscle stabilization and shaped distal bony contour appropriate to improve prosthetic function and cosmesis. The amputation is low transcondylar, still retaining full distal weight-bearing characteristics. The quadriceps mechanism is reconstructed. The small reduction in femoral length permits centering of the axis of knee movement more nearly level with the opposite intact limb and the inclusion of intrinsic prosthetic knee mechanisms.

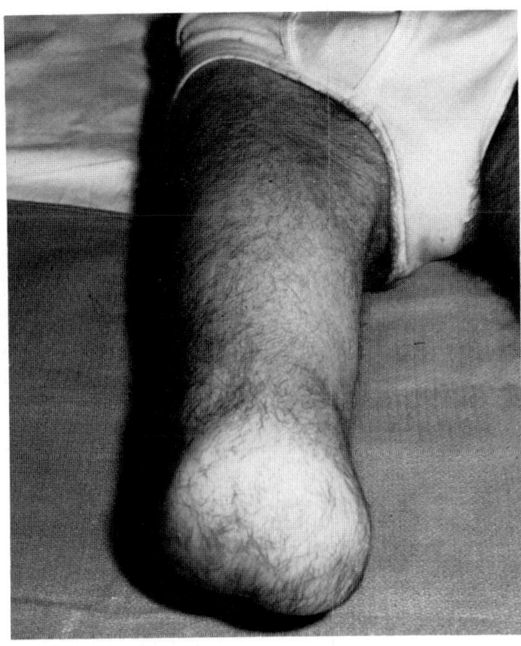

Fig. 3.5. Knee disarticulation amputation with thigh muscle stabilized, patellar removal and quadriceps repair. The condyles have been contoured to improve prosthetic socket fit.

A wide array of outstanding prosthetic knee disarticulation substitutes are available today. These include hydraulic, six-bar linkage and safety-knee mechanisms. A higher level of thigh amputation is not justified when satisfactory knee disarticulation can be carried out. This applies specifically to the young, vigorous amputee regardless of sex.

ABOVE-KNEE AMPUTATION

Until recently, amputation through the thigh was the level of choice for peripheral vascular disease. Healing could be expected in a relatively high percentage of cases. Effective rehabilitation terminated upon firm healing of the wound and instructing the amputee how to manage wheelchair and crutch living. Only a small percentage of these individuals became successful prosthetic users. Often at the insistance of the patient and family, a prosthesis would be fitted only to remain unused after a short and unsuccessful rehabilitation effort.

The younger and more vigorous above-knee amputees commanded the attention of prosthetists and rehabilitation personnel. The many young men and women throughout the world who sustained leg loss through the thigh in World War II expected better prostheses than were then available. Response to their needs was prompt. Suction suspension was developed in Germany. Quadrilateral socket design was developed in the United States. A wide array of knee mechanisms emerged and hydraulic control of both knee and ankle joints followed. Modular endoskeletal systems reduced prosthetic weight allowing more geriatric above-knee amputees to successfully walk.

The remarkable improvement on above-knee prosthetics brought pressure to bear on surgeons to improve amputation techniques. It soon became evident that muscle stabilization was an absolute prerequisite for physiological amputation through the thigh. A strong, cyclindrical stump can be obtained only when thigh muscles are stabilized to prevent migration of the distal femur and to capture muscle activity for prosthetic control. Persons with above-knee amputation now have the opportunity for a high degree of cosmetic and functional restoration (Fig. 3.6).

Appropriate surgery is the first of a series of events leading to full rehabilitation potential. The principles of this surgery are: 1) conservation of length; 2) muscle stabilization whenever feasible; 3) plastic skin and scar management; and 4) retention of free, active hip movement and strength. Even when suction is used as a suspension mechanism, the stump contacts the inner wall of the socket everywhere. The position of the scar is unimportant provided it is not adherent and tender. The ideal above-knee residual limb is cyclindrical, muscular, strong, nontender, and with minimal fixed flexion or abduction at the hip. Total socket contact with some end weight-bearing capacity is present.

Increasing use of below-knee amputations for peripheral vascular disease has made through-thigh amputation less important statistically. It remains, however, the second most frequently performed major amputation.

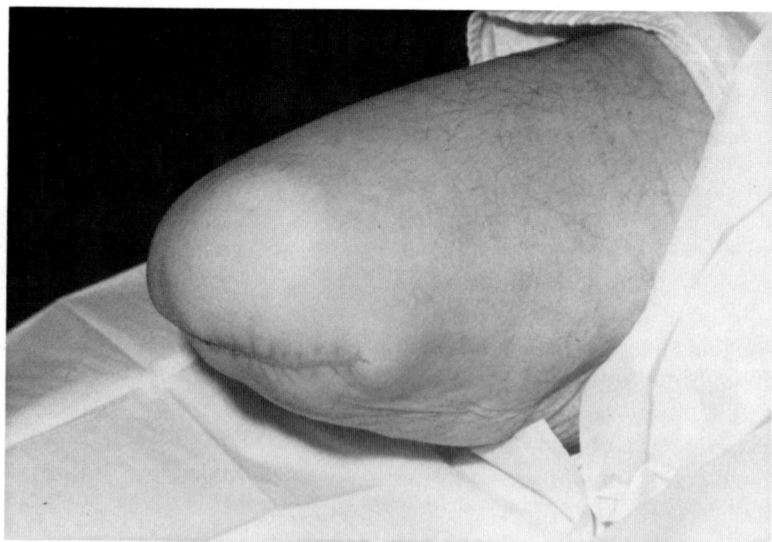

Fig. 3.6. Physiological above-knee amputation with muscle stabilization. The femur is well centered. The skin flaps are closed in the conventional anteroposterior plane. A sagittal skin closure is equally effective. It may allow more effective muscle stability and prevent lateral femur drift.

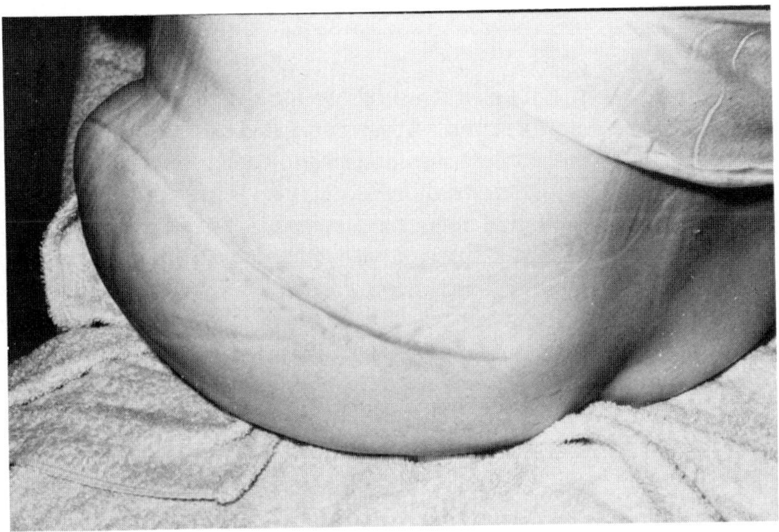

Fig. 3.7. Hemipelvectomy for malignancy. This level of amputation can only infrequently be fitted with a prosthesis.

HIP DISARTICULATION AND HEMIPELVECTOMY

Amputations at the level of the hip joint and through the pelvis are required occasionally for malignancy, extensive trauma, severe and uncontrolled infections and as a conversion operation for congenital deformity. We have performed a number of hip disarticulations for severe vascular disease.

Surgical techniques are well established. Modifications of standard procedures may be required to eliminate adjacent malignant growth; less often for other conditions. Well motivated individuals with good strength manage quite well with the excellent available prosthesis. Rehabilitation to regular prosthetic use is painstaking and may be discouraging. It should be forcefully pursued early following amputation when the individual is a potential walker (Fig. 3.7).

REVISIONS AND SPECIAL AMPUTATIONS

Staged amputations are used frequently in the presence of infection and trauma. The combination of infection and ischemia is often encountered in the presence of diabetes and may require initial surgery to localize and control infection, then definitive amputation at the lowest appropriate level for primary healing. We frequently have performed open ankle disarticulation in the presence of a septic, ischemic, diabetic foot and a few days later successfully carried out a definitive, closed below-knee amputation followed by an uneventful postoperative course. Staged amputations of this type are appropriate under a wide variety of circumstances when infection is present (Fig. 3.8).

Fresh traumatic contaminated wounds are handled in a somewhat similar manner. All viable skin is saved. After careful debridement, the bone is prepared for a definitive amputation at the indicated length. The wound is lightly packed, drained and immobilized. A few days later, secondary soft tissue closure is accomplished forming a suitable, definitive stump. Maximum conservation of limb length consistent with surgical circumstances remains the basic necessity. Staged amputations of this type have largely replaced earlier guillotine-skin traction methods. When preservation of length is critical and control of infection may be prolonged so that skin grafting or other plastic innovations may be required, then guillotine-skin traction is used instead of the delayed flap early secondary closure technique. Antibiotics and other measures for modern infection management are responsible for these improved techniques when staged amputations are necessary (Fig. 3.9).

The importance of seeking to obtain low levels of amputation in ischemia, and, specifically, knee salvage will result in an occasional failure at the primary selected level. The failure may be due to ischemia, infection or a combination of both. Judgement, experience and precision, as well as

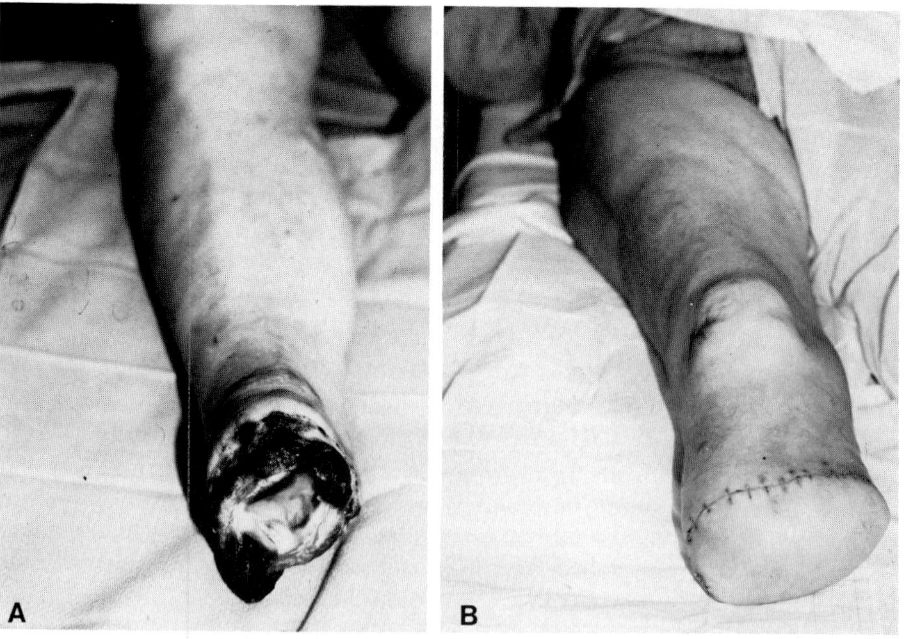

Fig. 3.8. A diabetic patient with a two-stage below-knee amputation for ischemia and severe infection. *A*, infection was controlled with open ankle disarticulation. *B*, a closed below-knee amputation was performed 5 days later.

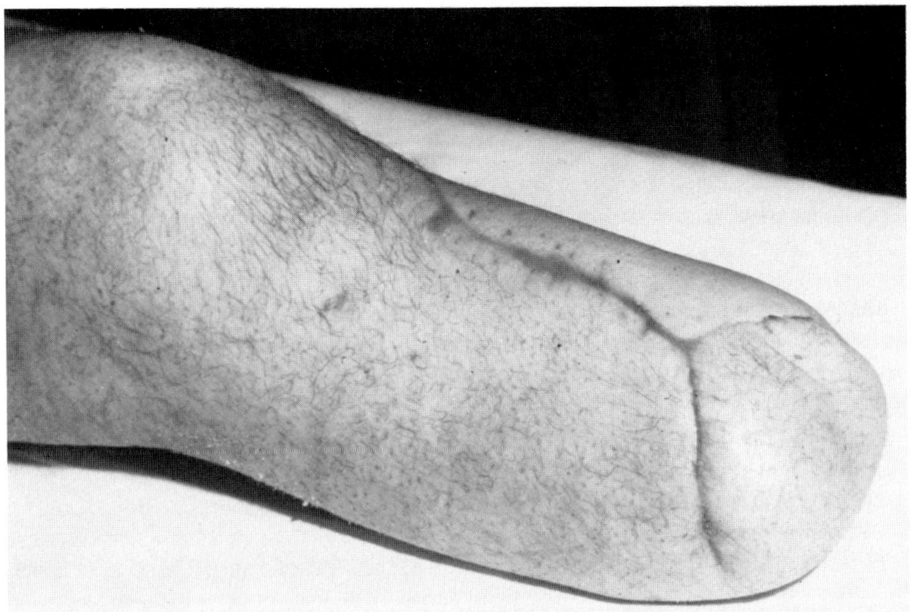

Fig. 3.9. Below-knee amputation for gas gangrene. Surgery staged with secondary closure following initial infection control. Scars are placed in consideration of prosthetic needs.

objective laboratory means for assessing skin viability here come into play. Even though local marginal necrosis occurs, a proximal revision from the below-knee level to a higher level, yet still below the knee, may heal. These decisions call for keen surgical judgement. Elderly, unhealthly patients tolerate multiple surgical procedures poorly. The patient may not be a candidate for ambulation so that primary healing is the main consideration with the level of amputation relatively less important. Proximal severe joint contractures, hemiparesis, bilateral limb loss and mental confusion exemplify contributing circumstances which weight the surgeon's decision.

Certain specialized amputation techniques are available when their use will provide a more physiological residual limb. Among these are tibiofibular osteosis (Ertl) at the below-knee level. We reserve this technique for children and younger adults when it can be used without sacrificing important stump length and when the prolonged healing time does not interfere with achieving maximum rehabilitation. Muscle and tendon transfer are occasionally required; coincident with the amputation, skin plastic procedures, including a wide variety of full and partial thickness grafts, may be necessary. Amputation in the burned and scarred extremity require the cooperative experience of plastic and reconstructive surgeons.

Anesthetic skin is not infrequently encountered at the amputation site as in meningomyelocele, spinal cord damage, peripheral nerve injury and leprosy. Critical prosthetic socket fit together with graduated increments of interface pressure against anesthetic skin, scar and skin grafts will gradually build up tolerance permitting prosthetic use. Skin grafts over pliable soft tissues frequently do well within a prosthetic socket. When the skin graft or scar is placed over and is adherent to bone, tendon and fascia, and when it is in an area of significant pressure, friction and then shear breakdown can be expected (Fig. 3.10).

Upper Limb Amputations

Most amputations through the upper limb result from trauma, tumors, infections and congenital deficits. The person involved is usually young and in good health. The relative percentage of upper limb amputations is low since peripheral vascular disease seldom leads to major upper limb amputation. Arterial thrombosis, emboli, neurovascular dystrophy (Raynaud's disease) and acute vascular trauma encompass most of the ischemic states requiring surgery. Excluding the fingers and thumb, less than 10% of major amputations occur through the upper extremity.

The hand has been described as the extension of man's eyes and brain. It's versatile sensory and motor function is indescribably complex. Volumes have been written on the anatomy and functional performance of the human

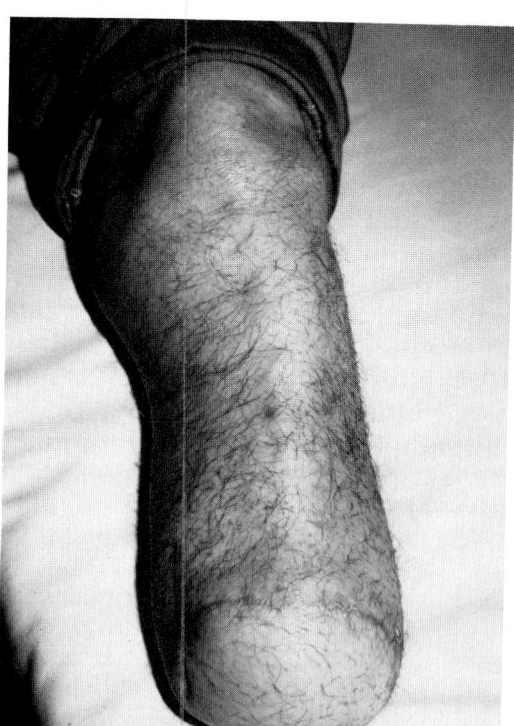

Fig. 3.10. Long below-knee amputation for trauma. Muscles are stabilized and some degree of end bearing is attained.

hand. Hand surgery is a large and distinctive speciality necessitated by the biomechanical and aesthetic importance of the hand and upper extremity. Because of its unique value to man, loss of any portion becomes a significant functional deficit.

Conservation is fundamental to amputation surgery in the hand and in the entire upper extremity as well. Nonetheless, we can function with considerable effectiveness and move about our environment freely when only one upper extremity remains. This contrasts to the lower limbs where, without a prosthesis, one becomes, in essence, immobile and dependent on the upper extremities for assistive walking when one or both legs are lost. Bilateral upper-limb loss, however, is critically disabling, even more so than blindness. For these reasons, unilateral upper-limb amputees frequently reject functional prosthetic substitutes particularly when the amputation is high. Conversely, bilateral upper-limb loss drives the recipient to herculean efforts to obtain substitute function through prostheses.

LEVELS OF AMPUTATION

Since conservation is the fundamental principal with upper limb surgery, there are no elective levels of amputation; all length is saved consistant with providing a comfortable residual limb tolerant of the prosthetic substitute.

Amputations Through Fingers and Metacarpals

Most function of the upper limb centers around function of the hand. Just as the operator of a large power shovel or crane sits high above its mechanism in the small cab and moves the various hinged elements to position and work the terminal unit, so the brain positions the upper limbs for motor and sensory hand function. There is no real reserve or overlap in hand function. Loss of even a single phalanx is important. Reconstructive hand surgical techniques such as transplantation of digits, polycization and neurovascular pedicle transfer exemplify the importance of each ray in its entirety. This same attitude of maximum conservation applies to amputations through the fingers, thumb, and metacarpals. Painful, scarred, immobile and gangrenous digits should be removed but needless loss of any functional tissue is avoided.

Amputations through the fingers and metacarpals rarely require prosthetic replacement. Prosthetic thumb substitutes have some value when reconstructive surgery cannot compensate for the deficit.

Transcarpal Amputations

Levels of amputation between the wrist joint and the metacarpals are useful when wrist function remains. There is no partial hand substitute as valuable as the remaining proximal hand with sensation and a strong moveable wrist joint. The remaining hand element can stabilize independently as well as provide a significant degree of bimanual function. When wrist function is lost, a wrist disarticulation can be advantageous under special circumstances. Reduction of extremity length to wrist level permits use of a prosthetic terminal device without excessive limb length. Each case is individualized; decision to remove the remaining portion of the hand is made only with the full knowledge of available prosthetic substitutes as well as the functional potential of that segment under consideration for removal.

Wrist Disarticulation

Amputation through the wrist is preferred to any higher level when the soft tissues are adequate for good skin cover. Distal radial ulner joint function must be retained to permit radial rotation. The radial and ulner styloid processes are moderately contoured without disturbing the distal radial ulner joint. The skin scar is placed dorsal and volar skin with its soft tissue pad is retained for distal coverage. Reattachment of major forearm muscle tendons which cross the wrist joint will improve residual limb function. Selected tendons can be stabilized under appropriate tension to periosteum or to bone near the amputation site. Muscle stabilization is particularly important when myoelectric forearm signals are planned to control the terminal prosthetic device.

Forearm Amputation

Amputations through the forearm conserve all length. The site of election is the lowest level consistent with good surgical management. Limited, local use of skin grafts can be used to save length when circumstances dictate. At the time of surgery, care is taken to retain rotary movement of the radius avoiding synostosis. Even though only a small portion of retained pronation and supination may be translated into prosthetic positioning, that motion is important (Fig. 3.11).

The principle of distal muscle stabilization applies in the forearm as well as at other amputation levels. Myoelectric signals and proprioceptive feedback are enhanced when maximum muscle activity is retained. To this end, ingenous and thoughtful surgical planning will be directly rewarded in terms of function whether or not myoelectric devices are used.

A short forearm amputation is functionally superior to elbow disarticulation. The biceps tendon can be divided at its insertion into the radial tuberosity to increase functional length, leaving the brachialis muscle as the effective elbow flexor. The sectioned biceps tendon can be stabilized into the distal humerus or used to reinforce the brachialis muscle above the elbow.

Elbow Disarticulation

Elbow disarticulation is preferred to a higher above-elbow amputation. Muscle stabilization is routinely performed, and moderate contouring of the humeral condyles is carried out, just sufficient to remove sites of pressure intolerance against the socket yet retain sufficient enlargement and contour

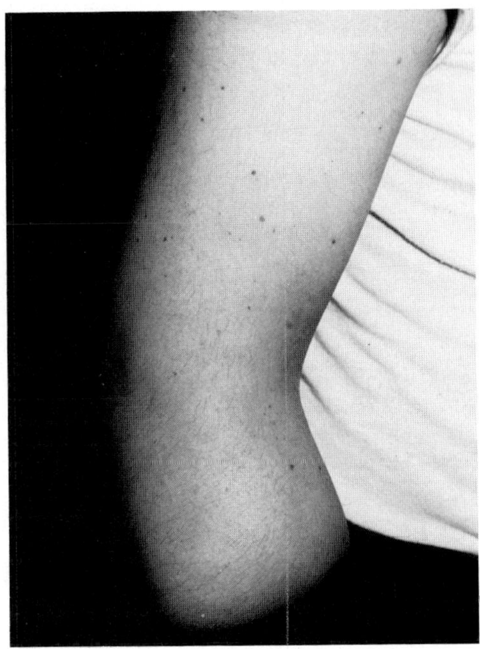

Fig. 3.11. Muscle stabilized forearm amputation resulting from trauma. Myoelectric signals are effective through retained active stump muscles.

to provide stability within the prosthesis, a major advantage of both wrist and elbow disarticulations.

Above-Elbow Amputation

Above-elbow diaphyseal amputation through the humerus is carried out at the lowest surgically feasible level. The bone end is moderately rounded and muscle stabilization is accomplished whenever possible. The very short above-elbow amputation is preferred to shoulder disarticulation even though little useful shoulder joint function is retained. The added surface and shoulder contour provided by the retained head of the humerus simplifies prosthetic fitting both functionally and from the cosmetic standpoint.

Shoulder Disarticulation and Forequarter Amputation

Shoulder disarticulation and forequarter amputation present no unusual problems and the surgical techniques are well documented. The general principles that have been outlined for ablative surgery apply. Unilateral amputees frequently reject the cumbersome prostheses except for appearance.

Immediate Postoperative Management

The rigid dressing with immediate postoperative prosthesis (IPOP) is particularly useful with upper-extremity amputations. Under proper circumstances a remarkable degree of functional terminal device control can be expected early in the postoperative period. Wound healing is enhanced by the rigid pressure dressing. Since no weight bearing is involved, stress on the wound is minimal. It is not unusual to see a midforearm amputee fitted with an immediate prosthesis at surgery able to open and close a conventional terminal device easily and comfortably the day following surgery. This same rapid rehabilitation is present when a myoelectric pickup and electrically controlled temporary prosthesis is applied. Psychological and physical advantages of the IPOP technique are dramatically evident with upper extremity amputations.

It is important to mobilize and exercise proximal joints and muscles whatever postoperative management system is used. Neck, shoulder, shoulder girdle, and remaining arm muscles are exercised immediately following surgery within the limits of pain. Good ranges of motion and muscle activity can be expected by the 2nd or 3rd postoperative day. The amputee is impressed with the fact that the remaining shoulder, arm, and neck muscles will be his means of prosthetic terminal device control. Successful use of the substitute limb will depend on this function.

Prompt rehabilitation to functional definitive limb use is the goal of upper-limb amputee rehabilitation. Following amputation, any significant time without prosthetic fit increases rehabilitation difficulty. The unilateral amputee quickly learns to compensate with the remaining arm so that the struggle to learn and refine prosthetic function is onerous especially at the higher levels of amputation. For this reason alone, the immediate fit technique carried through directly to definitive limb fit has many advantages.

Amputation through the upper limb is nothing less than creative reconstructive surgery. The person with arms handcuffed behind the back is instantly aware of an unbelievable degree of loss of environmental relationship. Functional substitution by prosthetic replacement intrigues the engineering and prosthetic professions. The surgeon, likewise, must accept the challenge to reconstruct the remaining part in a manner allowing the full potential for environmental contact.

The quality of life of individuals coming to amputation, young and old, depends on decisions of the type outlined. These decisions were less relevant when physical medicine and prosthetic rehabilitation were modestly effective. The surgeon is now committeed to a level of reconstructive technical responsibility matching other contributors to functional restoration.

Immediate Postoperative Fitting

Following surgery, quiet uneventful healing of the operative wound will depend to a significant degree on the physical environment. Tissue rest, edema control, temperature, humidity, unconstricted fluid and metabolite exchange are physical forces over which the surgeon influences some degree of control. These extrinsic environmental forces join the intrinsic genetic cellular and nutrition responses for healing to occur.

Vitality, the power to live and go on living, best expresses in one word the healing process. The process fascinates surgeons for it is the essence of their science and art. We in medicine are constantly observing, experimenting, modifying those parameters under our control to assist the body to heal its wounds.

The amputation is in many respects, the ideal clinical laboratory for the study of postsurgical wound healing. The operative site is at the end of the limb; there is no distal tissue to be considered. The operative site is in its entirety available for external environmental manipulation. This fortunate circumstance permits near ideal postsurgical care based on the known facts about wound healing.

SOFT DRESSINGS

Wrapping the wound with sterile soft dressings does little more than minimally protect it and keep it clean. These are the only advantages other than easy access for dressing changes and unrestricted mobility of the limb. Compressive wrapping adds support, some immobilization and a degree of pressure depending upon how the bandages are applied. Elastic bandages are useful if wrapped carefully, well supported, and frequently observed. Pressure under these bandages is, however, difficult to control and proximal limb constriction commonly occurs. Heat and humidity at the wound site may be unfavorable. Well suspended, tapered stump stockings of appropriate material such as cotton or orlon are usually more effective. In either circumstance, distal pressure can be favorably influenced by a pressure interface material such as reticulated polyurethane or carefully fluffed gauze placed between the wound covering and the pressure wrap or stocking.

RIGID DRESSINGS

Rigid and semirigid dressings allow much greater environment control. The wound is put at rest during the early days of healing. A compressible distal interface material combines pressure with wound support by the rigid dressing. The patient now moves about freely and more comfortably. When the immediately proximal joint is immobilized, as with the knee in the below-knee amputation, undesirable joint flexion is eliminated in the early, postoperative period. For these reasons, the use of rigid dressings following amputation enjoys worldwide use (Figs. 3.12–3.15).

When properly fabricated and applied, the rigid dressing can be used as a provisional socket for a temporary upper or lower limb prosthesis. The physical and psychological benefits of early prosthetic function are well known; the individual again becomes bimanual and bipedal. Precautions must be taken consistent with wound stress particularly in the lower limb. Prompt, primary, uncomplicated wound healing is the first step in the rehabilitation process. When wound healing is tenuous, as in the ischemic limb, we allow no weight bearing until the first cast change, usually 10 days

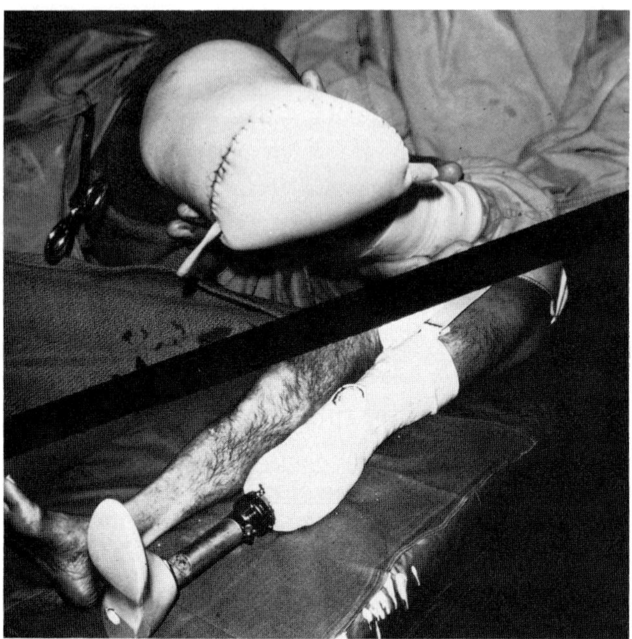

Fig. 3.12. Below-knee amputation fitted with a rigid dressing (*top*) and temporary prosthesis (*bottom*) at the time of surgery.

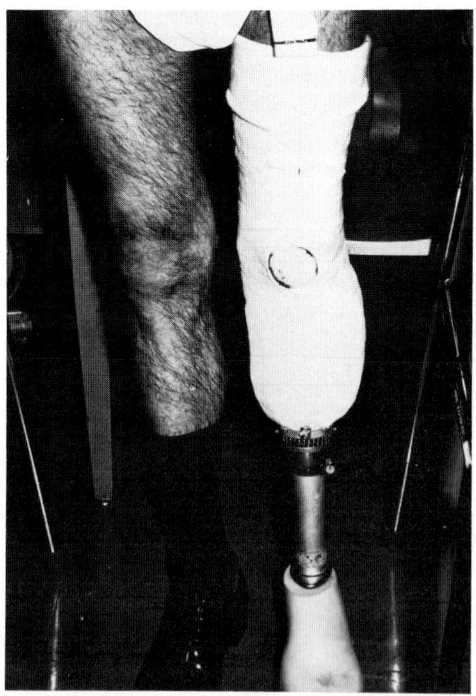

Fig. 3.13. Limited weight bearing in an immediate postsurgical prosthetic fitting.

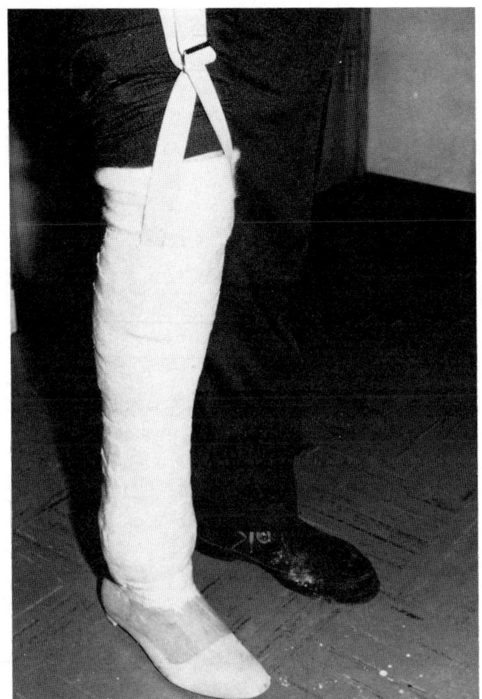

Fig. 3.14. Immediate postsurgical prosthesis for a Syme amputation.

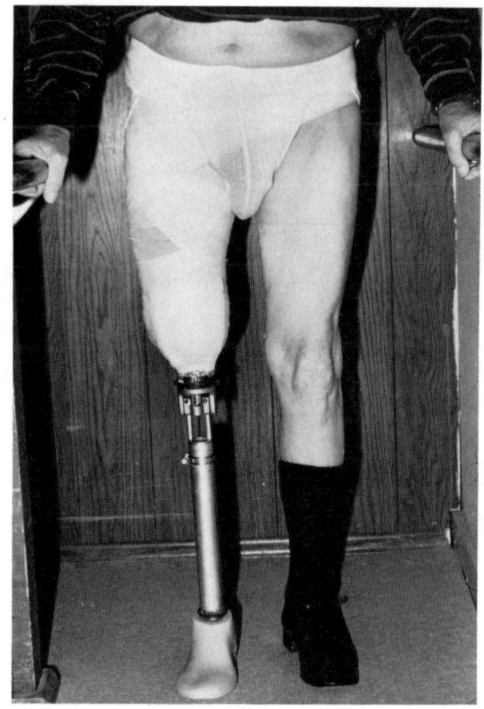

Fig. 3.15. Immediate postsurgical prosthesis for the knee disarticulation and above-knee amputation. The spica portion of the dressing is semirigid.

to 2 weeks after surgery. Early terminal device function with all of its advantages cannot be allowed to compromise wound healing.

The immediate postsurgical prosthetic technique dates back to World War I. It was revived and standardized by Berlemont (4), Weiss (29), and ourselves (5–8). It can be used for open as well as closed amputations. Demonstrated advantages make immediate postoperative rigid dressing, with or without prosthetic fitting, the routinely recommended method of choice when properly applied.

A variety of materials are available for the rigid and semirigid dressings. These include elastic plaster of Paris, conventional plaster of Paris, thermolabile plastics, Unna paste and related semirigid dressings. Improved materials will continue to be introduced. Rigid dressings and immediate postsurgical prosthetic fitting management depend on knowledge of their use and detail in application.

AIR BAG AND CONTROLLED ENVIRONMENT SYSTEMS

Redhead and his associates at Roehampton, England, have developed an innovative air pressure system for immediate postoperative amputee management. This is referred to as Controlled Environment Treatment (CET). The residual limb is placed inside a sterile polyvinyl bag. Pressure, humidity, temperature, sterility and gas composition are all controllable through an attached console. It is possible to observe the wound at all times. Immobilization and the ability of the patient to be sitting up and standing are both less effective, however, than the rigid dressing technique. Immediate postsurgical airbag systems developed in America and Australia will allow limited weight bearing through the dressing bag. The advantage of the CET air boot is its proximal venting characteristics, a modified hovercraft design. It is essentially a flow-through system rather than simply a dressing bag containing air under pressure. The CET method has been used to treat a wide variety of pathological states in the arm and leg as well as amputations. These include stasis edema, posttraumatic edema, hand surgery, postvascular reconstruction in the intact ischemic limb and others (Fig. 3.16).

General Postoperative Care

The elements of good patient care apply to those individuals undergoing amputation as with other surgery. Elderly and debilitated persons whose limbs are being amputated for ischemia are particularly subject to postoperative complications. Diabetes control, pulmonary support, adequate nutrition, proper electrolyte balance and early patient mobility present self-evident need. It is important to give sufficient medication for adequate pain control particularly during the first 2 or 3 postoperative days. Stump pain and phantom sensations tend to linger on when pain in the immediate postoperative period is not well controlled. Rigid dressings, in particular, permit early patient mobility. Supervised physical therapy should begin

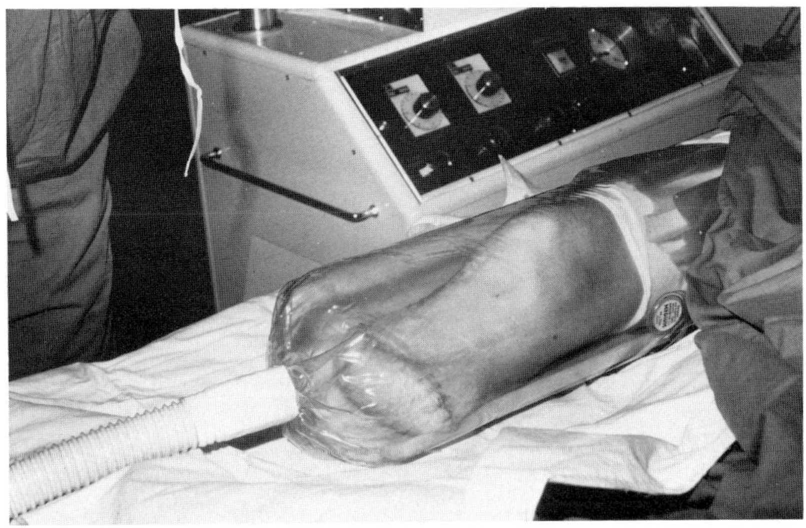

Fig. 3.16. Controlled Environment Treatment (CET) dressing envelope for a below-knee amputation immediately following surgery.

preoperatively where possible and resume on the first postoperative day. Good psychological support is mandatory.

Amputations due to trauma including burns are not uncommon in a patient who is multiply injured. It may not be possible to carry out early postoperative amputee rehabilitation as effectively as desired. It is nonetheless necessary to proceed aggressively from the outset. In this way, complications and delays can be avoided.

Two conditions require specific emphasis. The first of these is the young person, often in the second decade of life, whose amputation results from malignant neoplasm. The threat of death from the tumor combined with the psychic and physical trauma of limb loss not only call for sensitive management but specifically for rapid postsurgical rehabilitation to prosthetic use.

The second circumstance involves congenital amputation and limb deficit. Parents are devastated by the disaster that has befallen them and their newborn child. An understanding, strongly supportive, amputee team will help them through this difficult period.

Wound Maturation and Prosthetic Fit

Time is particularly important in amputee rehabilitation. The cycle includes surgery, wound healing, stump maturation and definitive limb fit. Time required for each stage is kept to the minimum. The rigid dressing—immediate postsurgical prosthetic management is particularly effective for early rehabilitation. The empty sleeve and the empty pantleg are to be avoided. While no specific time limits are set, certainly most patients will proceed from surgery to definitive limb fit in a few weeks rather than months. When the process is routinely prolonged it should be critically reviewed and errors eliminated.

Conclusion

Excluding a small number of congenital amputations not requiring surgical modification, all amputations are the result of surgical treatment. Amputee rehabilitation begins with the surgery, in fact, whenever possible rehabilitation begins in the preoperative period. The patient is less than well served when the surgeon is primarily a technician and completely delegates immediate postoperative and long-range rehabilitation to other members of the team. The failure to share continuing responsibility denies the surgeon opportunity through observation to improve and more fully understand his contribution. Amputation surgery requires this commitment.

The quality of life of individuals coming to amputation, young and old, depends on decisions of the type outlined. These decisions were less relevent when physical medicine and prosthetic rehabilitation were modestly effective. The surgeon is now committed to a level of reconstructive technical responsibility matching other contributors to functional restoration.

REFERENCES

1. Achauer, B. M., Black, K. S., and Litke, D. K. Transcutaneous PO_2 in Flaps: A New Method of Survival Prediction. *Plast. Reconstr. Surg.*, *65:* 738–745 1980.
2. Anselmo, V. J., and Zawacki, B. E. Multispectral Photographic Analysis: A New Quantitative Tool to Assist in the Early Diagnosis of Thermal Burn Depth. *Ann. Biomed. Engr.*, *5:* 179–193, 1977.
3. Barnes, R. W., Shank, G. D., and Slaymaker, E. E. An Index of Healing in Below-Knee Amputation: Leg Blood Pressure by Doppler Ultrasound. *Surgery*, *79:* 13–20, 1976.
4. Berlemont, M. *et al.* Ten Years of Experience with Immediate Application of Prosthetic Devices to Amputations of the Legs on the Operating Table. *Prosthet. Orthot. Int. 3:*1969.
5. Burgess, E. M., and Zettl, J. H. Immediate Postsurgical Prosthetics. *Orthotics Prosthet.*, *21:* 105–112, 1967.
6. Burgess, E. M. and Romano, R. L. The Management of Lower Extremity Amputees Using Immediate Postsurgical Prostheses. *Clin. Orthop. Relat. Res.*, *57:* 137–146, 1968.
7. Burgess, E. M., Romano, R. L. and Zettl, J. H. The Management of Lower Extremity Amputations. TR 10-6, United States Government Printing Office, 1969.
8. Burgess, E. M. Immediate Postsurgical Prosthetic Fitting: A System of Amputee Management. *J. Am. PT Assoc.*, *51:* 139–143, 1971.
9. Burgess, E. M. Wound Healing After Amputation: Effect of Controlled Environment Treatment. *J. Bone J. Surg.*, *60A:* 245–246, 1978.
10. Burgess, E. M. General Principles of Amputation Surgery. In Atlas of Limb Prosthetics Surgical and Prosthetic Principles, (AAOS), pp 14–18. C. V. Mosby, St Louis, 1981.
11. Burgess, E. M. Postoperative Management, In *Atlas of Limb Prosthetics Surgical and Prosthetic Principles*, (AAOS), pp 19–23. C. V. Mosby, St. Louis, 1981.
12. Fee, H. J. Friedman, B. H., and Siegel, M. E. The Selection of an Amputation Level with Radioactive Microspheres. *Surg. Gynecol. Obstet.*, *144:* 89–90, 1977.
13. Golbranson, F. Immediate Postsurgical Fitting and Early Ambulation. *Clin. Orthop. 56:* 119–131, 1968.

14. HOLLOWAY, G. A., AND WATKINS, D. W. Laser Doppler Measurement of Cutaneous Blood Flow. *J. Invest. Dermatol., 69:* 306–309, 1977.
15. HOLLOWAY, G. A., AND BURGESS, E. M. Cutaneous Blood Flow and Its Relation to Healing of Below Knee Amputation. *Surg. Gynecol. Obstet., 146:* 750–756, 1978.
16. HOLLOWAY, G. A. Cutaneous Blood Flow Responses to Injection Trauma Measured by Laser Doppler Volocimetry. *J. Invest. Dermatol., 74:* 1–4, 1980.
17. KEGEL, B. Controlled Environment Treatment (CET) for Patients with Below Knee Amputations. *Phys. Ther., 56:* 1366–1371, 1976.
18. KERSTEIN, M. D. Utilization of an Air Splint after Below-Knee Amputation. *Am. J. Phys. Med., 53:* 119–126, 1974.
19. KOSTUIK, J. P. *et al.* The Measurement of Skin Blood Flow in Peripheral Vascular Disease by Epicutaneous Application of Xenon[133]. *J. Bone J. Surg., 58A:* 833–837, 1976.
20. LASSEN, N. A., AND HOLSTEIN, P. Use of Radioisotopes in Assessment of Distal Blood Pressure in Arterial Insufficiency. *Surg. Clin. North Am., 54:* 3–55, 1974.
21. MATSEN, F. A. *et al.* Transcutaneous PO_2 Measurement in Peripheral Vascular Disease—A Preliminary Report. *Surg. Gynecol. Obstet., 150:* 525–528, 1980.
22. MOORE, W. S. Determination of Amputation Level by Measurement of Skin Blood Flow, (Letter to editor). *Arch. Surg., 109:* 124, 1974.
23. MOORE, W. S. Determination of Amputation Level. Measurement of Skin Blood Flow with Xenon[133]. *Arch. Surg., 107:* 798–802, 1973.
24. RABISCHON, P. Personal communication, 1974.
25. SARMIENTO, A. *et al.* Lower Extremity Amputation: The Impact of Immediate Postsurgical Prosthetic Fitting. *Clin. Orthop., 68:* 22–31, 1970.
26. SHER, M. H. The Air Splint. An Alternate to Immediate Postoperative Prosthesis. *Arch. Surg., 108:* 746–747, 1974.
27. WAGNER, F. W. The Diabetic Foot and Amputation of the Foot, In *DuVrie's Surgery of the Foot,* edited by R. A. Mann, 4th ed., pp. 341–380. C. V. Mosby, St. Louis, 1978.
28. WAGNER, F. W. The Syme amputation, In *Atlas of Limb Prosthetics Surgical and Prosthetic Principles,* (AAOS) pp. 326–334. C. V. Mosby, St. Louis, 1981.
29. WEISS, M. Myoplastic Amputation, Immediate Prosthesis, and Early Ambulation. Department of Health Education and Welfare, United States Government Printing Office, Washington, D. C.

4

Prosthetic Fitting and Components—Lower Extremity Amputees

J. FOORT

Prosthetic fitting is the process of making a replacement of a missing part of the body, or a prosthesis, of the right measure, shape and size. Components are the parts of the prosthesis of which it is composed. The manner of fitting and the components selected depend upon the characteristics of the person to be provided with the prosthesis. Among characteristics that affect prosthetic fitting and component selection are the age of the person, the sex, the reasons for amputation, but especially the level of amputation. The level of amputation affects how the person will function, how easy or difficult rehabilitation will be, the ease with which the cosmetic and functional needs will be met and the frequency of return for follow-up care. Therefore, the discussion will proceed on the basis of level of amputation, starting where amputation becomes significant. Amputation becomes significant at the place where control offered by the ankle and support of weight offered by the foot are reduced or affected. The significance is both cosmetic and functional.

Transmetatarsal Amputation

In this amputation the foot is divided through metatarsal bones and, as such, ankle function is fully retained. The amputee needs a toe filler—preferably mounted on an insole. Special attention should be given to the stump-toe filler interface. One can expect significant friction at this interface during push off, which could cause skin breakdown.

Lisfranc's Amputation

Lisfranc's Amputation of the foot divides it between the *tarsus* and the *metatarsus*. What is left is referred to as the *stump* or, in more modern terms, which will be used in this discussion, the *residual limb* or *residuus*, the part remaining or the remnant (Fig. 4.1).

A sense of what will happen when the foot is amputated at this level can be gained as we imagine the changes that will occur upon removal of these structures. Because the natural arches of the foot are undermined, the residual foot seems flat. It can be rightly concluded that, while there is a loss of both function and cosmesis, this residual limb segment will easily support body weight, even one-legged, and even permit careful jumping and running.

PROSTHESIS

To deal with the prosthetic requirements, it is sufficient to *fill* the shoe with any material that is nonabrasive and which will not impose significant leverage against the front or talar surface of the amputation site. Wool, cotton or silastic foam, a synthetic rubber, has been used to fill the gap in the shoe at the toe end. More elaborate constructions also have been used for preserving function, improving cosmesis or protecting the residual limb. But the simpler provisions usually are suitable for the functions required—to prevent the foot from sliding forward in the shoe and to support the shoe for a more natural appearance. Like the shoe, such fillers must be replaced periodically.

Chopart's Amputation

The foot is said to be *disarticulated*, between the talus and the remaining bones of the forefoot. This amputation level results in severe impairment of ankle function. The strong calf muscles pull upward on the calcaneous with little opposition from muscles in front of the ankle joint. Also, the extension

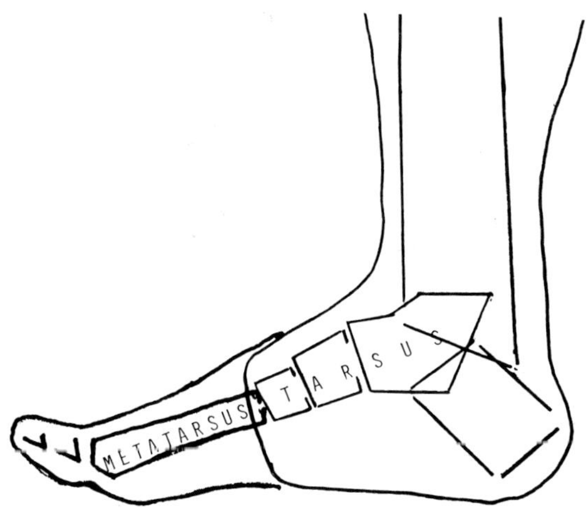

Fig. 4.1. Diagram of Lisfranc's amputation.

of the calcaneous toward the back causes even the weight borne on it to exert a moment which also forces the calcaneous up. The consequence is that there is a tendency for the residual foot to point downward, or to take what is called the *equinus* position. This exposes the amputation site, which may be tender, to the prospects of pressure from the prosthesis. The weight-bearing potential, on the other hand, is more than adequate when the residual foot is correctly stabilized within a prosthesis. Both the area of support and the ruggedness of the support surface are suitable.

PROSTHESIS

When dealing with Chopart's amputation in terms of fitting a prosthesis and selecting components, it is most often best treated as though the ankle joint was nonfunctional. Otherwise, the prosthesis must grip the calcaneous in order to make control by the ankle possible against the actions of the prosthetic forefoot when weight is supported on it.

Accepting that the ankle will not be functioning, then, the first requirement is that the support surface of the prosthesis at the sole be shaped to allow comfortable transmission of weight of the body to the prosthesis.

In addition to a surface which will transit support surfaces comfortably, the prosthesis must be shaped to link it comfortably and securely to the residual limb so that control forces can be transmitted.

FITTING

To make the impression of the residual limb, one can either wrap plaster of Paris bandage around it to the required level—usually to the inferior or bottom edge of the patella—making the impression sectional for easy removal, or use dental impression material, *alginate*, which can be cast around the residual limb placed within a container of appropriate size. This latter method is convenient to both the prosthetist and the amputee.

When the alginate impression has been withdrawn from the container, it can be split with a tongue depressor or something similar so that the residuus can be easily withdrawn. The mass is then returned to the container with the stockinet adhering to it. Thus supported, the plaster of Paris model can be poured up in it. The model is made as soon as possible after the impression has been made because of the tendency for the alginate to shrink.

The plaster model will include the whole residual foot volume and the shank to the level of the knee cap. The model of the residual limb must be shaped to improve it for use as a mold in construction of the plastic socket. Such shape changes are made to improve weight-supporting characteristics of the socket, and to improve control over the prosthesis.

SOCKET

The sort of socket to be constructed over this model can vary. It is usual to proceed as though the amputee had disarticulation of the ankle which means that the socket will extend upward almost to the tibial tubercle level. Occasionally the socket will extend higher if the residuus is not tolerant of bearing any weight. Then weight is borne on the regions of the shank below the knee crease all the way around, and an enclosing top end of the socket will be required. Otherwise, the socket is split down each side and across the back at the bottom to form a trap door which can be removed for entry or removal of the residual limb. This is illustrated in Fig. 4.2.

For such a socket to be effective, it must be sufficiently rigid to resist the forces imposed between it and the residual limb. At heel contact of walking, the force pattern will be something like that in the illustration. Toward the end of stance phase, the force pattern will be reversed. This is obviously a simplification of what is occurring. Forces are in fact moving about and changing in magnitude as the step proceeds. It is possible to sense, now, how carving material from the model of the residual limb can affect the socket so that the forces are concentrated on appropriate areas, as for example, against the anterior (front) surface of the proximal (top) end of the tibia.

There are reasons why I have emphasized the Chopart's amputation and prosthesis. Although the amputation is held in poor esteem by most, observations are that, in fact, these amputees are infrequent visitors for repairs, adjustments and replacements once they have been dealt with adequately by the prosthetist. They are difficult to fit, it must be admitted, and the forefoot section must be custom made. But it is the role of the prosthetist, and each team member, to save function for the amputee even when it poses problems for those who assist him if, in balance, this enhances the quality of his life.

Syme's Amputation

The Syme amputation is nearly equivalent to ankle disarticulation. The procedure results in a shortening of the residual limb by approximately 7 cm. The discrepancy of length in the Syme's residuus does not prevent weight bearing directly against the floor with the residuus. This capacity to bear weight on the end is not universal among these amputees. Results seem to range from very good to poor. But many have weathered years of satisfactory function—even 30 or more.

PROSTHESIS

The Canadian plastic Syme's prosthesis, or one of its variants, is used universally. In the original form, it consisted of a plastic socket which was split along the medial and lateral sides and across the bottom at the equator of the bulbus section so that the bulbus end of the residual limb could enter upon removal of this trapdoor. The trapdoor is hinged and secured with a strap as was indicated for use with Chopart's amputation. The foot used is a specially adapted Solid Ankle Cushion Heel (SACH) foot. The SACH foot

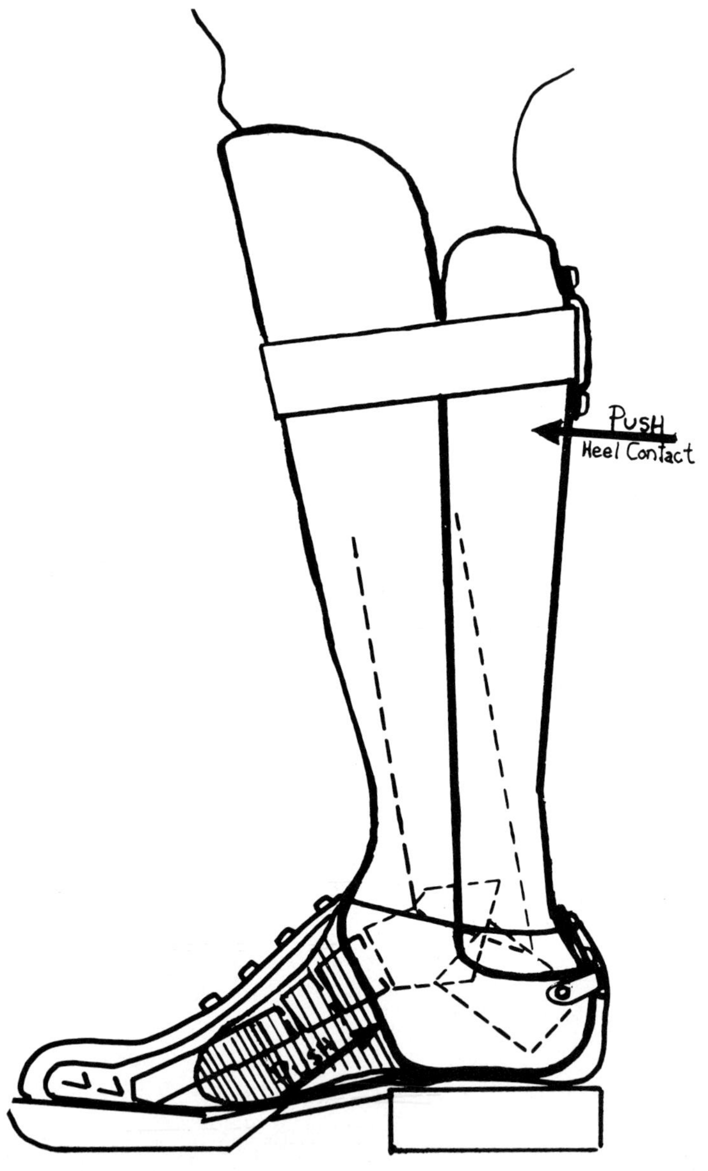

Fig. 4.2. Cutaway view of a foot socket prosthesis with hinged trapdoor and strap, useful in Chopart's amputation.

acts as a rocker, and knee function supplements foot movement for a normal-appearing gait. *Figure 4.3*, a cutaway view of the Symes prosthesis, illustrates how the residual limb fits into the socket and how the SACH foot is constructed and attached. It also shows the adjustments which must be made to the top of the foot to accommodate the bulbous lower end of the socket.

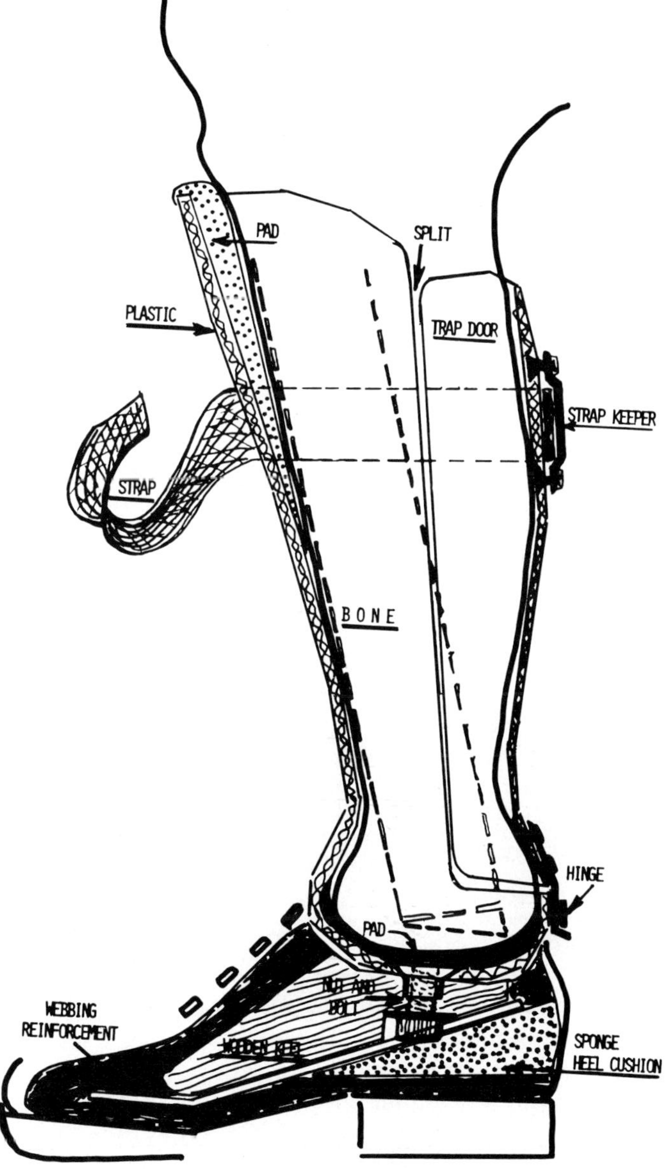

Fig. 4.3. Cutaway view of a Syme's prosthesis and a Solid Ankle Cushion Heel (SACH) foot construction.

FITTING

As with Chopart's amputation, either the alginate or the plaster cast method may be used to make the impression. The plaster cast method involves making a plaster cup over the end and extending it up the anterior surface of the residual limb to the lower edge of the patella and backward approximately to the midline on each side. Edges of the front and end section are thickened and lubricated before the posterior section is laid on. Once completed, the sectional impression is removed for reassembly and casting of the residual limb model within it, just as was done for the Chopart's procedure. By overlapping sections and marking reference lines across, reassembly can be done accurately. In fact, if the impression is made carefully, the second section being worked in around the first, positioning of the parts is quite obvious.

The sort of remnant being discussed here is quite like the others already discussed in that it bears weight directly on the end, and all shank muscles are intact. But, as there is little stimulus for their maintenance, the shank muscles shrink markedly. The narrowness above the weight-bearing end caused by this atrophy accentuates the bulbus nature of the weight-bearing end providing a configuration which permits easy suspension of the prosthesis. However, when the socket fits close to the shank along its full length, the narrowing increases the difficulty of getting the prosthesis on the residual limb. Procedures have been devised to overcome these difficulties. The maleoli, or ankle bones, can be surgically trimmed to narrow down the end so that the prosthesis, the socket totally enclosed, can be entered directly from above. The cosmetic advantages are obvious. Such a prosthesis can be shaped externally to appear more natural. Otherwise, either the posterior opening or side opening type of socket would be used. The difference between the posterior opening socket and the side opening socket is that the latter is much stronger. The former, on the other hand, permits the socket tightness to be adjusted. This is an advantage, since the residual limb tends to fluctuate in volume in the course of the day.

SOCKET

A recent development is the Tucker prosthesis which has a socket with windows on either side and a consistency more pliable than other types. The socket can be entered from above. There is no closure over the side windows. The foot designed for the Tucker prosthesis provides the same rocker action as other SACH feet, but is uniquely designed to solve the problem of aligning the foot under the socket and adjusting the length of the prosthesis. The keel of the foot is a stiff synthetic rubber which is much more pliable than usual for SACH feet. (A complete procedural manual has been prepared by the inventors, Tucker and Cochrane, 800 Sherbrook St., Winnipeg, Manitoba Canada, R3A 1M4).

Some say that a closed ring at the top, fitted to support weight at the knee level, is required because so few of these amputees are end bearing. For those who are not end bearing, the prosthetist has no alternative; to make that procedure standard, however, may be to encumber the Syme's amputee needlessly.

When the bulbus end has been trimmed, as in the newer surgical procedures, the prosthesis can be suspended by inclusion of sponge rubber sections within the prosthesis which will form in snugly against the residual limb when it is in place in the socket. The end results can be quite cosmetic.

Below-Knee Amputation

Persons who have been amputated through the shank make up the largest proportion of the amputee population. Below-knee (BK) amputations are now so frequent, as compared to other types, that it is reasonable to expect that of amputations being performed at any time, 75% will be of this type. Contrast this to the practices of even 20 years ago when amputations were more often done above the knee in many of the situations in which BK amputations are now done. The reasons are worth considering. The attitude that life saving was the purpose of amputation has given way to the attitude that function must be conserved if amputees are to be rehabilitated back to a life worth living.

HISTORIC

Some of the factors in this viewpoint can be considered. The concept of rehabilitation now receives more emphasis. Some surgeons who have made amputation surgery a major interest have helped encourage the change in attitude from viewing amputation as defeat to the view that amputation is reconstructive surgery. Considerable credit also must go to prosthetists and researchers who improved prosthetic practices. An example of the impetus given to BK prosthetics is Radcliffe's gathering of about two-dozen people in the field to review what was being done and to assist with the planning of strategy to make improvements in practices. Others were experimenting with various techniques and designs which would directly aid in establishing improved prosthetic procedures which would conserve function. Canty was experimenting with total contact sockets. Inman and Loon were experimenting with end bearing for BK amputees. Levy and Barnes, who were looking into problems of skin damage, helped establish the rationale for total contact sockets for the containment of distal tissues. Sockets so designed were intended to combat edema in the tissues that might lead to their eventual breakdown—a prospect of serious consequences for the amputee with vascular disease. At the same time, a number of influences were at work to enhance the chances for more conservative surgery for the preservation of function. There was a concentrated effort at the university level to improve practices through education in new techniques of teams which included prosthetists, therapists and surgeons. At the same time, the prosthetists were strengthening their associations and were increasing their efforts to upgrade their profession. Behind all this, government agencies, such as the Veterans' Administration in the United States, exerted strong pressure to ensure that research was done and that the results reached the population of disabled.

BK amputation was further encouraged by concentrated efforts to use "immediate postoperative prostheses," prostheses which are fitted in the operating room directly after the surgery is finished. The technique suited BK amputations especially. It had been introduced initially by Berlmont and later by Weiss of Poland and carried forward in America by Burgess who did much to popularize it. It was introduced into practice through special education programs for teams, which included up-to-date information derived from various research projects which were generating ways to improve prosthetic practices. Out of the drama of immediate fittings came acceptance of the "rigid dressing" for the residual limb after surgery. Such a dressing offered protection, confined edema and provided a link to the body which might later be used to initiate early ambulation. All of these influences coincided with the increasing numbers of amputees from cardiovascular problems and the desire to see more of these people recover some of their independence.

PROSTHESIS

Currently, there are two basic types of prostheses for the BK amputee. One is the *patellar tendon bearing below-knee prosthesis* (called the PTB prosthesis). The other is a variant which includes a thigh corset and side joints. This latter type is a leftover from the system which was originally used for virtually all BK amputees except for the few who were provided with "muley" prosthesis, forerunners of the PTB prosthesis. Such changes as have been included with its use are: principles of alignment developed for the PTB prosthesis, methods of fitting, and use of the SACH foot. The design of the corset and the side joints used are basically unchanged from the original system. In a setting where prosthetic practices are advanced only a few amputees are equipped with corsets and side joints. The infrequency of their use accounts in part for the limited changes that have been made in those elements of it which are not used in the PTB prosthesis. The difference between the two types is that supporting structures of the PTB prosthesis pass only a short distance above the level of the femoral tibial junction at the knee; the joint and corset BK prosthesis supports above the knee extensively, even extending to the pelvic level (ischial-bearing BK prosthesis) under some circumstances, such as when the residual limb is fragile in areas which would typically support weight, or when the knee joint itself is unstable, or the femur is nonweight bearing as in the case of fracture (Fig. 4.4.)

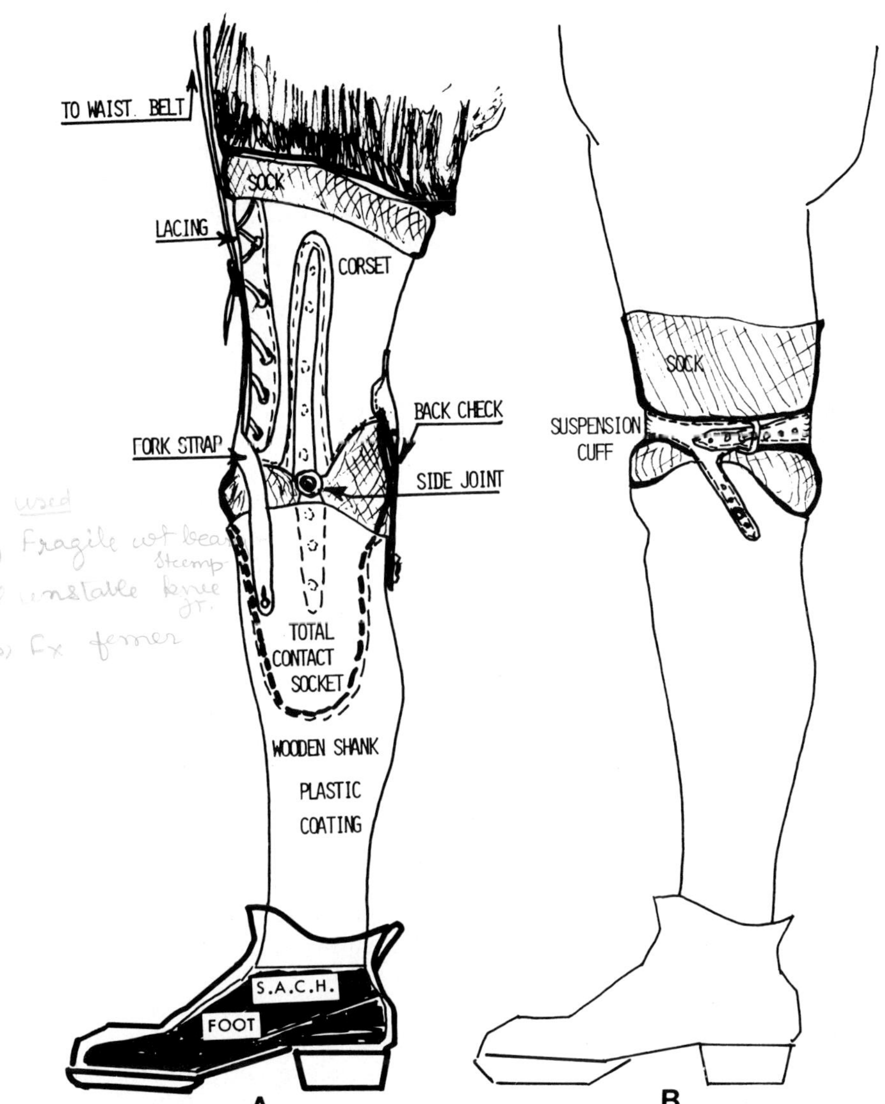

Fig. 4.4. *A*, side joint and corset prosthesis. *B*, patellar tendon bearing (PTB) below-knee (BK) prosthesis.

CRITERIA

Given that the residual limb may have to be fitted with the joint and corset type, there are simple and definite criteria on which to base a decision. They are:

1. When the amputee needs the prosthesis stabilized against rotation around the long axis of the limb for periods when the knee is bent. (Stair climbing under strenuous conditions or ladder climbing are examples.)
2. When the amputee must do heavy lifting over a significant period of time. The thigh corset can be temporarily tightened to give the extra support needed through the thigh and, when the knee is bent, considerably more support is derived from the back surface of the thigh corset.
3. When there are instabilities within the anatomical knee. If the instability is from side-to-side (as in some injury cases and in the case of some congenital amputees) the side joints will be intimately fitted and linked rigidly to reduce flexibility of the side irons at the thigh for more effective transmission of the needed support forces. If the instability involves hyperextension of the knee, then a link called a "back check" or "check strap" can be fastened between the bottom edge of the back surface of the corset and the back of the shank at any convenient level to prevent the knee from hyperextending. The side joint and corset system also can control dislocations.
4. When the amputee is unable to support body weight on the below-knee residual limb; in that case, support on the thigh alone will not be sufficient. At the top end of the corset, a cuff sufficiently rigid to be effective for weight bearing and shaped for the purpose must be used. (The appropriate shape will be discussed in considerations of sockets for amputations above the knee.)
5. When the amputee has poor judgement, to ensure that the prosthesis will be correctly donned. Some people are dependent on others to put on a prosthesis or to assist them in putting it on. When side joints and corset are included on the prosthesis, the way to put it on is more obvious.
6. When the amputee expresses a definite preference for the joint and corset type of prosthesis. If the person has been wearing such a prosthesis for many years, the condition of his muscles may make conversion to a PTB prosthesis difficult if not impossible. This will be especially so if the thigh has been used extensively for weight bearing and a back check has been used to control knee extension. He could be tried for conversion by having him wear the new socket-foot system without the thigh corset attached and then he could have the corset joint system added if trials were not successful.

If these criteria are adhered to, no one who needs or wants the additional support and stabilization offered by the joint and corset system will be denied it. Experience suggests that fewer than 1% of the BK population would be candidates for a joint and corset type of BK prosthesis. For people who sit a great deal, (elderly people, for example), the joint and corset type of prosthesis is contraindicated because of the constrictive effect at the back of the prosthesis where the bottom edge of the corset pinches bunched up tissues against the top edge of the socket.

Some people will feel that the length of the residual segment of the limb is a factor in deciding whether or not to fit side joints and corset. The implication is that if the residual segment is short, then the joints and corset are required for weight bearing and stabilization of the prosthesis on the short residual segment. But such short residual segments can be fitted adequately with the PTB prosthesis. In fact, the criteria given to define who should get the joint and corset type of prosthesis effectively identifies who would get the PTB type.

RESIDUUS

Let us consider the residual limb now. In comparison to the various amputations around the foot and ankle, the striking difference is that end bearing is not possible in most cases. Even the residual segments specially prepared by either plugging the medullary cavity or by making a bridge of bone between the fibula and the tibia at the end to enhance end bearing are not suitable for more than a minor amount of force through the end. (Probably, in part, due to movement between the prosthesis and the residual limb.) Only those amputees who have a high level of BK amputation which passes through cancellous bone have the capacity to bear considerable weight on the end. Total contact sockets which completely enclose the residual segment over the end, are not for end bearing, but to enhance circulation, improve stabilization of the prosthesis on the residuus and to improve proprioception, or the amputee's sense of where the prosthesis is in relation to space. In fact, the socket usually must be made with extra space provided to ensure clearance of the tibial and fibular ends in the socket. The soft tissues posteriorly and toward the end are what will be snuggly contained by the typical, well fitted, total contact socket.

WEIGHT BEARING

Without the capacity to bear weight through the end of the residual segment, every other potential area of it must be utilized, and every aid to effectiveness provided because of the severe wedging effect that the supporting socket of the PTB prosthesis can exert on the segment. The term "PTB" is derived from "Patellar Tendon Bearing." It is not accurate as a description of what actually takes place, but at the time of naming it, it was believed that a distinctive and descriptive term was needed to emphasize this structure as a weight-bearing surface, and to distinguish the prosthesis from all others. Besides the function of the patellar tendon as a support structure, the medial or inside buttress of the tibia is a major support surface. It extends from the medial midline of the residual segment around toward the back surface, even beyond the medial hamstring tendon which is so easily identified bridging the knee at the back when the knee is flexed. A well fitted socket forms in against this surface purposefully, and sweeps around the corner defined by the bridging medial hamstring tendon to flatten out, more or less, against the back surface of the residual segment. In many sockets, a deep relief channel is made for the medial hamstring tendon, designed to reduce or prevent pressure on it. If the patellar tendon is a good weight-bearing structure, one must wonder what is different about the other tendons. A better practice is to omit such channels in the socket, (including one for the lateral hamstring) but to flare the back lip of the socket generously so that the tendons at the back will be comfortably supported when the amputee sits, and such weight-bearing capacity as the back of the residual limb might have will not be lost. Another typical feature of many BK sockets is the extension of the back wall of the socket high into the space between the medial and lateral hamstring tendons. This, coupled with the channels for the hamstrings, often gives such sockets the appearance of having a probe directed into the knee crease behind. What is the merit of abandoning potential in the tough tendonus structures in favor of pressure into the area of the knee through which major blood vessels pass? An additional feature often seen is a bulge into the popliteal region between the tendons in the same region. This is to be deplored. Any of these features mentioned can contribute to a choking effect on the residual segment which produces a painful sensation at its end, even throbbing and perhaps edema.

So far, we have identified the patellar tendon, the medial tibial flare extending around to the back surface, and possibly the hamstring tendons as potential weight-bearing areas. It is likely that some support also is derived from a general wedging effect, especially against the section which includes the surface of the tibia in front. One can visualize the combined action of the wedged anterior feature of the socket and the flattened posterior surface combining to provide support. It may be, too, that support is derived from the femoral condyles. In fact, that is probably why the patellar tendon is so successful as a weight bearing structure, being backed up by the femoral condyles. Also, this could be why flexing the knee is a positive factor during weight bearing in the socket. The tibia anteriorly, the femoral condyles, and the tendon would gain from this.

Many prosthetists are now discarding modifications along the crest of the tibia and around the tibial tubercle. They reason that they lose surface, and with regard to the tubercle of the tibia, the pressure on the patellar tendon forces this structure away from the socket anyway, except during sitting.

SOCKET

The use of every available residual limb surface for support and stabilization requires that a parallel concern be given to how the socket is constructed. Many people use soft socket liners or inserts rather than fit hard sockets. These soft liners are intended to help make the socket conform to the residual limb so that the forces are more evenly distributed on the residuus. Lining the socket in this way gives the prosthetist a margin of safety and, also, he can make adjustments underneath so that the surface contacting the residual limb is not spoiled. Thus, he can grind material from the supporting socket shell or he can cement in liners which will increase pressure on selected areas of the residual limb. A well fitted hard socket can be just as comfortable, as has been confirmed frequently by converted users. A thin-walled socket which has no liner will be cooler, cleaner, lighter, more pliable and more cosmetic. The lower frictional forces which it will exert also can be of value in reducing shear of the skin or of underlying tissue layers which work against each other. Such a socket also assists in reducing the relative movements which inevitably occur between the residual limb and the socket. One part of this relates to how the prosthesis is held on, suspension, and the other part relates to stabilization against bell clapper actions between the residuus and the socket.

SUSPENSION

Let us consider the ways in which suspension can be achieved. In the original PTB prosthesis, a suspension cuff which encircled the limb above the knee was recommended. It had downward directed tabs which angled toward the back and which were attached to the socket, posterior to the midline of the socket on either side and at about the level of the tibial femoral junction. Attachment there was to buckles or buttons fastened to the socket. This is still a common way to hold on the PTB prosthesis. Sometimes a belt is linked to it by a strap that attaches to the top edge of the cuff in front. This is frequently elastic in part. Use of it permits the amputee to wear the suspension cuff more loosely and this is helpful if he sits a lot or has circulation difficulties. It also improves control over the prosthesis for walking. For some users, a simple strap looping over the top of the knee and attached at either end to the prosthesis toward the back is sufficient to hold on the prosthesis. Some prosthetists fit the socket over the knee in front. This is very effective as a suspension method when carefully done, and is especially useful for persons who have very short residual segments. It is an encumbrance to others, however. This particular method is called *suprapatellar* suspension. It is not generally used alone, but in combination with extensions on either side of the knee which grip the femoral condyles. This method of side extensions is called *supracondylar* suspension and was first used in the United States by Woodall. These extensions above the knee greatly increase stability of the prosthesis on the residual limb in all directions by placing more of the residuus within the socket. The cosmetic effect can be quite good. The added surface can be used to improve the gradient of forces between the various areas of the socket and the supported residuus so that shear between tissue layers is reduced or prevented (Fig. 4.5).

Supracondylar suspension is sometimes achieved by means of wedges inserted between the socket and the knee on either side. This technique from Germany involves building spaces in the socket for the wedges and then setting the wedges in place once the residual limb has been inserted. The wedges prevent easy withdrawal of the residuus. The best way is to fit supracondylar extensions which are an inherent part of the socket. These extensions must be springy to permit entry of the residual limb into the socket. Thus, the socket is made fairly thin. Failure of the built-in extensions to hold on the prosthesis usually lies with not having narrowed down the mouth of the socket sufficiently, and not having made the narrowest section sufficiently high to pass beyond the space needed by the femoral condyles during flexion of the knee.

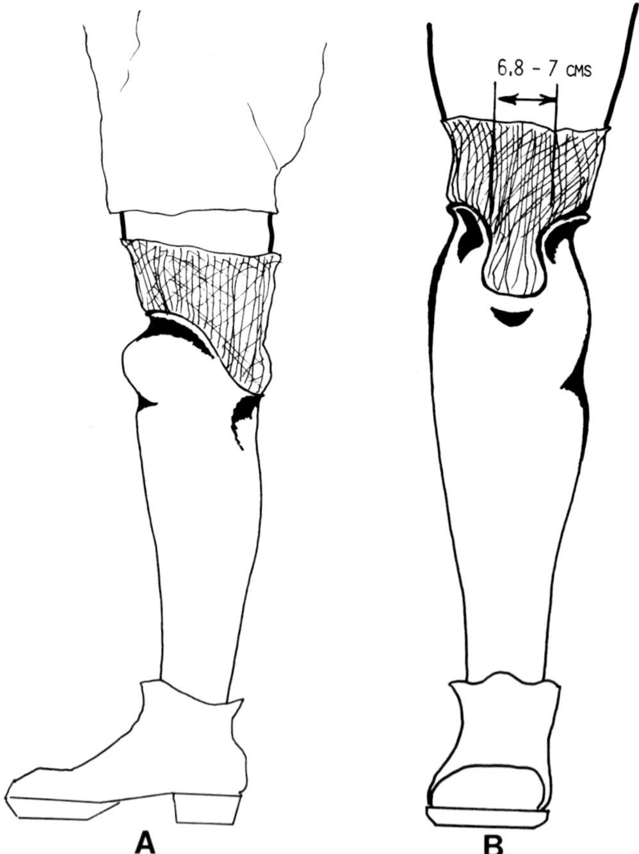

Fig. 4.5. *A*, suprapatellar and *B*, supracondylar suspension prosthesis for below-knee (BK) amputation.

The common problem of suspension is the tendency of the moving knee to feed the prosthesis off the limb. This tendency is minimized when necessary movements are least constrained by the prosthesis and unwanted movements are most effectively blocked. These requirements have led some to use suction suspension. For maintenance of suction, a valve is set into the socket, as is done for the thigh level amputation prostheses, and the residual limb is in direct contact with the socket. Then, because the forces in a BK socket are so high, maintaining skin health is the greatest problem with suction suspension. Galdik of San Francisco used it extensively during the 1950s. He had the amputee grease the residual limb segment and forcibly insert it into the prosthesis. The quality of this type of suspension is certainly high, but the consequences of fluctuations in segment volume can be great, and a suitable tissue cover over the skeletal anatomy is a requirement.

In the residual limbs resulting from more recent surgical procedures, muscle bulk is retained, and the amputee is encouraged to maintain it by exercise of the muscles. With muscle bulk available, he can bulge the muscle to aid in suspension of the prosthesis. This clinging effect was called the "adherency technique" in Germany. Blevins in the United States had tried to stimulate such a suspensive technique by placing sponge rubber buns between socks over the posterior aspect of the residual limb near the popliteus and having the prosthesis put on with these in place.

Summarizing, the ideal prosthetic socket would be suspended from the femoral condyles, have suspension from the patella region added if the residuus were short, be in total contact with whatever reliefs were needed for bony prominences, have generous flares or gradual pressure gradients between various parts which transmit forces for support of the body or for stabilization of the prosthesis on the residual limb, be free of padding or insulative linings, be thin walled to allow distortion under load and to reduce bulk and reduce heat retention, allow inclusion of a sock over the residuus, and utilize every available surface of the residual limb for the transmission of support and stabilizing forces.

ALIGNMENT

The fit of a socket cannot be entirely isolated from the responses which accrue from the movements imposed by ambulation. The magnitude of phasic forces at critical moments and their direction of action are anticipated as nearly as possible in the fitting of the socket, but how the component parts of the prosthesis are positioned (aligned) in relation to one another has an important effect. This "alignment" factor is related to two things: 1) the tilt of the foot, or its angle with respect to the socket, and 2) the position of the foot with respect to the socket in transverse directions. The length of the prosthesis is assumed to be correct.

Because of the intimate relationship between fit and alignment, a knowing prosthetist never adjusts the fit of the socket until he has tried to optimize comfort by means of changes or adjustments to the alignment. The significance of alignment as a source of discomfort even when fit of the socket is adequate can be appreciated by considering how forces can be increased or decreased by alignment changes. To examine this, let us consider what effects on the residual limb follow the gross displacement or the gross angulation of the prosthetic foot. It may help to imagine that the prosthesis can pivot against the end of the residual limb as though it were a ball in a socket. Thus, all the tilting will be seen in terms of displacements between the top edges of the socket and the adjacent areas of the residual limb.

If we move the foot far forward, as indicated in Figure 4.6 *A*, there is a long lever effect now toward the front. There will be a continuous resistance to knee bending and a forceful tendency to knee extension during weight bearing on the prosthesis. There obviously will be a high force against the patellar tendon region and a similar high force at the bottom of the socket against the residual limb at the back. The tissues there will be compressed while there will be gaping between the back top edge of the socket and the residual limb and a corresponding gaping between the end of the tibia and the socket in front. This illustrates what is called a "force couple." Force couples indicate what the conditions are and how to change these conditions. Placing the foot in an extreme backward position without a change in foot angle with respect to the residual limb segment, obviously will have the opposite effect in terms of where the forces will be. The knee will now be forced to bend, or failing that, will suffer high forces at the back of the knee and distally against the front of the tibia. Extreme shifts of the foot to the inside or the outside can be visualized in the same way. Always, there will be a force couple or some body action which will nullify it (Fig. 4.6 *B*).

Foot angle changes have an effect on timing of the forces against the residual limb as the stride proceeds. Consider first an excessive downward tilt of the foot from some optimal position. Imagine that the heel hardly makes contact and immediately thereafter the support force shifts to the end of the forefoot at the ground. There will be a tendency to force the knee into extension, or to prevent it from flexing. Again, the patellar tendon will be heavily pressed soon after heel contact and a counter force toward the end of the residual limb will be against its back surface. If the amputee were able to overcome the tendency, this could result in a sudden bending of the knee and a complete reversal of the force pair of the residual limb. When the foot is tilted upward, the heel contact period during the stride, weight bearing on the prosthesis, is prolonged. The reverse force couple prevails. The knee will yield, or failing that, there will be a force couple which presses hard behind the knee and hard against the distal tibia anteriorly. This illustrates a common difficulty which can be overcome by teaching the BK amputee to relax the knee on the prosthetic side until the foot is flat on the floor after heel contact, or by setting the foot at a greater plantarflexion angle (Fig. 4.6. *C*).

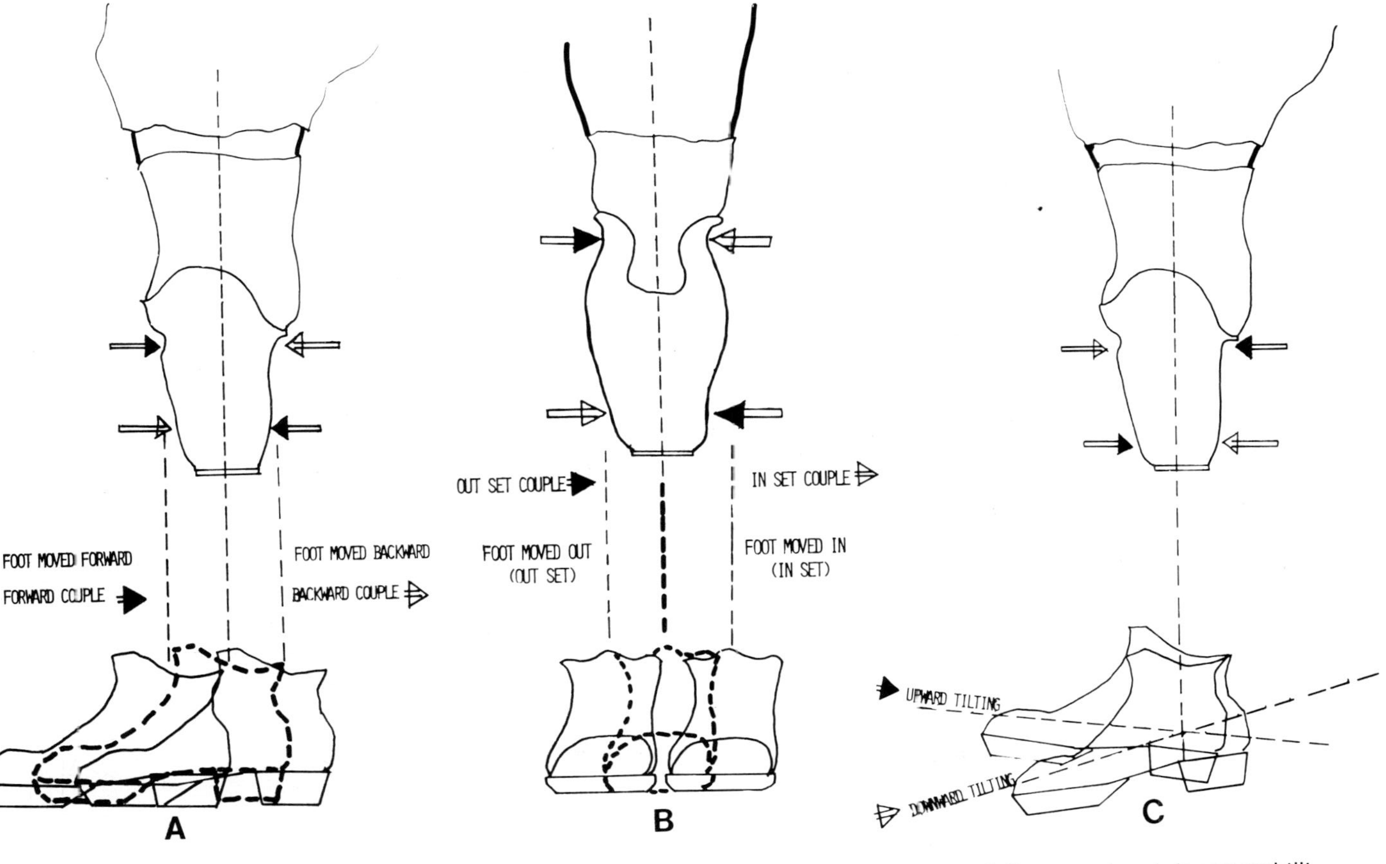

Fig. 4.6 Prosthetic foot alignment. *A*, forward and backward; *B*, out set and in set; and *C*, upward and downward tilt.

Besides the motions which occur between the prosthetic socket and the residual limb as clues to needed alignment changes, one can check the residual limb for markings imprinted on it by the socket due to these forces. There may be the print of the sock, abrasions, or redness.

Because quite small changes in alignment can have detectable effects on comfort, "adjustable legs," devices which can be used to adjust the position of a socket over the foot and its inclination in trials, have been designed. Many prosthetists have become accustomed to relying on such devices. In more recent times, prosthetic components of a knob and tube nature have been designed which include alignment capabilities within them. With these devices, it is possible to tilt segments of the prosthesis, to shift positions of segments and to adjust the length. These systems are referred to as *modular*. They permit assembly of the structural elements of prostheses from prefabricated parts. In BK prosthetics, their main value lies in these inherent adjustable features which remain in the prosthesis for any subsequent changes that might be needed. It would be valuable also to have the capacity in these devices to make quick replacement of the socket possible. A soft cover dresses up the system.

ROLE OF FOOT

Typically, the foot used in the PTB prosthesis and in the joint and corset type also, is the Solid Ankle Cushion Heel (SACH) foot. Other types of feet with articulated joints also are used. With these, alignment changes can be made by adjusting the "bumpers" or "stops" which limit and control the articulations. The SACH foot can be rotated around its attachment bolt, but for angular changes in the plantardorsiflexion directions, some alignment coupler at the foot must be used. A similar device is needed under the socket to shift the position of any prosthetic foot. A more detailed discussion of components will follow under Prosthetic Components.

Knee Disarticulation Amputation

As prosthetic procedures have improved and the variety of options in terms of components have increased, a new interest in knee disarticulation amputations is discernable. This is heartening. Let us look, however, at what can be done for these amputees under the best conditions. There is no argument about the functionality of the typical knee disarticulation residual limb. It is accepted now that the mediolateral flaps can be used to save the condyles when very short BK amputation is contraindicated. The amputation is less traumatic than other types in the same region. Designers could solve the problems associated with the hardware. Prosthetists know that the end-bearing feature, once adequately fitted, serves the amputee well over long periods of time with fewer needs for attention than below-knee or above-knee amputees.

The great, broad articular surface of the femoral condyles at the knee is so obviously capable of total weight bearing that no more needs to be said. Also, if the condyles are left intact the flares, which so easily hold on the BK prosthesis although the muscles and joint actions would drive it off, easily can suspend the knee disarticulation prosthesis against the passive femoral end. When the condyles have been trimmed away in the interest of cosmesis or to improve the tissue cover, then the suspensive feature is diminished and such alternatives as suction suspension may be required.

NEEDS

Let us consider just what it may be that the knee disarticulation amputee needs:

1. A socket which provides a comfortable platform against which the condylar surface will fit with a minimum of motion and with an even distribution of pressure;
2. A socket which fits close to the femoral shaft on the lateral side, and which secures it from in front and behind against tilting actions centered on the articular surface as pivot;
3. A secure fit on the medial side to establish the necessary force couples associated with tilting actions between the socket and the residual limb which must be blocked;
4. An intimate fit against the femoral flares at the knee for retention of the prosthesis without impingement on boney prominences;
5. A port of entry into the socket which will not undermine other functions required of the socket;
6. Swing phase control over the shank so that he/she can take full advantage of the strength and stability of the residual limb for getting the most out of the prosthesis;
7. Cosmetic restoration to a degree which will not undermine acceptance of the functional advantages expected of this type of amputation;
8. A joint action which allows easy sitting and arising under normal conditions, such as at table, in buses or cars;
9. A foot which acts to make the passage over the prosthesis natural and free of discontinuities;
10. The capacity to pivot during weight bearing on the prosthesis without experiencing high torques on the residual limb from the prosthesis (especially desirable because of the potential for high activity levels and the bony nature of the residual limb);
11. The prosthesis to be light weight;
12. The prosthesis to be cool.

FITTING

Starting with the fitting technique at the point of taking an impression, the technique of Wilson, formerly at the Biomechanics Laboratory, University of California, Berkeley, is good. The end of the residual limb is first fitted with a plaster of Paris cup made up of small strips of plaster bandage, each worked carefully against the condyles until they are enclosed to a level which ensures retention of the end impression on the residuus. This is made strong enough to carry the weight of the amputee so that he can bear down on it while other sections of the impression are being made. Next, the section covering the lateral surface of the residual limb is laid on, overlapping the cup, and shaped in against the femur to catch it in a channel. The impression extends up to the greater trochanter or hip joint level. This can be secured in place by plaster bandage which is wrapped around the remainder of the thigh as the layup adjacent to the femur hardens. A single thickness is sufficient. Finally, the medial surface, somewhat flattened like the base of a triangle with apex at the femur, is laid on, overlapping both of the previous sections sufficiently to allow reassembly of the impression. The medial section is not only flattened somewhat, but is flared outward as it approaches the adductor mass, terminating at the crotch. The length of impression obtained is greater than needed for most cases and enough for any. Control over the tissues can be enhanced during this phase of making the impression if the end-bearing cup is set into a sling, as in the Northwestern University Suspension Casting system, and the other two sections are made against the supported thigh.

The three sections of the impression are lubricated at each step as required to ensure their separation for removal. Marks to ensure accurate reassembly of the sections also are made.

If the residual limb is mature, little needs to be done to it other than the addition of reliefs to the plaster model. If the limb is not mature, then model adjustments must be made to reduce bulk over areas which correspond to soft tissues. Those amputees who have not matured can be expected to need more than one socket, as do new amputees in general.

SOCKET

The socket should be made thin walled to enhance the cosmetic effect, help keep it cool and allow some limberness in appropriate areas so that it is easy to get on and off. The socket need extend no higher than the level which will allow good control. Reports of amputees preferring to have the socket extend to the ischial tuberosity level so that the top end will be anchored may be correct, but had the socket been fitted intimately enough such an extensive socket would not have been needed. This is an area for experimentation. A socket no deeper than 20–24 cm measured from the weight-bearing surface to the top edge laterally should provide a socket of adequate depth. Such a socket will be lightweight; it will be cool; and it will cling to the residual limb. Cosmetic effect will be optimized. It will be strong and flexible where required. It will be structurally suitable when glass cloth strips are interspersed between 10 layers of nylon tricot so that the glass cloth is shingled toward the top edge of the socket and toward the front and back of the area over the femur, with the maximum thickness adjacent to the surface to which the joint system will be attached. Only tricot will cover the medial surface where the port of entry will be made. The port of entry will be flexible with this layup, and if it can be overlapped, the socket can be adjusted for girth. Whatever base is created for attachment of the hardware should not require additional layup of plastic after fabrication of the socket. Such a second step could spoil the function of the socket. Instructions offered by the manufacturers should be modified to realize this aim. It is assumed that a polycentric joint system will be used. Such a system is attached to the socket on a sloping surface at the back, somewhat toward the bottom. If an anchor plate happens to be part of the joint system, this would be included within the socket when it is made. Alternate ways of dealing with the knee disarticulation amputee in terms of socket design include the use of soft sockets, sockets with rubberized liners, sockets which can be pushed into against sponge rubber inserts mounted inside the socket to act as grips for suspension and "open frame" sockets comparable to those advocated by Woodall for above-knee amputees at one time, one of which has been used successfully for a case with fractured femur. The socket style to choose for the standard knee disarticulation residual limb, i.e. one which has not been trimmed and which has the patella in an unobtrusive position with respect to the weight-bearing area, is that which meets the sorts of criteria outlined. It is hard to imagine a better socket than one which is directly and intimately fitted and of a construction which is selectively pliable and stiff to ensure achievement of the desired effects.

PADDING

As for padding in the bottom of the socket, space would be made for it by including it on the model of the residual limb at the time of laminating the socket. It should be thin, durable and fairly dense foam, such as would be used on a soft-soled shoe. Then the residual limb will not sink in during weight bearing on it. A better practice is to fit with sufficient care that no pad will be needed. Then the sock worn over the residual limb will give enough protection. Suction suspension is inappropriate for such a capable residual limb unless the condyles have been trimmed extensively enough to undermine them as areas in which to carry suspension forces.

KNEE MECHANISM

Polycentric knee mechanisms now available are based on the work of Lyquist of Denmark and were derived from studies of Radcliffe. The device chosen should have the option of using either hydraulic or pneumatic swing phase control units within it. If the level of activity to be expected is low, pneumatic control is sufficient. Otherwise, the hydraulic control will be used if one durable enough is available.

The system referred to here will be modular. Thus, a cosmetic cover will be part of the system. If a rotator is to be included to reduce torques on the residual limb, it will be attached in the prescribed way to the foot. The foot of choice is the SACH foot, correctly selected for the appropriate heel cushion density, either medium or soft.

ALIGNMENT

The foot would be aligned carefully with respect to its plantardorsiflexion angle. As with other long-levered residual limbs, alignment is not nearly as critical as for other levels. The shorter the socket is made, however, the more exact must be the alignment of the prosthesis. Because of the way in which the knee mechanisms of the polycentric designs are organized for attachment, the forward-backward position of the knee unit with respect to the socket is essentially preestablished, as also would be the side-to-side position of the foot. Forward or backward placement of the foot through lengthening or shortening of the swing phase control mechanism is available. For other adjustments, only wedging between the knee unit and the socket can be suggested. It can be expected that with the ability to shift the foot and change its angle pertaining to the side view, and the ability to adjust length, all the changes that might be needed to improve on careful bench alignment can be made.

Above-Knee Amputation

Above-knee (AK) prosthetics was for a long time a strong focal point for research activities and design and development work on equipment and techniques. In the course of over 28 years, which included the United States experience during which a number of developments were undertaken at the Biomechanics Laboratory of the University of California, there are a number of significant factors which can be identified. During that period, the emphasis shifted from AK to BK prosthetics owing to the trend toward conserving function. In the early part of that period, work was being done for a younger group of amputees, many of whom were above-knee amputees. As the change came, the sort of person who became central was the elderly amputee, usually a person with multiple problems of which amputation for circulatory troubles was one. In the earlier time, such an amputee would have been amputated above the knee to preserve his life. Now he would be amputated below the knee in all likelihood. As a result of the changes in the population needing devices, some of the work in the AK field dropped to a lower priority.

Highlights in AK prosthetics based on North American experiences are as follows:

1. Establishment of biomechanical principles in relation to AK prosthetic fitting and alignment;
2. Design and entry into use of the SACH foot;
3. Use of adjustable equipment for prosthetists to use to determine the alignment of prosthesis prior to making the artificial limb. (Included was equipment for duplicating alignment into the final prosthesis from the adjustable one.);
4. Establishment of education programs for prosthetists which the Veterans' Administration required persons to take if they would fit veterans;
5. Development of fitting equipment and techniques;
6. The design and introduction of temporary sockets for use on new amputees during their early training phase;
7. Increasingly strong distribution centers which mass-produced components and disseminated information to the trade;
8. The resolution of the use of suction suspension as a means of suspending AK prostheses generally, rather than for particular application;
9. Increasing participation of medical specialists in the evolution of improvements;
10. Transfer from research environments of concepts now manifest in various designs referred to as "modular";
11. The shift in emphasis from equipment to the amputee as clinic teams emerged to foster mutual education of their members;
12. The internationalization of activities pertaining to prosthetics in general.

The devastating effects of loss of the knee, the usefulness of end bearing, the value of conserving length, and some of the biomechanical features of fitting sockets and aligning prostheses have received attention. This discussion will supplement what has been said and identify what is different about the AK amputee as compared to other levels already covered.

One feature of AK prosthetics which is abundantly clear is that there is a welter of equipment pertaining to it: knees, swing phase controls, fitting equipment, suspension methods, artificial feet, modular devices, rotators, adjustable legs, duplicating jigs, valves for suction sockets, and balms for the residual limb. A single thoughtful comment that can be made is that when there are multiple options for a particular problem, it can only be that either the problem is not solved or considerations of the market place predominate. Both of these factors are true with respect to AK prosthetics. What has to be done here is to keep free of the details and work through it in a way that will reduce uncertainty, if possible.

TEMPORARY SOCKETS

Early ambulation can be initiated using modular components which permit length and alignment changes to be made easily as needs change, and which are compatible with the installation of temporary sockets. Also, the system used should offer functional options, be suitable for cosmetic restoration, not rob the prosthetist of space he needs to make a good cosmetic effect for sitting, and be sufficiently durable to serve the needs of the particular person who will use it. Most pertinent among adjustable features is that which permits adjustment of foot angle, because one of the needs of such an amputee is prosthetic knee joint stability, and foot alignment in the plantardorsiflexion directions has a telling effect on this stability. The foot of choice is the SACH foot with a soft heel cushion. As for the socket, it would be valuable to have a prefabricated socket system which allowed adjustment for shrinkage in the soft tissue areas. However, we are stuck with what is available and such adjustment is not adequately allowed for. What can be said is that temporary sockets can be confidently used if this principle is adhered to: *The prefabricated socket will be of a size and shape which is compatible with the person who will use it and appropriate for the level of activity at which the user will function.*

Reason for success can be predicted:

1. The activity level of the user is low; therefore the chances of his being harmed by it are remote if not impossible.
2. There is competent supervision as it is being used.
3. The environment in which it is used is protective, *i.e.* he is in a rehabilitation setting.
4. The residual limb is well padded with tissues and perhaps bulky with edema.
5. The prosthetic components and their alignment are appropriate.
6. The suspension system is optimal for control of the prosthesis by the amputee. (Do not overlook shoulder harness, nor feel like a heretic for using it.)
7. The shape and size of the socket used is appropriate.
8. The necessary skills for using the system are available to the amputee.

The system can only fail if:

1. The person for whom it is used is inappropriate for the available system.
2. The system is unsatisfactory.
3. The required skills to use the system are not available.

Adequately dealt with and worn as fully as possible throughout the day, even if only for sitting, the temporary socket on a modular system will:

1. Protect the residual limb;
2. Control edema;
3. Accustom the amputee to the feel of a socket on the residual limb;
4. Allow early initiation of rehabilitation on a prosthesis;
5. Provide a means by which an amputee's potential as a wearer can be assessed;
6. Offer a means by which an amputee can be kept walking while a definitive limb is being made or adjusted;
7. Serve as a therapeutic tool for conditioning or reconditioning an amputee.

The only other alternative to a temporary socket is a fitted one. Since it is time-consuming and expensive to provide a socket which is fitted, there is no sense in preparing one that is marginal. This is particularly important when the new amputee who has to be fitted is lean, bony and likely to have a low activity level. Such a person needs every advantage to realize a worthwhile level of performance.

FITTED SOCKET

For the person who has reached the stage of needing a fitted socket after successful conditioning on a temporary one, or for the lean bony person, just mentioned, there are a few primary requirements. The fitted socket must:

1. Not impinge on the groin as the patient sits;
2. Be easy to put on;
3. Be comfortable standing;
4. Be secure against rotating out of place on the limb;
5. Not be so bulky that it is hard to get into clothing;
6. Stay in place as patient sits or stands;
7. Be cosmetically acceptable;
8. Be easy to clean and basically hygienic.

If the residual limb is unlikely to shrink, or is lean, then a fitted socket should be used right from the start if possible. A number of techniques are available. The sockets obtained divide into two groups, wooden or plastic.

FITTING TECHNIQUE

When a plastic socket is to be made, as is now the more common practice, the main steps are 1) to make an impression of the residual limb; 2) to cast a model of the residual limb in the cavity obtained; 3) to adjust the shape of the model by adding or removing material until it is suitable to use as a mould for making the socket; and 4) making a plastic socket. These are the same now familiar steps which pertain to any impression-based socket preparation. There are these ways in which impressions can be made:

Hand Casting

Plaster of Paris bandage is wrapped around the residuus as the amputee stands, and when the material begins to set, the hands hold it in a way that provides finger indentations at areas where weight-bearing features and flares will be developed during the adjustment (modification) of the shape of the model. This is the best technique for persons with lean boney residual limbs, or special shape problems, such as found in some congenital amputees.

Adjustable Brim Fitting Method

(Berkeley brims or Hosmer brims are names interchangeably used to identify the equipment.) In this procedure, quadrilateral brims which can cover the top few inches of the residual limb in the same way as the socket will, and which can be adjusted to change the front-to-back widths independently on the medial and lateral sides, serve as jigs for the fitting procedure. The required brim is selected, either left or right, from a set of 10 for the given side and attached to a stand. The amputee stands weight bearing down into the brim which is then checked for size, substituted for another if necessary, and finally adjusted to the correct front-to-back widths. Then, a plaster of Paris wrap is made around the portion of the residual limb which protrudes beyond the brim, and the wrap is made to include the lower border of the brim to link brim and impression together. The resulting cavity is then used to make the model. While the original method was to have the amputee stand, an alternate method is to have him lie on the natural leg, residual limb up. The brim is held in place by an assistant as the plaster impression is made. This is a way of preventing engorgement of the residual limb which may otherwise occur due to the constrictive effect of the brim. Also, it is much less strenuous for older or feeble people. Figure 4.7 shows the typical manner in which impressions are made.

New York University Technique

This method also involves use of a jig as part of the impression making procedure. The jigs are based on the previous method, but this method varies in that there are only three brims for each side of the body. The brims have a flexible lateral section to compensate for the lower number of jigs. All other parts of the procedure would be essentially the same as for the adjustable brim fitting technique. More work may be required to adjust the model than with the previous technique, but the final result should be comparable.

Veterans Administration Prosthetics Center Technique

The equipment is designed to be left-sided and right-sided so that only two jigs are required. Also, the manner of using the system is different from

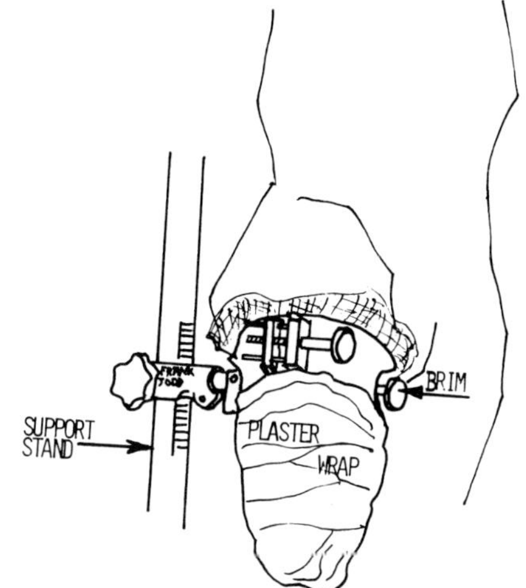

Fig. 4.7 Adjustable brim fitting technique for hand casting an impression of residual limb in above-knee (AK) amputation.

the previous two methods. The plaster is laid on the residual limb after the jig has been sized on the residuus. Then, the clad residual limb is inserted into the jig and held to shape as the amputee stands down on it. When the plaster is hard, the amputee removes his limb, and the cavity is used to pour up the plaster model. Considerably more work is required to adjust this shape than with the other two techniques, but less than for the hand casting method.

SOCKET INSTALLATION

Once a socket has been obtained by any of these methods, it is attached to the adjustable leg if a wooden shank-knee set-up is to be used, or is set up directly onto the modular components if that system is to be used. The socket will be mounted on the prosthetic components with thigh and shank lengths appropriate, and the knee axis in the required position. The socket will be placed so that the hip joint of the residual limb will be in enough flexion to allow the amputee to impose a backward impulse to the prosthesis when he/she is standing upright on it. This provides him/her with voluntary control over it. A balance must be struck between how much voluntary control or how much alignment contributes to the overall stability the patient has, with or without a stabilizing device at the knee.

STABILITY

Looking at the factor of stability at the knee, we must consider it in terms of 1) the amount contributed by alignment; and 2) the amount that the hip can contribute. As already indicated, alignment factors are those which involve the positions of the different parts of the prosthesis relative to the residual limb. How elements are organized is based on the effects we expect from the forces operating between the prosthesis and the environment, including the body at the socket end and the ground at the foot end. As we saw in discussions of the BK amputee, moving the prosthetic foot forward or backward with respect to the residual limb has consequences on the forces directed transversely upon it and on the direction of resistance to movements tending to occur at the knee. For the AK amputee, gross forward placement of the prosthetic foot makes the knee of the prosthesis very stable. Such stability makes initiation of swing phase difficult unless the amputee unloads the prosthesis first. Also, any attempts to make the knee bend impose high forces at the end of the residual limb in front, and at the top behind. Setting the foot back excessively makes the prosthesis unstable at the knee so that a backward action from the residual limb is required to maintain stability if it can be maintained at all. The extending action imposes forces on the top at the front and on the bottom at the back as far as the residual limb is concerned. These ideas are given to assist the prosthetist with conceptualizing what can happen. The fine details watched for by the prosthetist as he aligns the prosthesis when the amputee is on the adjustable components pass so quickly and are so small, even for the practised eye, that he has to proceed by trial and error until he has brought the prosthesis into the required alignment. The relative movements between the prosthesis and the body at one end and between the prosthesis and the floor at the other give him his clues.

ALIGNMENT

AK prosthesis alignment will be considered in terms of gross alignment changes so that the effects of changes will be clearer. As before, we look at the alignment in terms of what happens as a result of specific changes in relative position of the parts which affect function with respect to the residual limb.

Any change in alignment will be reflected in the patient's gait and comfort in walking. Alignment changes can be considered under the following conditions:

1. Conditions of low load which pertain to the time when the prosthesis is swinging through space, called the *swing phase*;
2. Conditions of high load which pertain to the time when the prosthesis is supporting the amputee, called the *stance phase*;
3. Conditions of stance phase when *alignment stability* predominates;
4. Conditions of stance phase when *voluntary control* of *stability* is possible.

Let us consider now what happens for certain extreme situations when changes are made to the prosthesis according to the items below.

1. *Length*—length changes due to shortening or lengthening of any of the structures longitudinally, but it also changes when the knee angle

or the foot angle is changed. Let us assume that the knee and foot will remain optimally placed for consideration of the effects of length changes. 1) The prosthesis is made too long. (a) The amputee will rise up (*vaulting*) on the normal foot to prevent the prosthetic foot from scuffing in swing phase as he walks with the prosthesis correctly placed under him. His control over the prosthesis most likely will be reduced and he will use more energy to walk because of the rising action on the normal foot which elevates his center of gravity; or (b) he will swing the prosthesis out in an arc (*circumduction*) to clear the foot on the prosthetic side, without necessarily rising up on the natural foot, and lean over the prosthesis as he bears weight on it. The amount of leaning will depend on how strong a lateral impulse he gives to the prosthesis. The impulse will be strong if he chooses to remain erect (*side sway*) and it will be weaker if his choice is to compensate by leaning (*list*). What he choses depends on comfort factors. If he were to get directly over the prosthesis he might experience discomfort in the crotch and also on the distal end of the femur laterally, or he might experience energy costs which would lead him to modify the action in preference for leaning outward over the supporting prosthesis. Figure 4.8 illustrates these actions. 2) If the prosthesis is short, the amputee will have better voluntary control over it, will usually shorten his stride, walk with a narrow base, but lean over the prosthesis. He also may have to bend the natural knee excessively to "let himself down" onto the prosthesis and, when his weight is supported by it, he might circumduct the natural leg to clear the natural foot.

A rule of thumb for judging what the length should be is that the prosthetic side and the normal side will be equal in length as the amputee stands only when the residual limb is also long—say supracondylar level.

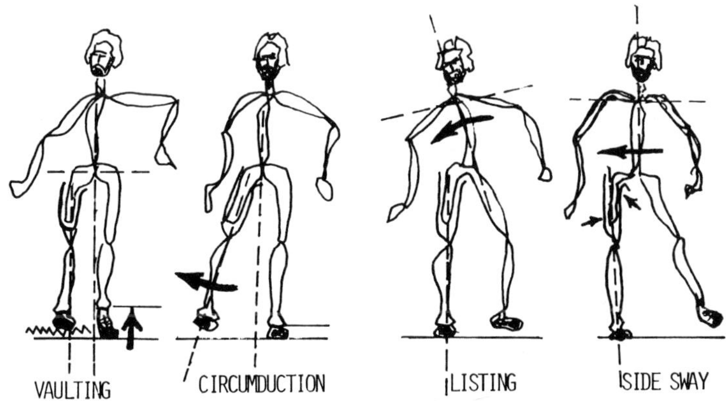

Fig. 4.8. Poor alignment actions when a leg prosthesis is made too long.

The prosthesis may be shortened as much as 2 cm for persons with very short residual limbs.

2. *Foot Position*—The foot can be positioned anywhere that the alignment system will allow within the base of a cone. Thus, positioning the foot to the front or rear, or to one side or the other side, will be considered. As changes are made, we think of the foot as a lever system. Such a lever system will have effects which the residual limb senses as forces imposed on it by the socket, as moments or bending actions are transmitted to it. 1) Moving the foot progressively toward the back as an alignment change will cause the stride on the prosthetic side to become progressively shorter. 2) Moving the foot progressively forward with respect to the residual limb will have the opposite effect, or progressively lengthen the stride on the prosthesis. 3) Moving the foot inward with respect to the residual limb can have a variety of effects. a) The amputee may maintain the hip adducted and walk with a narrower base (feet closer together). This will cause gaping between the top of the socket and the body near the hip joint and discomfort at the crotch level and at the distal end of the residual limb on the lateral side. These areas are subjected to pressure from the force couple to be expected when the body is using the abductors to stabilize the pelvis to prevent excessive drop on the natural leg side as it is in swing phase. A well fitted socket will remain comfortable under these conditions *if* the residual limb is sufficiently long to permit such pelvis stabilization by the abductors. This is by no means a universal capability among amputees. The force couple is produced by force upward from the ground and force downward from the center of gravity of the body, which would tend to make the prosthesis bend to displace the prosthetic knee laterally if it could. The hip joint can function to modify such affects, and it will if there are discomforts. If the discomforts are sufficient, the period on the prosthesis will be shortened, *or* b) the patient will abduct the hip, thus moving the foot laterally (outward) for weight bearing on it, and lean over the prosthesis for control, again dividing the action between leaning and giving his/her body a lateral impulse as he/she comes to full weight bearing on the prosthesis. The choice always depends on comfort and energy costs. Since the aim is that the patient walk with a narrow base and with the body erect for the sake of a more normal appearance, it is clear that the first option (*a*) can only be realized if the socket is comfortable under these conditions. Comfort depends on the magnitude of the forces imposed on the residual limb by the socket, the area of support available between the socket and the residual limb, and the relative movements occurring as the loads are transmitted between the socket and the residual limb. The magnitude of the forces which provide the mediolateral

stability associated with erect and narrow-based gait depends on the distance between the force couple acting to stabilize the system within the socket and the area over which the constituent forces act. Both of these factors are dependent on the size of the residual limb, the areas available for force transmission and the distance between the resultant points of application. Length is also a factor in movements between the prosthesis and the residual limb. We can conclude, then, that length is going to be an important factor in determining whether or not an amputee can walk erect and with a narrow base. 4) Lateral or outward shift of the foot also has a variety of possible consequences. a) The amputee may compensate by moving the foot inward as he/she walks by adducting the hip on the prosthetic side. From this the patient gains the narrower base of walking, *or* b) the patient will leave the foot out set and gain balance over the prosthesis during stance phase by leaning over it, *or* c) leave it placed outward as he/she puts weight onto it, giving the body a lateral impulse from the push of the normal leg to shift himself/herself over the prosthesis, thereby reducing or eliminating list over it. The degree of list compared to sway provides an indication of what actions are taking place.

The results related to inward or outward positioning of the foot are under some degree of voluntary control. The response which the person makes to the different mediolateral foot positions depends on the muscular strength, the vigor with which they walk, the length of the residual limb, the tolerance of tissues to the forces which must be borne, their weight, other alignment factors which make demands on the reisdual limb (flexion-extension control for example), length of the prosthesis, and such things as the components used. Any failure to achieve a comfortable, natural appearing gait will be evidenced by such deviations as listing over the prosthesis, side sway, and such other manoeuvers as might moderate discomforts and enhance control for the least amount of effort compatible with a gait acceptable to him.

3. *Foot Angles*—Tilting the foot in the major direction (plantardorsiflexion) has a great effect on comfort, stability and control. Tilting the foot in the minor direction (inversion-eversion) has little effect on anything but cosmesis. Rotating the foot on an axis parallel to the long axis of the residual limb (toe-in toe-out) has important effects equivalent to insetting or outsetting the foot with respect to the axis according to the instantaneous position of the prosthesis in the stance phase of walking. But the position selected is dictated by cosmetic considerations and for the purposes of this discussion can be neglected. This leaves us with angular changes in the plantardorsiflexion directions to consider. 1) *As the major axis of the foot increasingly inclines downward, the stride on the* natural side *is*

progressively shortened. 2) *As the major axis of the foot is progressively inclined upward, the stride on the natural side is progressively lengthened.* These effects, especially the effect of shortening stride on the normal side, can be seen easily when such changes are made to the feet of prostheses of elderly or weak persons. When the resistance of the forefoot is felt, the natural limb will descend to bear weight no matter where it is. Substitution of a passive foot has the immediate effect of lengthening stride on the natural side. (This suggests that a foot for the geriatric category of patients might be better with *no* forefoot action at all.)

The aim of the alignment procedure is to organize the angular position of the foot relative to the residual limb axis so that the *timing* of the action of forces at the foot is optimal. The requirements relate not only to the length of stride, prosthesis or normal, but also to stability and control during weight bearing on the prosthesis. One requirement is that the natural limb also be supporting weight when weight is transferred to the heel of the prosthetic foot. Under these conditions, any backward action at the hip joint of the residual limb exerted to control the prosthesis will be effectively transmitted to the prosthesis as the prosthetic foot anchors it to the ground and the normal foot anchors the pelvis. Thus, at the moment of heel contact on the prosthesis, forces for stabilizing the prosthetic knee and for impelling the body forward over it are effective. Once the natural foot leaves the ground, momentum carries the body forward, and alignment factors dominate prosthetic knee joint stability. When the foot angle is optimally set, the prosthesis is programmed to provide the balance between voluntary control and alignment stability which is compatible with the least use of energy and a natural appearing gait. For stability and control to be optimized (and it is safety that is in our minds), the foot angle selected will ensure that the line of action of support forces will fall in front of the knee axis once voluntary control is lost by initiation of swing phase on the natural side. This is a simplified view. Arm actions contribute to shifts in the center of gravity which can alter the direction of the line of action of support forces, and this represents a form of voluntary control. Nor are the forces acting on the prosthesis fixed throughout the walking cycle at the socket end. At heel contact, the prosthesis is pressed anteriorly at the brim. Toward the end of the stance phase on it, the pressure is posterior on the socket brim. Thus, as the action point at the foot moves from the heel to the toe, the action point at the socket end moves in a reverse direction. At some point along the prosthesis there will be a little deviation of the line of action's distance from a point on the prosthesis (Fig. 4.9). Since this will be in the region of the knee, moments on the prosthetic knee joint are probably fairly constant throughout the stance phase of walking on the prosthetic side. Thus, when

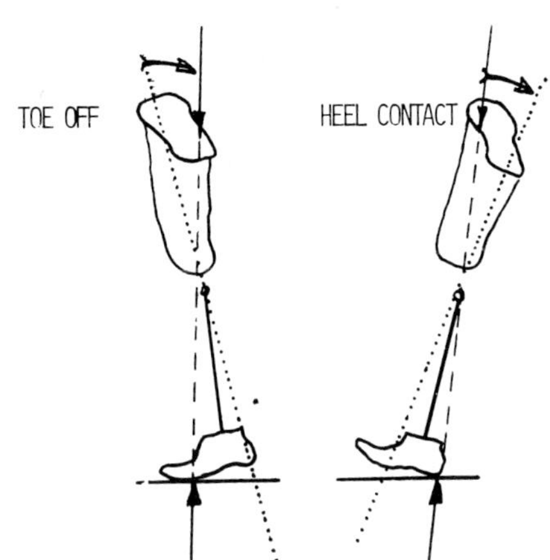

Fig. 4.9 Shifting action line between prosthetic socket end foot.

the foot is properly aligned, stability from alignment and voluntary actions are in good balance.

Because the distance along which the ground reaction action point moves between heel contact and full support on the toe is greater than the distance the action point at the socket moves, in all probability the foot has greater influence over stability of the knee than has the socket. This would explain the common experience in which knee stability is increased when the prosthetic foot is plantarflexed. In Germany, the system of alignment is based on this idea. The AK amputee is set up so that he/she essentially walks on the end of the forefoot throughout most of the stance phase on the prosthesis. This ensures that stability is high during the early period of the stance phase, and allows stability to diminish as the step proceeds so that, at the end of the stance phase, the prosthetic knee can be overbalanced for initiation of the swing phase. The diminution of stability comes from the increasingly posterior position of the support forces at the socket. Stability of the prosthetic knee is "broken" when the amputee "sits down hard" (Tubersitz Method) on the prosthesis, simultaneously flexing the residual limb hip. In German prostheses the foot is typically further toward the back than in the prostheses set up by others. The result to be expected (Foot Position, 1)) is that the stride would be short, and that is so.

The significant effect that alignment of the major axis of the foot has on comfort, energy use and cosmetic effect is known to prosthetists who use feet with articulated ankles. The results required can be obtained by adjustments to the stops or bumpers of these articulated feet. When the SACH foot is used, the best results are obtained when there is an alignment coupler such as some modular systems include. Otherwise, inserts in the shoe or wedging between the foot shank junction must be done.

WEIGHT BEARING

This discussion of alignment has been required as a prerequisite for the discussion of socket design. There is such an intimate relationship between the fit of a socket and the alignment of a prosthesis that one cannot be considered apart from the other. One can think of the socket as a "sloppy link" which transmits forces for 1) support of body weight and 2) control of the prosthesis by musculature. The support forces are typically higher than the control forces. Thus, an examination of the residual limb anatomy in relation to support forces is of prime importance. Possible weight-bearing structures are:

1. Ischial tuberosity;
2. Hamstring tendons;
3. Gluteus maximus;
4. Posterior aspect of the greater trochanter;
5. Posterior surface of the femur (with the hip joint flexed);
6. Lateral surface of the femur (with the hip joint adducted);
7. Inguinal crease area;
8. Tendon of adductor longus;
9. Pubis symphasis;
10. Ischiopubic rami;
11. Muscles, especially when tensed;
12. Fluid mass acting hydraulically;
13. Other pelvic areas, even to the contralateral (other) side.

Obviously, the potential of some of these possible support areas will be greater than others. None should be ignored when analysis is made, especially when a difficult condition is being dealt with. It is better not to get stuck on such ideas as "ischial bearing," but to tailor each socket to what the person presents as potential and needs. I recall a person whose hamstring tendons had been stripped from the ischium. Neither structure could tolerate force. The socket was fitted to use mediolateral wedging between the lateral surface of the femur and the medial aspects of the residuus in the crotch for weight bearing, along with gluteal shelf support coupled to support from the anterior brim flare over the inguinal crease. This represented a good and durable solution.

SOCKET DESIGN AND MODIFICATION

For the usual well padded person with sound anatomy, the quadrilateral socket is most typically used. The quadrilateral shape applies not only to AK amputees but also to BK amputees who must be provided with proximal support (ischial-bearing prostheses) and to brace wearers with normal anatomy, such as people with fractures. The socket type derives its name from the boxlike shape it has as one looks down into it. When the anatomical cross-section of the residual limb at the crotch level is examined, there may seem to be less logic in the shape than there is in fact, especially if one relates it to the skeletal anatomy. Then one will see the ischial tuberosity, the tendon of adductor longus and the greater trochanter as stable landmarks around which the socket must fit. These landmarks define the *basic triangle* around which to design the shape of *any* socket at this level and levels immediately below. Deviations from the basic triangle at the proximal levels of the AK socket occur to accommodate the tissue volume adjacent to the sides of the triangle. These tissues include the tendon, muscles and subcutaneous fat (Fig. 4.10).

This viewpoint differs markedly from the usual. A further deviation from the usual is the designation of the lateral surface of the femur as a weight-bearing surface. *The lateral surface of the adducted residual thigh is a*

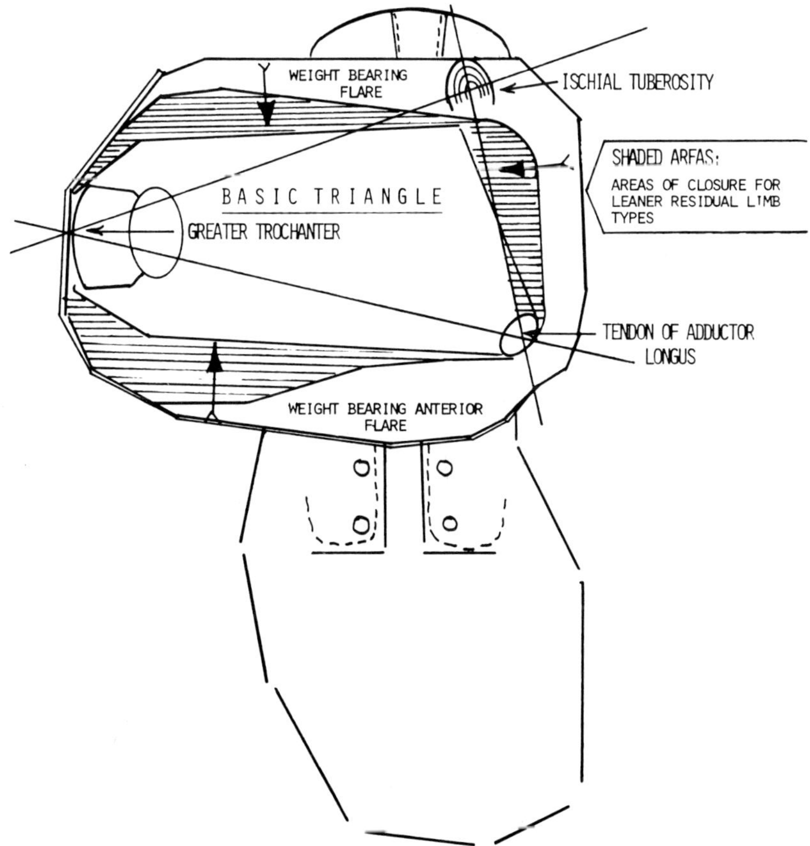

Fig. 4.10. Looking down into a socket for an above-knee (AK) amputation shows the basic triangle design.

major *weight bearing surface as well as a potential force transmitter for pelvic stabilization through actions of hip abductors for persons with midthigh or more length.* Use of the sloped lateral side of the thigh remnant for weight bearing demands a corresponding surface in the socket, including the brim of the socket at the crotch. There are different ways to shape the socket to obtain the required counterthrust from the medial side: 1) the front and back walls of the socket can converge toward the medial side; 2) the flare of the medial brim can slope inward, be broad and be fitted against any tolerating resistant surfaces; 3) the socket can be shaped to load the medial surface more distally; and 4) for residual limbs with end-bearing abilities, the end can be secured to stabilize the femur against the socket surface for weight bearing.

The role of the posterior brim always has been adequately acknowledged with respect to weight bearing. Less frequently has the role of the anterior brim been acknowledged (UCLA (University of California Los Angeles) functional long leg brace). *The inguinal crease area and posterior aspects of the residual AK limb combine as the major weight-bearing structures acting together in alternating pattern to transmit forces between the body and the prosthesis in the socket.* At the beginning of stance phase on the prosthesis, the inguinal crease area absorbs the thrust of the body against the socket. As the step advances, the support forces are shared increasingly with the posterior structures of the residual limb. By the time the stance phase is nearly ended, all of the force is supported by the posterior structures.

The thrust of these arguments is in the interest of greater flares with more generous radii of curvature over those areas of the socket which transmit these support forces. The posterior brim, for example, is often not curved nearly enough, but thrusts abruptly into the gluteal fold. Would it not be an improvement to shape the posterior brim for a progressive shift to the back of the forces supported by the posterior brim? The posterior wall of the socket can now be seen in terms of its support function when the hip is in the flexed position. Much more detailed treatment of this whole question of how the residuus bears weight would be a worthwhile undertaking. It would lead to much improved temporary sockets, for example, or even the *modularization* of sockets. But a general principle can be stated: *wherever there are high forces concentrated at the brim of the socket, the radii of curvature must be generous so that the forces are as broadly distributed over the supporting surfaces as possible, and so that the gradient of forces across a surface will be as gradual as possible.*

The four *corners* of the typical AK socket of the quadrilateral type differ from one another according to their functions. The curvature around each corner of the quadrilateral socket at the top is such that suction suspension can be maintained without imposing stress on underlying tissues. The groove in the anterior corner is shaped to fit the tendon of adductor longus comfortably. The posteromedial corner varies in its size according to the volume of the residual limb and the degree to which it supports the tendons for weight bearing at the top brim. It also is affected by the firmness of tissues contained by it. The leaner the person is the more obtuse is the angle between the posterior and medial walls of the socket at the top, and the less pronounced is the radius in this corner. For the very lean person, this corner can be positioned so far toward the axis of the residual limb that the ischial tuberosity will be positioned quite medial to the inside corner. The usual belief is that the ischial tuberosity should be positioned lateral to this corner as an invariable rule. Situations have been observed in which the ischial tuberosity hung outside the socket while the hamstring tendons supported weight. Such observations help to confirm that more than the ischial tuberosity is involved in weight bearing.

Although emphasis must be placed on the role of the upper sections of the AK socket in providing support, the lower regions also play a part both in supporting weight and in bearing forces which stabilize the prosthesis on the residual limb. Here there are great variations in shape because the shape relates to musculature and other tissues more than to the firm, invariable bony, tendonous structures. Only generalizations can be made: *within the socket, the walls will be contoured to allow forces to be evenly distributed across the broadest possible areas for stabilization and support.* One of the commonest failures in AK sockets fitted by the adjustable brim fitting technique is bulging below the level corresponding to the bottom edge of the fitting brim. Such a shape tends to choke the residual limb proximally *unless* it is a high level amputation. Then, the bottle-like shape is an asset for the retention of suction for suspension. Another difficulty arises because the front brim of the socket made using this equipment impinges on the anterior superior spine when the amputee sits. Some prosthetists merely cut the brim level down. This produces an edge which exerts increased pressure on the inguinal crease area. Folliculitis or even boils can result. When the socket is further adjusted to avoid contact with these, the problem is compounded. The proper thing to do is to fit the socket with a generous flare that will not impinge on the anterior superior spine during sitting. Otherwise, the socket brim, when adjusted, should be lowered without a reduction in the curvature over the edge or the area of support.

Often the *total contact* feature of the AK socket is ineffectual. *The socket must be shaped to give space for a sensitive or sparsely covered femoral end toward the front, back and lateral sides while the soft tissues medially toward the end are compressed upward and inward by pressure from the socket.* The soft tissues will often fill up spaces created for protection of the bone end.

The total contact socket has been a boon to the amputee. This is not only in terms of reducing the pressure gradient between the top and the bottom of the residual limb in the socket which lessens the tendency toward edema, but also in terms of proprioception provided by contact between the tissues and the socket distally. No doubt stability of the residuus in the socket is increased, as also might be weight bearing distally. Sometimes the amputated end is poorly padded and downward pull of the prosthesis in swing phase is supported over too small an area for comfort. The discomfort experienced is a stinging sensation caused by the suction drawing on too small an area of the residual limb end. Fibrous material can be used as an end pad to spread the area available for support of the negative pressure of the suction socket. Otherwise, the free volume under the end of the residual limb must be increased. Bony impingement with the socket at the bottom requires a check of alignment, and then, if warranted, enlargement of the socket distally to obtain clearance or, if the condition is due to sinking in, reestablishment of the weight-bearing characteristics of the socket to give the required relief.

The well fitted socket reflects the major role played by the femoral remnant as a control link and weight-bearing structure. With regard to its function of controlling the prosthesis, this generalization can be made: *since the hip joint is the main control point and the femoral remnant the link through which control forces are passed to the socket, the femur must be secured in the socket throughout its active phase of support and control.* It will be caught in a triangular trough with the apex along the length of the remnant. As indicated before, the end is protected on three sides.

VARIANTS

An endless stream of details is possible concerning the effects of variations in residual limb shape, size and measure as well as the functionality of the remnant in terms of firmness and musculature, but discussion can be limited to those observations whigh might be useful to prosthetists regarding particular residual limb types:

1. Short residual limbs must have sockets which extend high enough to enclose parts of the pelvis for weight bearing and control. There must be belling out of the walls of the socket below the brim level so that tissues can be trapped to assist retention of the prosthesis by suction. Distal tissues on the medial side should be compressed upward and inward to aid in filling the spaces provided.
2. Persons with long residual limbs must be fitted more loosely, proximally, and sufficiently snuggly below, so that the force gradient along the length of the residuus will be as low as possible as a precaution against edema formation.
3. A socket which is snug mediolaterally must be looser in a compensating way anteroposteriorly. The converse also holds. The choice is between weight bearing on the medial and lateral structures as opposed to the anteroposterior structures.

4. Bony above-knee residual limbs tend to have sockets which are shaped more like the triangular plug fit type of socket. Persons with heavy tissues and more normal musculature tend to have sockets which are more quadrilateral in shape. Variations between the extremes of residual limb types have comparable variations in the shape of the socket if the sockets are well fitted.
5. Having the amputee lie on the sound side while an impression is made of the amputated side is superior to having him stand weight bearing in the apparatus or against the support of the hands when the impressions are being made by any method.
6. Female amputees require a higher lateral brim than males so that fatty tissues can be enclosed in the socket for cosmetic purposes. Also, they may require a lower medial brim or, better still, one generously flared so that the downward inclined ischiopubic rami can be comfortably included within the socket and formation of a tissue roll be obviated.
7. Persons who have been amputated at an early age often have thin, inward bowing, tapered femoral remnants which are short and hooked. Fitting the proximal regions for weight bearing in this sort of residual limb results in a bell-like shape generously flared on three sides, but somewhat hooked over the trochanter on the lateral side. As with the shorter residual limb, such a residuus must often be fitted higher onto the pelvic regions to obtain the required degree of control and support.
8. The quadrilateral shape suits small children well. They are hardly a problem in any event because of their light weight and speed of repair. Consideration must be given to the changed shape needed as maturation proceeds. There will be a gradual shift away from the quadrilateral shape unless the amputation was done at a fairly advanced stage of life.
9. Persons with congenitally affected limbs have to be treated as they present because of the wide variety of possibilities in their form. Often a factor is joint instability. The shape of a socket for such a person should add stability between the prosthesis and limb by adding stability to the joint when the joint is adjacent to the top of the socket. This can be achieved by fitting higher onto the pelvic region of the AK residuus. Such an extension also can be used for the attachment of control straps. A strap similar to a Silesian bandage can be made to act as a gluteus medius for the amputated side. Overzealous attention to "normalizing" through the application of a limb prosthesis to a severely affected person before he has had a chance to adapt naturally to his situation can be a disadvantage.

In this discussion of AK prosthetics I have concentrated on clinically relevant material which has included discussions of fit and alignment. I have left components for discussion in a subsequent section because, with hip disarticulation and hemipelvectomy amputations, the full range of components comes into view. Also, in discussions so far, a new way has been used of looking at alignment in which the residual limb is the basis of the reference system, and a new view of weight bearing has been submitted. The intention was to diverge from the existing approaches so that something would be added and a better result might be gained for such amputees presenting for solutions to their problems. In the discussions concerning hip level amputees, the sum total of what has been learned, and some new elements will emerge.

Hip Disarticulation and Hemipelvectomy Amputation

Loss of the entire limb through disarticulation of the hip or approximate disarticulation, and more particularly, removal of half the pelvis, are severe losses. However, such amputees do wear prostheses effectively as a matter of routine. An important determinant in whether or not such an amputee becomes a prosthesis wearer is how soon after amputation he is initiated into use of a prosthesis: *Use of a prosthesis must be initiated as early as possible for hip and pelvis amputees to forestall development of dependence on crutches if use of a prosthesis is planned.* Once these amputees experience prolonged use of crutches, conversion to use of a slow and confining prosthesis is unlikely, even though the amputee may reconsider from time to time. Only when the hands are affected seriously by crutch use will a more serious effort be made by the amputee to master a prosthesis. Use of modular components for this level of amputation is desirable because of the adjustable features and functional options which are available. Whatever components are used, the basic design is the same. The name of the prosthesis used for either level is the *Canadian hip disarticulation prosthesis.* Differences between the two categories of amputees relate to the design of their sockets and the manner in which suspension of the prosthesis is achieved (Fig. 4.11).

PROSTHESIS

The Canadian hip disarticulation was first used in 1952 when, in response to a request that he make design changes to the original single axis side joint used until then, McLaurin developed the alternate approach which was to use a broad anteriorly placed joint on the socket which could be gravity stabilized rather than lock stabilized. He and Hampton fitted a paratrooper with the first model within 2 weeks of its conception. Changes made since then relate entirely to details rather than principles. In the original prosthesis, a standard wooden knee-shank set-up was used, with a second set-up inverted and stripped to supply the hip joint and thigh section assembly. The socket consisted of rigid fiberglass. It gripped the pelvis under the iliac crests on both sides and provided a rigid platform for weight

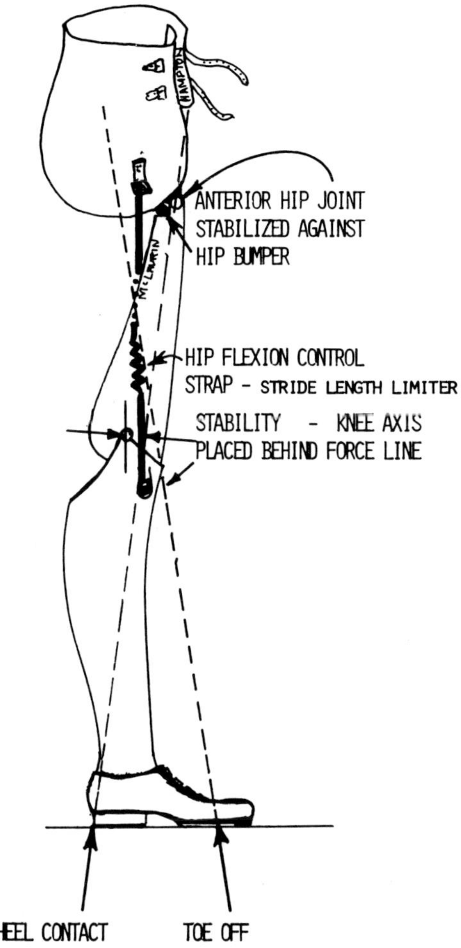

Fig. 4.11. Canadian hip disarticulation prosthesis.

bearing and a junction in front for mounting the hip joint. The one-piece plastic socket was held in front by a crossed strap latched to one side. A strap joined the socket and knee to act as a check on the length of the stride. In alignment, the line joining the hip axis and point of contact of the heel passed 2 cm in front of the hyperextended knee axis. A single-axis foot was used. Suspension was from the area over the hips below the crests, and from the sacral region behind. Stability of the knee was maintained by gravity throughout the weight-bearing period of the stride on the prosthesis. As in this original design, all subsequent variants have the hip joint stabilized shortly after the double support time by a hip joint bumper or stop, which transmits forces from the thigh to the socket so that the line of action of the forces from the top end shifts behind the joint upon activation of the hip stop. Meanwhile, the ground reaction point moves forward countering the posterior shift at the socket so that the knee stability is maintained. A hard "sit" into the socket accompanied by a rotation of the pelvis unstabilizes the knee for initiation of swing phase. The knee flexes first and, as the knee reverses its direction of bending, the hip joint of the prosthesis flexes. After the shank reaches full extension, there is a short period of swing from the hip joint followed by a snubbing action from the stride length control strap, readying the prosthesis for the next step of the weight-bearing phase. For sitting, the same manoeuver is used to break the knee, and the hip joint folds to allow descent to the chair. This manoeuver can look very natural.

In more recent applications of the system, the hip joint is set as low as can be done and as far back toward the midline of the body as possible. The advantage is that there is a more cosmetic distribution of the length of the limb between the thigh and shank sections. Also, forces on the hip stop are lower and the heavy "bumping" action sometimes seen as the hip stop engages is less.

In aligning the prosthesis, the best practice is to place the structural elements (foot, shank, thigh) as close to the body midline as possible. The hip joint axis should be inclined to make the prosthesis below the joint swing away from the midline or to diverge from the line of progression. This aids clearing of the natural limb with the swinging prosthesis as well as setting the foot in a good position for weight bearing.

Actions of the prosthesis are fairly natural if there is limited flexion at the prosthetic knee in swing phase and if most of the forward displacement of the foot comes from hip flexion. This is why amputees provided with stiff knees such as those with hydraulic dampers, do so well. Also needed, but not available, is a kicker for the thigh so that the period of the prosthesis is shorter for a quicker step. As it is, the prosthesis is irritatingly slow, a big factor in amputee rejection.

SOCKET

The socket of the hip disarticulation amputee is a form-fitting plastic pelvic container which has a broad base for weight bearing through the ischium and gluteus. The support surface must extend well past the midline of the body initially to ensure that the ischial tuberosity will be supported inside the socket. Trimming can be done later if the surface is too extensive.

Various forms of the socket have been tried, including various positions for opening it for entry, various degrees of stiffness of the laminate used, and various methods of suspension. Typically, the socket encloses both iliac crests for suspension. The joint axis is placed as low as possible on the socket and close in to the socket. The position is set prior to laminating the socket so that the required base is preestablished. A pad inside the socket is allowed for by including it on the mold over which the socket is made. The pad serves to cushion the support surface of the body and to cover the hardware included inside the socket when an anchor plate is used to secure the hip joint assembly. A well fitted socket could dispense with the pad.

The layup of the plastic socket I make includes nylon tricot up to about 10 layers interspersed with glass cloth in the joint attachment area and across the weight-bearing platform, extending laterally halfway up the socket. Approximately 20 layers of carefully placed glass cloth are included, shingled toward edges by variations in the sizes of the pieces and staggered in the layup. In the crotch flare area, dacron felt, not glass cloth, is used so that the edge can be trimmed and smoothed. Also, the felt has a stiffening effect. Extension of the glass cloth into flexing sections invites shearing of the material and failure of the socket. All excess resin must be expressed from the laminate for the best result. The aim is to produce a socket with some give in it, pliable for entry and stiff in the weight bearing and hip joint support areas. The socket should be springy to reduce shock during walking.

The original socket which clipped to the pelvis like a large pant clip locked below the crests of the ilia was closer than many subsequent designs. The diagonal socket which the designers proposed cut the socket away over the crest of the ilium on the amputated side, substituting the suspensive feature of the enclosing socket by a simple loop which hung against the crest. On the opposite side, the socket extended higher than the normal crest. The aim was to optimize containment of the force couple which is low on the amputated side and high on the normal side viewed from the front or back as the amputee bears weight on the prosthesis. The effect of the force couple was overestimated in this design and the design was extravagant for that reason. The usual method now is to include both crests and to fit the socket tightly. Entry can be made through an opening in front, to the side, or even at the side toward the back. The advantage of the front opening is that the socket can be loosened during sitting or after distension following a meal. The side-back opening is more secure for walking.

The difference between the socket for a hemipelvectomy amputee, as compared to that for a hip disarticulation amputee, stems from the fact that weight must be borne on the gut, on the natural ischial-gluteal region and on the rib cage. Also, the limb must be suspended from the shoulder. The "diagonal" socket just discussed has been used for this level, but the support offered by bilateral fitting of the rib cage is too valuable to sacrifice. When it is used, the prosthesis offers better support of weight and better stabilization of the prosthesis on the body. The difficulty such an amputee has is that he can slip out of the proper position in the diagonal socket. A lateral extension on the natural side against the thigh helps prevent lateral displacement toward that side in the socket.

Even when the fit of the hemipelvectomy amputee's socket is optimal, there will be considerable pumping and a periodic need for him to readjust his position in the socket in order to maintain good function. Such challenges have not prevented some hemipelvectomy amputees from being successful wearers. To attempt rehabilitation on such a prosthesis for this level is not to be discouraged. Once fitted, these amputees seem to be less problematic than some hip disarticulation amputees as regards abrasions and discomforts. It may be that they are less vulnerable because of the support obtained from the gut when the lungs are full and the diaphragm held. Such action allows some adjustment to pressure.

As we consider components which can be used, their application to all levels of amputation will be covered. As with amputation levels, the discussion of components will start at the foot and work up.

Prosthetic Components

FOOT

Feet can be described in terms of the number of degrees of freedom offered by their joints. The joints include the ankle or whatever is the substitute for it, and the "break," is the point at which the functional forefoot ends. For our purposes, discussion will be limited to the ankle joint. The maximum number of degrees of freedom offered by any foot is three. These include the ability to tilt the major axis relative to the residual limb, to tilt the minor axis and to rotate around the axis of the limb. The major axis tilts give a normal appearance to the gait, reduce stresses on the shoe, allow adjustment of the plantardorsiflexion angle by means of adjustment to the bumpers which limit the range of motion at the ankle. These feet usually have motions which are discontinuous so that actions are not totally smooth as the weight is borne on them through the full arc of the stride. Figure 4.12 shows representations of the functions of prosthetic feet.

For elderly amputees, for whom a very limber foot is an asset, such a foot

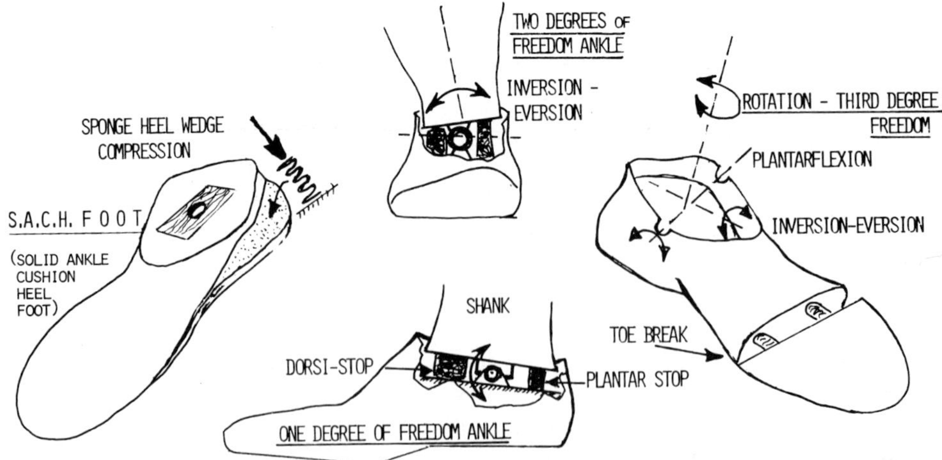

Fig. 4.12. Functional features in a prosthetic foot.

as one with three degrees of freedom would be suitable if the bumpers were soft. More functions than are required are included, so that use of a foot with less function would be in order. A factor to consider in the provision of any foot is its weight. For vigorous amputees the possibility of greater need for maintenance would be a consideration. The more moving parts, the more there is to go wrong. Noise then would be a problem. A foot with three degrees of freedom should work well for any level of amputation considering it only from the functional point of view. A requirement for the hip level amputees is that the heel bumper (plantarflexion resistance) be low and the front bumper be resistant. That combination allows the foot to comply with the ground at heel contact for a cosmetic effect, and offers a stable base on full load as the front bumper engages. With such an arrangement, also the point of action at the forefoot moves rapidly toward the end for improved stabilization of the prosthetic knee. A typical AK amputee would have similar needs. The heel bumper would be stiff enough to prevent foot slap at heel contact. Knee disarticulation amputees can be included with these for the purpose of designating the needs at the prosthetic foot. The BK amputee could be excluded because the gains would be small. Only the rotation function would be desirable, as for any other level. This feature reduces shear on the residual limb during such manoeuvers as pivoting. It is also of value for ordinary walking because of the rotary element inherent in walking. Hip disarticulation level amputees often display a rotary movement which appears as slippage between the foot and the floor when the forefoot supports weight. Complaints of instability would indicate that use of the rotator was contraindicated or that the unit being used was too limber.

The inversion-eversion function can improve cosmesis by allowing the foot to conform to the ground when unevenness is encountered or on slopes. It also may reduce, in some small measure, shock that can result from stepping on small lumps with one or the other side of the foot.

A foot with two degrees of freedom at the ankle will probably not include the rotary function. It could be provided by adding a rotator. Existing rotators are heavy and, until now at least, durability has been a problem. That the function is appreciated by amputees is a fact. Without that function, the two degrees of freedom foot still is a valuable system and, as with the other, allows alignment adjustment to both the major axis and minor axis tilts. A foot with a single direction of tilt, such as the usual conventional foot was the most common type of foot until advent of the SACH foot. Alignment changes can be made to the major axis angles, of course. Durability, as with any device with moving parts and constraints, and the attendant noise of dysfunction, can be a problem. A special case of such a foot is the one used as an integral part of the hydrocadence prosthesis. The foot action is interlinked with knee action to allow easy conformation of the foot to the floor even when extreme angles, as would be a part of sitting with the knee highly flexed, are performed. This function permits the amputee to fit into tighter spaces than would otherwise be possible. Clearance under tables, in cars, and so on, is improved.

The SACH foot is not really a "no degree of freedom" foot! It is better thought of as a device which is jointed at the toe-break or at the end of the forefoot. Thus, the heel wedge which compresses to provide a simulation of plantarflexion at heel contact is equivalent to the heel bumper of any other foot. The compliance of the toe section does give the foot some degree of inversion-eversion action. Little rotational function can be expected. If this function were required, a separate rotator unit would be installed at its top surface. The SACH foot, acting like a rocker, gives the smoothest transition over the full range of a step when it is correctly aligned and the heel wedge is correctly selected for the weight and vigor of the user. It is particularly suitable for BK amputees who can easily use the knee to regulate forces imposed by actions of the prosthesis emanating from the foot. For hip level and thigh level amputees who are lightweight (such as women) or who have a low activity level due to frailty, a soft, even a very soft, heel wedge is best. Heavier people and more active people require heel wedges which are more resiliant. The stiffer the action the more definite is the supporting action. Such resiliant feet would be preferred by bilateral amputees who need a more sure base of support. Not all SACH feet are the same. Some manufacturers make the wedges small and relatively ineffectual. Flatness at the sole reduces function, for example. The degree of adjustment of alignment possible in articulated feet is not present in the SACH foot, which must have an alignment coupler attached or be angled or wedged at the attachment point to the shank. As with most other feet, toe-in and toe-out can be adjusted. Another way of adjusting the foot by inserts between the sole and the shoe, already has been referred to. Trials intended to identify alignment changes which might be needed are sometimes made by strapping raises to the shoe of the SACH foot to simulate the effects of plantar or dorsiflexion changes.

The Grissinger foot provides three degrees of freedom, *i.e.* plantardosiflexion, eversion and inversion, and rotation. This foot is ideal for the young athletic amputee, but maintenance is high.

Whatever shank assembly is used, the mode of attachment of any foot is a bolt system. In the case of the SACH foot, for example, a single central bolt of high quality steel is used. Breakage of the bolt relates to loosening followed by bending of the bolt and its eventual fatigue and failure. Putting in a larger bolt is not the answer, but rather maintaining tightness of the bolt—which should be periodically checked. Enlarging holes for a larger bolt merely makes other component parts weaker.

SHANKS

From the structural point of view it really doesn't matter what structural element goes between the foot and proximal components. Two main systems exist: 1) exoskeletal or crustacean structures which, as the terms suggest, support loads through their outer shell. Wood has been the most common material used, and is still very widely employed. Other systems have used plastic shells, even laminates of wood or fiber, and still others have used shaped aluminum, which is still in use to quite a degree but less and less so. The main advantage to aluminum is its light weight for high strength. Its disadvantage is the difficulty of working it. 2) endoskeletal or pylon structures which lie central to the prosthesis and which must be "dressed up" with some form of outer cover. Outer covers have included rigid plastic shells, prefabricated foam covers and, more recently, sculpted foam covers which form a single coating to the base of the socket, bending as the knee bends. Endoskeletal systems are seen in all the *modular* systems. Alignment couplers plug on to tubing in these systems and the couplers are bolted to adjacent components such as the foot or socket in a BK prosthesis. The tubular section allows adjustment of shank length.

Which of these systems is used, the exoskeletal or the endoskeletal, depends on such factors as durability, cost, cosmesis availability, speed of assembly and established practices or prejudices. There will be a gradual transition to modular systems for those situations which suit it, a fact already in evidence. Frequently a modular system which has the one piece cover is used for women. Such systems, if they were competitive with wooden components would most certainly be used on elderly patients whose level of activity would not be sufficient to cause malfunctions. They would be used on growing children, especially those in the fast growing period even though frequent malfunction could be a problem.

They can be used for BK amputees very effectively because the cosmetic cover does not have to pass over a moving joint. The BK amputee is the first category of amputee for which the modular system is appropriate. The system includes a foot, probably the SACH foot, an alignment coupler (Fig. 4.13) the tubing to make up length, a second alignment coupler and the socket attached to the coupler. The cover, hollow for containment of the mechanical parts, is placed on and sculpted to the required shape. Contrast this to the use of wood. An alignment device is used, usually the Berkeley adjustable BK leg or the Gardner Staros coupler, to join a wooden base on the socket to the foot. Alignment is determined by the same methods as with other systems, and then the alignment device is removed and replaced by a piece of wood. The wood of the socket base, the wooden section which replaces the alignment device, and often, a wooden section attached to the foot are assembled in a jig which allows transfer of the alignment. The "rough" limb is then sculpted to shape as an exoskeletal shank, filler being used to bring all surfaces to an even level of the appropriate shape. The whole shank and socket assembly is then "reinforced" with plastic laminate to give the limb a coherent shape, color and texture (usually shiny) as well as to make it structurally sound. This is certainly a durable system. Alignment changes or changes in length require additional hand work. This is not

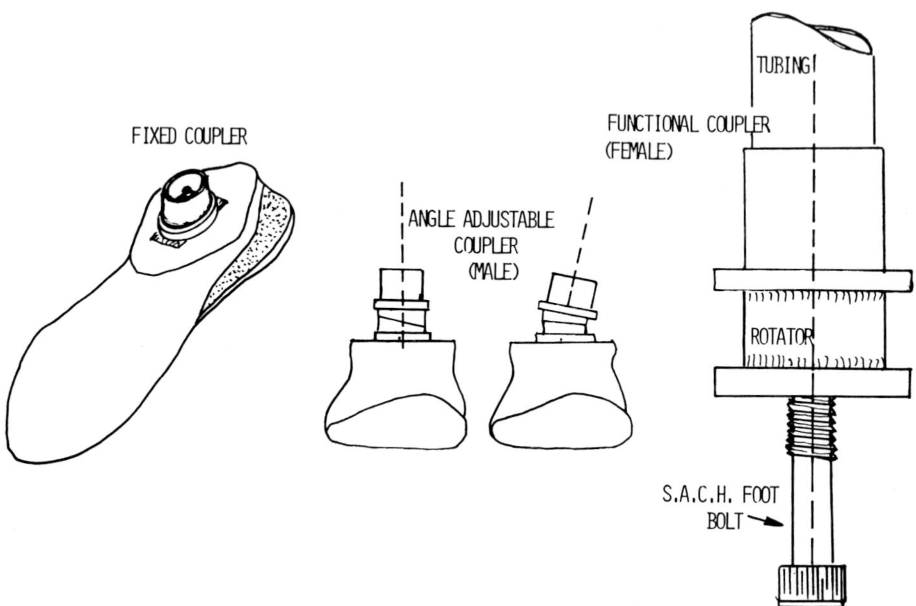

Fig. 4.13. Alignment couplers (adapters) for use between prosthetic shank and foot.

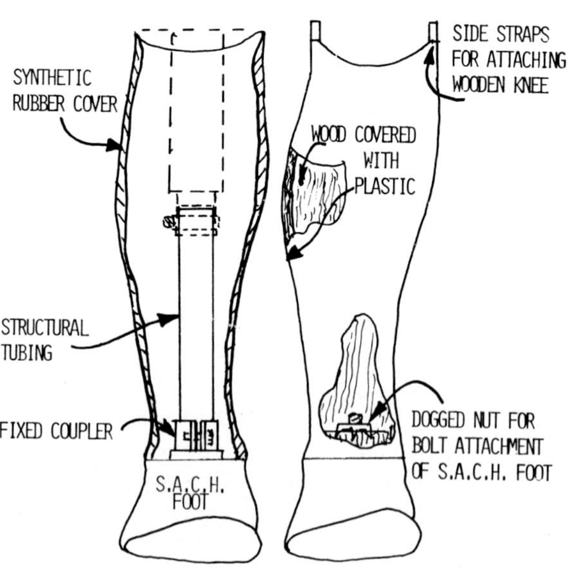

Fig. 4.14. Cutaway view of prosthetic shanks. Exoskeletal (*right*), and endoskeletal (*left*).

so much the case in a well planned and made modular BK limb. In some instances, it is not possible to use modular components because clearance between a component (such as the foot) and the residual limb (such as very long BK residuus) is insufficient for installation of the hardware. Then wood must be used. From the views of two shank sections (Fig. 4.14) one exoskeletal (*right*), and one endoskeletal (*left*), a clear picture of the systems can be gained.

KNEE JOINTS

Side Joints

At the knee disarticulation level, the missing knee joint function must be simulated. The need is for a pivot which provides the necessary cosmetic effect for sitting and swing phase, while allowing the amputee to do such things as kneel. In the past, and even now, the practice was to attach side joints such as are used on BK prostheses with a corset system to the shank, usually wood covered with plastic, and to attach the socket to the upper joint arms, using either plastic or leather sockets. Jigs to keep the joint axes of the side joints in alignment would be used so that joint wear would be less likely, and actions would be smooth. The upper and lower joint arms would be shaped to fit the adjacent prosthetic and anatomical parts. Plastic laminated over such joint arms make them unobtrusive to a point. Leather would cover the side arms at a leather socket. At the shank, and at the plastic socket, plastic laminate serves to reinforce the joint arms as well as to provide a cosmetic surface. For the knee disarticulation amputee, such a joint system poses both cosmetic and functional problems. The cosmetic problems arise because the side joint heads show through clothing and are hard on clothing. They make the prosthesis wide at the knee, even to the point of impeding entry of the prosthesis into pants for example. For women, even when the most meticulous attention has been given to installation of the joints and cosmetic treatment, the system falls short. Another side joint system has a double pivot. It is referred to as "polycentric." Such a system is too fragile for use in prostheses.

Polycentric

Now the practice is to use the "polycentric" knee joint. The principle on which the system is based is that the many centered link-pivot system can be tailored to cause the apparent knee axis to be in the optimal position at any instant. For the knee disarticulation amputee the systems are designed so that the socket can be attached to a plate which carries the pivots and links of the polycentric system. The links are pivotted in a way that makes the assembly fold up close to the socket at the back of the socket where the attachment is made through the plate. No protrusion upward or outward of the knee follows flexion, and a cap or apron closes around the knee to provide a cosmetic surface. A cosmetic cover is used over the tubular sections below the polycentric linkage and extends up over the linkage. The cover can be a standard one or a custom made one, depending on the system used. Whereas in the side joint system there could only be a kicker strap to aid swing control, and some attempts were made to include pneumatic and hydraulic systems, even friction systems, in the modular systems with polycentric links, all the elements of use in lower and higher level prostheses which pertain can be used in knee disarticulation prostheses. Such systems as pneumatic cylinders, hydraulic cylinders and spring assists are available. Controls fit between the links unobtrusively. Although problems of failure are reported, in fact, these systems should be used rather than the side joint system previously common. In the end, designers will develop what is needed in the face of demand. Such an amputee with a pneumatic or hydraulic swing phase control can set his own pace. Figure 4.15 shows knees schematically.

The polycentric system designed for use in knee disarticulation prostheses is just as valid for AK amputees, especially those with long residual limbs which are hard to match to components of another sort. But the system, set to a standard more in keeping with the cosmetic need than for such other functional results as can be obtained with polycentric linkages, has some rivals when it comes to the fabrication of AK prostheses. There are the previously established wooden components in a variety of forms as well as a variety of modular systems and components. One system is a hybrid between the wood and the exoskeletal systems which are entirely complete structurally. The hybrid system consists of metallic shank elements into which pneumatic and hydraulic controls can be installed. A wooden knee is used. A tubular section without alignment capabilities links the upper shank to the foot through an adapter. A shapable outer foam block is the basis for cosmetic restoration. No other hybrid system exists, and other knee mechanisms for the AK amputee's prostheses are what can be classed as truly modular in that all parts are prefabricated ready to use in the final prosthesis without modification by hand work. Other polycentric knees designed specifically for AK amputees fall into one or the other of two main categories: 1) those which are designed to enhance voluntary control, such as the University of California four-bar linkage system; and 2) those which are designed to provide stability, such as the Northwestern University system. Neither of these systems is in regular use, but similar systems will emerge in modular form eventually and, therefore, the functional differences need to be known.

Single Axis

Besides the polycentric knee already referred to, there are the single axis knees which can be divided according to whether or not they lock. The "free knee" is most commonly used. (This is true of wooden systems as well as

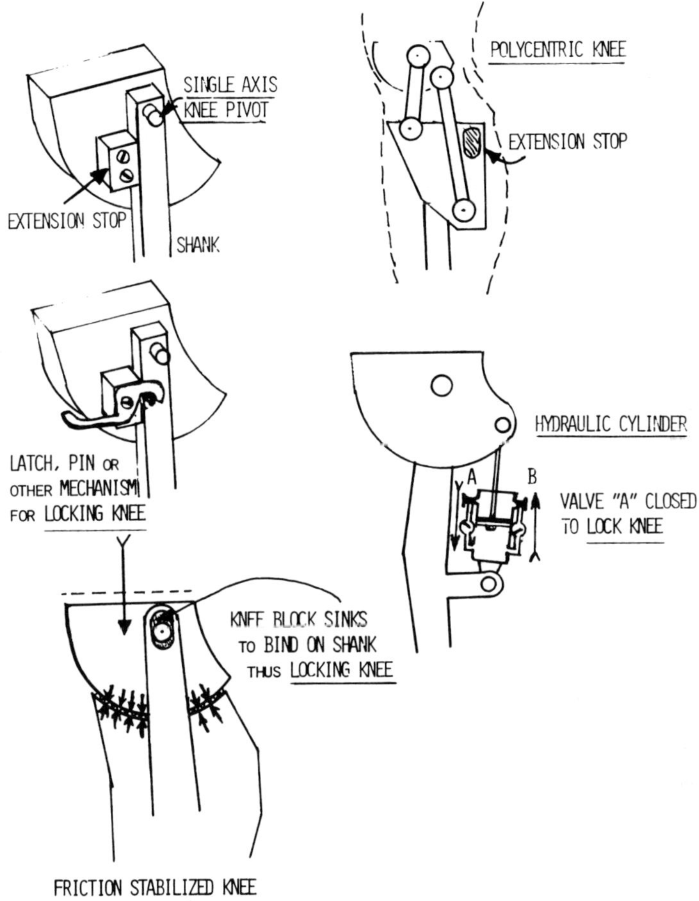

Fig. 4.15. Prosthetic knee joints.

modular systems). If the locking technique is examined, it will be found to be of three types: 1) the knee locks due to friction, either band friction or friction created between mating surfaces when the thigh section moves downward on a crank against the shank section, for example; or 2) the knee locks through hydraulic resistance when a valve is closed so that the piston cannot move; or 3) a latch or pin is used to lock the knee manually. Other types of links have been tried, but they lead back to the design of polycentric systems.

SWING CONTROL

A variety of methods have been used to control the swing of the shank. The most common system is the band friction system used in wooden knees. When the bands are tightened, they allow actions of the hip controlling the prosthesis to pass beyond the knee to the shank, as flexion of the knee is resisted. Speed control is limited with such a system, and keeping the friction adjusted is a constant problem for the vigorous user, especially. Other friction systems which have been designed but which are almost irrelevant now that modular designs are advancing into service, include intermittent friction, disc friction and bar friction. Attempts to make systems which were more responsive to the actions of the user were responsible for design of such systems, but none has been a match for the piston type controls even though costs were more modest.

Piston type controls, especially hydraulic ones, offer repeatable performance and a high degree of responsiveness to input from the amputee. Cost is admittedly high but, as use expands, the relative cost should be less because of the high costs related to hand fabrication of other elements of the prosthesis. The principle on which they work is to pass fluid from one side of the moving piston to the other through canals which are valved to regulate the flow, and hence the rate at which the shank can swing. The cylinder is attached to the shank as a rule and the piston is attached to the thigh. Thus, as the prosthetic thigh drives the piston up and down, resistance to flow of the fluid damps the action much like a door stop does. The dampening allows force from the hip to affect the prosthesis below the knee joint. The fluid is either air or oil. These swing phase control systems were originally designed for wooden prostheses, but now are in some modular designs. Because the length of the piston rod can be adjusted, there is control over the position at which the knee joint will stop extending. Thus, the position of the foot with respect to the axis of the residual limb can be set. The pneumatic system, while it provides less function than the hydraulic type, has the advantage that leaks are no problem. When air enters the hydraulic system on the other hand, the action becomes bouncy or even impossible. Figure 4.16 illustrates swing phase control methods.

THIGH

A difficulty in the use of some modular systems for AK amputees is that the space available between the end of the socket and the knee axis is such that a person with a long residual limb will be long thighed unless a special adapter is used. With wooden knees it has always been possible by special attention to shape the top of the knee to get the bottom of the socket right down onto the knee bolt. For such long residual limbs, the best practice would be to adapt the knee disarticulation polycentric system or to be sure to provide the space needed for any mechanism which might be preferred. Amputees with short residual AK limbs can have extensions included between the knee mechanism and the bottom of the socket in their prostheses to make up length of the thigh. The same extension method provides the thigh length needed in hip disarticulation prostheses. At the top of the extension, instead of the socket base as for the AK amputee, the hip joint

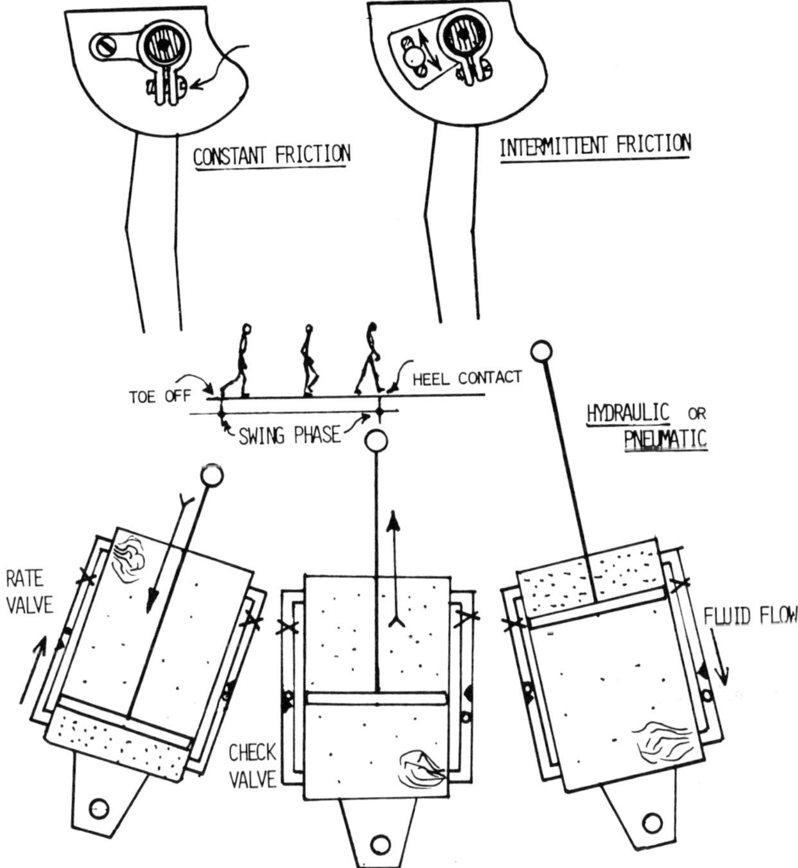

Fig. 4.16. Swing phase control methods for prosthetic knee.

assembly is attached for the hip disarticulation amputee. This assembly includes a bracket for attachment of the socket, the alignment coupler and the hip joint pivot, including stride control.

In the hip disarticulation prosthesis we see the most complete assembly of modular components found in any prosthesis. A variety of components is available because whatever is used at the other levels becomes available for use at this level. In addition to the modular designs, the standard wooden set-ups have components specifically designed for the hip level prostheses. Actually, the wooden components are still most commonly used. The sort of advantages inherent in them include robustness and the ease with which they can be cosmetically sculptured. The wear on clothing which they impose finally may defeat them for all levels of prostheses. Before that can happen however, modular systems will have become much more reliable and the cosmetic restoration more attractive and durable.

HIP JOINT

When a wooden thigh section is used for the hip disarticulation prosthesis, it is usually used with a hip joint such as the Northwestern University system. It allows alignment of the lower segments to be made *en bloc* from the hemispherical alignment coupler between distal parts and the socket. Once the lower elements have been set as required, the alignment system is tightened to lock it, the amputee tries it and, finally, when alignment (positioning of the foot with respect to the pelvis) is satisfactory, the adjustable unit is pinned in its final position. This arrangement, coupled with the ability to adjust foot angle, would allow complete assembly of the prosthesis and its final adjustment on the patient. Changes in the knee stop can be used to adjust back-forward knee pivot position relative to the pelvis. A check strap similar to the original is used for stride length adjustment. Friction knee control is contraindicated. A pneumatic control at the knee is to be favored because of the kicker action that can be obtained when the flexion resistance is high.

One still sees amputees being fitted with pelvic bands which include either a double or single pivot system between the band at the pelvis and the top of the socket of the AK amputee. Such systems will eventually be phased out. Amputees who are accustomed to them will continue to use them if their hip musculature has atrophied from disuse. No new amputee should be required to use one. A Silesian belt, which is a strap passing around the pelvis and anchored at each end to the socket at the lateral side near the hip joint, will certainly do as much as, for example, the double pivot pelvic band system.

Prescription and Assessment

As has already been said, prescription is a process until it is clearly established what it is the amputee actually needs. Then, there is no need for the intervention of every team member into the process of prescribing the prosthetic system. The prosthetist, involved as he should be in the planning of rehabilitation, will easily select the components which are appropriate to meet the needs of the amputee at a particular stage. The team's function is to spell out those needs as seen from the various points of view particular to the disciplines of the members. The amputee's requirements can be expressed in functional terms. It is no prescription to recite a list of components. Components are such an inconsequential element in prescription that it would be better to leave them out of discussions and leave their designation to the prosthetist. The aim of the clinic is to bring the members together so that everything pertinent to the patient's best management can be used to develop and maintain impetus of a good plan. At its best, the clinic is a problem-solving forum where learning as well as treatment is an aim. Such things as "Should a therapist adjust alignment?" or "Should a prosthetist give training?" or "Should a doctor prescribe prosthetic components?" only arise for discussion in weak teams. If each has a role so divided from his team mate that no overlap exists, then something is going to be left out for someone, and that someone will be the amputee.

As to examining patients to determine whether or not a prosthesis is satisfactory, I have used a simple quick checklist which I keep in my head and apply as I am confronted with a person in a clinical or review situation. There are eight factors to consider:

1. Have there been medical or social changes? Changes in life style, location, the weather or the season, sickness, a job change, or family difficulties are among changes that can affect how a person is performing on his prosthesis. A change in his physical or emotional state will definitely affect his performance. A teenager reaches a point when he will not tolerate a scraped and noisy prosthesis. A man with domestic problems will "lean" on his helpers. And so on.
2. What is the prosthesis like? An old prosthesis can be a better friend to an amputee than a new one until adaptation is complete. Or a prosthesis may show signs of neglect or, conversely, be well looked after and maintained. It may be suitable or unsuitable for the amputee. It may be past repair but have a good socket *shape*. What to salvage and what to discard are open for consideration. The socket shape can be transferred if it is good, and should be.
3. Is the gait pattern suitable? Good alignment, freedom from pain, mechanical parts in good order, adequate energy for the task of using a prosthesis; these are the sort of factors to consider as one views gait.
4. Can the prosthesis be adequately controlled by the amputee? Problems with the suspension, swing phase control problems, difficulties with stance phase control of stability, weight of the prosthesis and the skill of the amputee are factors.
5. Is the prosthesis correctly aligned? One should check to see if the position of the foot, its angular orientation, as well as the position of the knee pivot, including its inward-outward angle, are correct. For the hip disarticulation amputee, the position and angle of the hip joint assembly would be checked. Suspension and length would be checked for all.
6. Are there mechanical problems? These could be at the foot, knee or hip, or in the suspension system or the controls or the cosmetic system. There may be noises.
7. Are there problems with the residual limb? One should look for the effects of force couples, and recall the previous points found among the other items. Suspension, socket finish, constrictions, restrictions to muscles, or hygiene may be factors causing various stump disor-

ders. Look carefully at the flares of the socket. The prosthetic socket presents a hostile environment to the residual limb, especially a suction socket. A worn or scratched or absorbent surface can be a cause for such disorders. Any skin breakdown or disorder in underlying tissues will lead back to some factor in the prosthesis or a medical problem needing attention. Infections may not relate to the prosthesis at all, and the prosthetist must be alert to the need for such conditions to be reviewed by a medical person. Habits of bathing, allergies, and dermatitis from another source may be factors in such disorders. On the other hand, socket materials are often considered the source of allergies which in fact do not exist.

8. Are there defects in the socket? Tightness, looseness, roughness, constrictive forces, or resistance to free movement of muscles are some defects. Pressure points, free volume under the residual limb end, abrasions, pimples, corns or cysts are signs to look for in checking the suitability of the socket. Lack of distal support in itself may not be a problem if the limb is not held on by suction or if, in a suction socket, proximal forces are very well distributed. Edema or discolourations at the end spell defect. Even if the difficulty is that the amputee has put on weight, it is the socket which is now inappropriate!

When these eight areas have been properly considered, the points that need attention will be clear enough. Each section will bring some element into focus which is reinforced by what is found in other sections. Once the needs are established, recommendations must be made, and the necessary actions should be taken without delay.

In this presentation I have tried to deviate markedly from what can be obtained in other publications or from other sources. I have tried to provide information resulting from the use of the systems and methods mentioned which will directly affect the function and well being of amputees.

5

Prosthetic Fitting and Components—Upper Extremity

A. BENNETT WILSON, JR.

Although there are many references throughout the centuries in both the lay and professional literature to artificial hands and arms it was not until after 1800 that relative motion between parts of the human body was harnessed to provide power for operation of artificial arms. Ballif, a dentist, introduced this concept in Berlin about 1812 (2, 3) (Fig. 5.1).

The next major development in upper limb prosthetics seems to be the split hook powered by the Ballif harness designed, developed, and made available commercially 100 years later in 1912 by D. W. Dorrance, a bilateral below-elbow amputee (20).

At the beginning of World War II arm prostheses were generally made of a combination of wood, leather, and steel. Limb prosthetics was practiced largely by individuals who had learned the art on a tutorial basis, there being neither useful texts nor formal education programs available. Although many arm amputees were served well by prosthetists in that era, amputees returning to the United States from combat in World War II felt that the same engineering knowledge that produced the sophisticated equipment they used in war should certainly be applied to the development of artificial limbs to provide better function than those furnished to them by the Army and Navy.

As a result of these complaints, the Surgeon General of the Army, in 1945, sought guidance from the National Academy of Sciences of the United States in the provision of artificial limbs to amputees in the military service. A conference on the subject in February of 1945 led to the initiation of a nationwide government-supported research and development program in limb prosthetics that was coordinated by the National Academy of Sciences from 1945 until 1975.

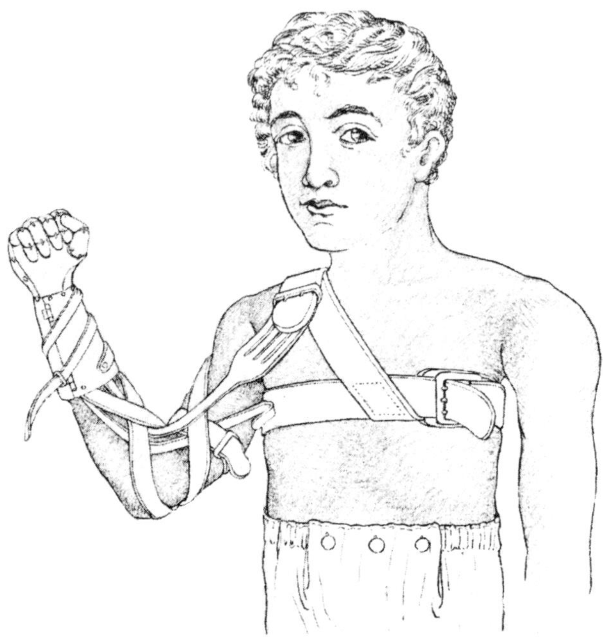

Fig. 5.1. Ballif arm (1812). The first example of the use of relative motion between parts of the body to obtain power for operation of an artificial arm. (Reprinted with permission from the American Academy of Orthopedic Surgeons (2).)

During the period 1945–1952, a body of knowledge based on research carried out at Northrop Aviation, the University of California at Los Angeles (UCLA), the Army Prosthetics Research Laboratory (APRL), and others was assembled by UCLA under the auspices of the National Academy of Sciences, and in 1952 the first formal courses in upper limb prosthetics offered in the United States were presented by UCLA to teams consisting of prosthetists, therapists, and physicians.

Aside from providing a logic for the design and application of sockets and harnessing, the research efforts had resulted in the development of alternating locking elbow units that could be activated almost imperceptibly through the body harness, voluntary closing terminal devices, techniques for the use of plastic laminates for sockets and structures, and specially designed connector units so that the "modular" concept could be used to provide patients with a combination of devices that would best meet individual needs. The new "armamentarium" permitted the prosthetist to provide the patient with a useful prosthesis at any level of amputation, and surgeons were urged to save all length medically feasible so that no function would be lost, as was often the case previously when long stumps and disarticulations were avoided because no satisfactory prostheses were available for those levels.

The manuals and educational programs at that time were restricted to prostheses using body power, but externally powered systems had not been overlooked by the research program. Indeed, testing of well designed electrical systems provided by the International Business Machines Corporation and Alderson, (1) revealed that the primary problem in the application of external power to upper limb prosthetics is the provision of sensory feedback, at least to the degree experienced by amputees using body-powered devices. As a result of these findings, the National Academy of Sciences recommended that priority in research efforts be directed toward sensory feedback rather than toward the design of more hardware (16, 17).

Unfortunately, no great progress has been made in upper limb prosthetics since the late 1950s when the concept of the use of electromyographic signals was proven to be practical by research workers in Russia (31). Since that time progress in clinical practice here and abroad seems to have been limited to refinements of concepts already proven.

Losses and Their Replacements

It is axiomatic, especially in body-powered prosthetics, that the higher the level of amputation, the less potential source there is for the provision of control and, therefore, the problem is compounded manifoldly as the level of amputation is raised.

Amputations through the upper limb (Fig. 5.2) are generally classified by level as:

Wrist disarticulation,
Long below-elbow,
Medium below-elbow,
Short below-elbow,
Very short below-elbow,
Elbow disarticulation,
Standard above-elbow,
Short above-elbow,
Shoulder disarticulation,
Interscapulothoracic or forequarter (not shown on diagram).

Figure 5.3 is a chart that shows the relationship between the functions retained and the functions lost at each level of amputation, and therefore reflects graphically how the problem of providing power and control for upper limb prostheses is compounded as the level of amputation is raised.

For the majority of upper limb amputees, the most important part of the prosthesis is the terminal device—hook, hand, or some specially designed gadget since it is the terminal device that usually provides the functions needed—prehension, pushing, pulling, etc. The other parts of the prosthesis are provided so that the terminal device can be placed where it is most

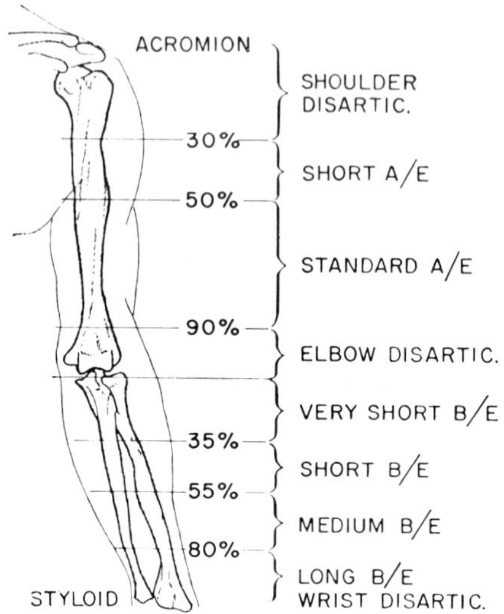

Fig. 5.2. Classification of levels of amputation through the upper limb.

useful and so that the body can provide the power and control needed for operation. The connection of the prosthesis to the body is, of course, a most important consideration, and is invariably an interdependent factor in any system.

Body-Powered Components Available

The major components of artificial arms are generally classified as follows:

- Terminal devices
  - Hands
  - Hooks
  - Devices for discrete functions
- Wrist units
  - Connection units that provide for passive control of pronation-supination
  - Connection units that provide for active control of pronation-supination
  - Connection units that provide for passive control of wrist flexion
- Elbow units
  - Below-elbow
  - Elbow-disarticulation
  - Above-elbow
- Shoulder joints

TERMINAL DEVICES

At one time the use of special terminal devices such as hammers, combs, forks, and knives as the most effective way of providing function was

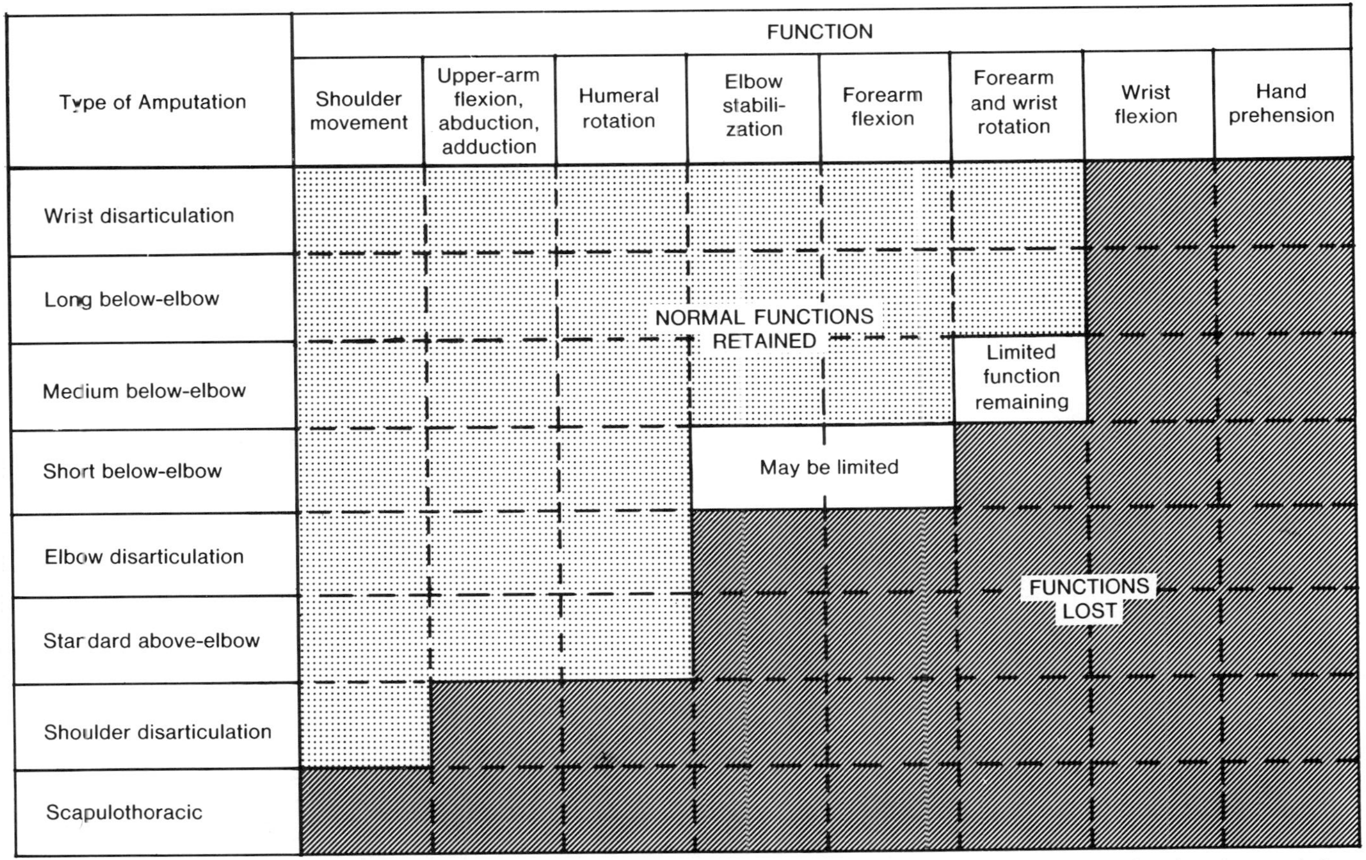

Type of Amputation	FUNCTION							
	Shoulder movement	Upper-arm flexion, abduction, adduction	Humeral rotation	Elbow stabili-zation	Forearm flexion	Forearm and wrist rotation	Wrist flexion	Hand prehension
Wrist disarticulation								
Long below-elbow				NORMAL FUNCTIONS RETAINED				
Medium below-elbow						Limited function remaining		
Short below-elbow				May be limited				
Elbow disarticulation							FUNCTIONS LOST	
Standard above-elbow								
Shoulder disarticulation								
Scapulothoracic								

Fig. 5.3. Diagram showing relationship between functions lost and functions retained at various levels of amputation through the upper limb. (Reprinted with permission from the American Academy of Orthopedic Surgeons (2).)

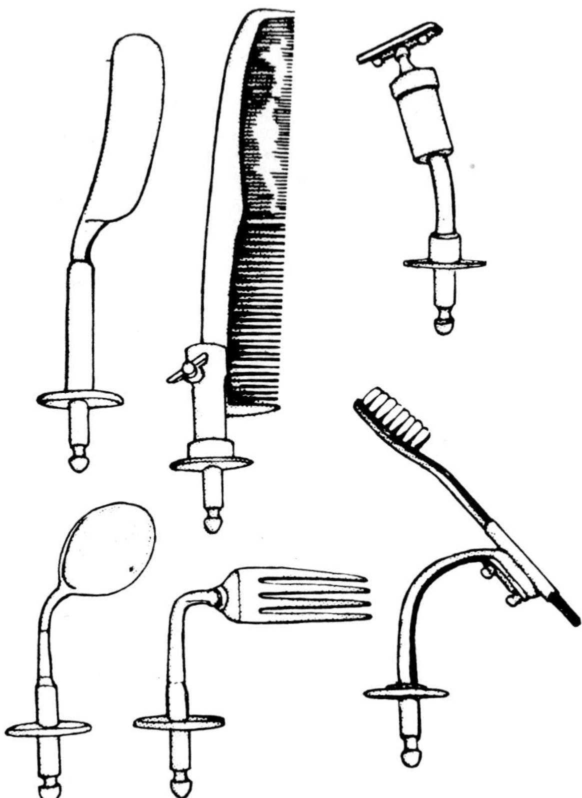

Fig. 5.4. Types of interchangeable terminal devices advocated from time to time. (Reprinted with permission from the American Academy of Orthopedic Surgeons (2).)

advocated strongly in Great Britain (2) (Fig. 5.4). Although the idea is re-offered from time to time, this concept has never been accepted in North America because of its obvious limitations, and terminal devices have been developed in Canada and the United States with the idea that they would be able to hold almost any instrument in a position of function. Individuals with specific vocational needs such as spray painters or assembly line workers often design special devices that fit their particular circumstances, but the needs are so special that it is not feasible economically for someone to make them available in large numbers. However, there are a few devices available such as a bowling "finger" (Fig. 5.5) and a device for use with a baseball glove (Fig. 5.6) (26).

Functional terminal devices can be classified as hands and hooks, which in turn are either voluntary closing or voluntary opening (VO) (Fig. 5.7). The voluntary opening devices employ a rubber band or a spring to close the fingers after they have been opened voluntarily by the amputee. The

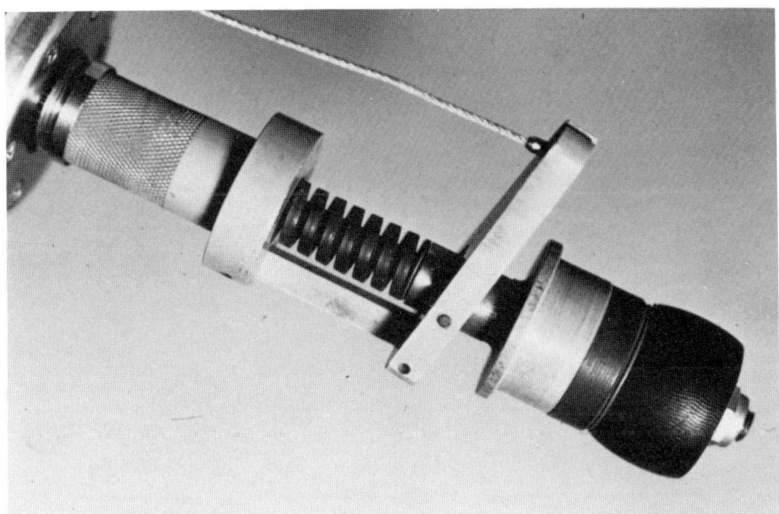

Fig. 5.5. Special terminal device for bowling by an upper limb amputee. The device is interchanged with conventional terminal devices. (Courtesy of the Veterans Administration.)

reverse cycle occurs in the case of the voluntary closing device, which was designed to provide an action that seemed to be more natural while making it easier to develop graded prehension. The disadvantages of the voluntary closing system with respect to the VO system are complexity and cost.

The 21 Hosmer-Dorrance *voluntary opening* hooks available are shown in Figure 5.8. There are three basic categories:

1. Standard functional models in three sizes,
2. Special utility models in four styles,
3. Infant and child models in two sizes.

The amount of pinch force is determined by the number of rubber bands used.

A two-load voluntary opening hook is also available (Fig. 5.9). The fingers on this hook are of the "lyre" shape, which has advantages and disadvantages with respect to the canted fingers used on most of the Dorrance designs.

When appearance is the only requirement, passive or purely cosmetic hands can be provided (Fig. 5.10). Passive hands usually consist of foam rubber molded over a flexible wire core covered with a cosmetic glove that can be tinted on a custom basis. The flexible core permits the patient to select finger attitudes to suit the occasion.

Several designs of voluntary opening hands (Fig. 5.11) are available. To increase the versatility without excessive body motion most of the designs use the "two-position" thumb (Fig. 5.12); that is, a thumb that can be placed

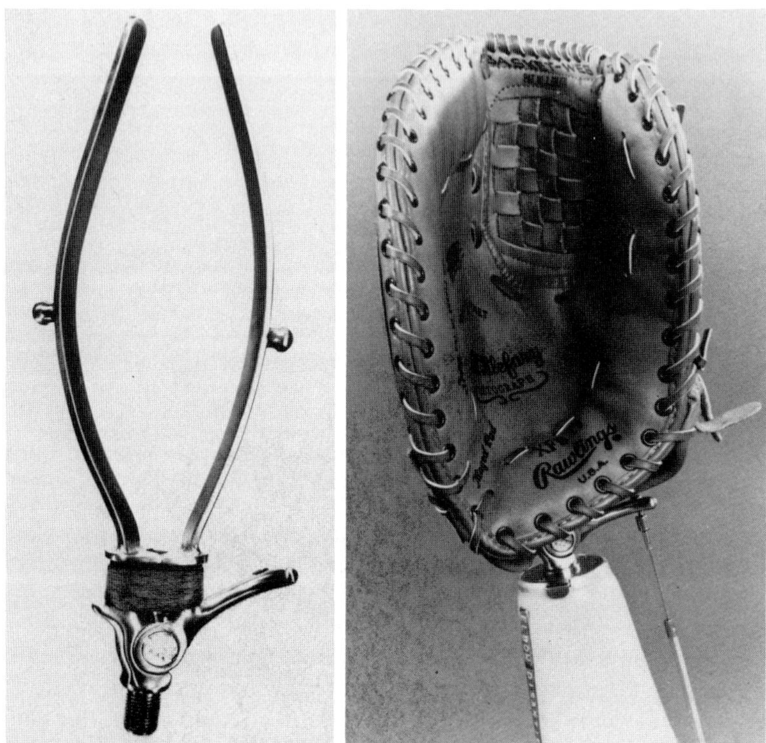

Fig. 5.6. Special terminal device for playing baseball. This device is a modified Dorrance voluntary opening hook. (Reprinted with permission from Hosmer-Dorrance Corp. (2).)

in an extended position so that a large object such as a drinking tumbler can be accommodated, yet an acceptable cosmetic effect can be maintained. The three-jaw chuck prehension pattern (22) is the most commonly used configuration for grasp.

The APRL voluntary closing hand (Fig. 5.13*A*) is a very sophisticated mechanical hand that employs an automatic lock to maintain the grasp applied to an object so that it is held firmly without effort by the amputee. Release is effected when the amputee applies the same amount of tension in the control cable that he used to effect the grasp. Unfortunately, the APRL hand is available in only one size.

The same type of function is available in the APRL hook (Fig. 5.13*B*) which is available only with the lyre-shaped fingers.

Artificial hands, almost without exception, are covered with replaceable cosmetic gloves, which are available in a number of shades and sizes (Fig. 5.14). The only acceptable material for cosmetic gloves for functional hands

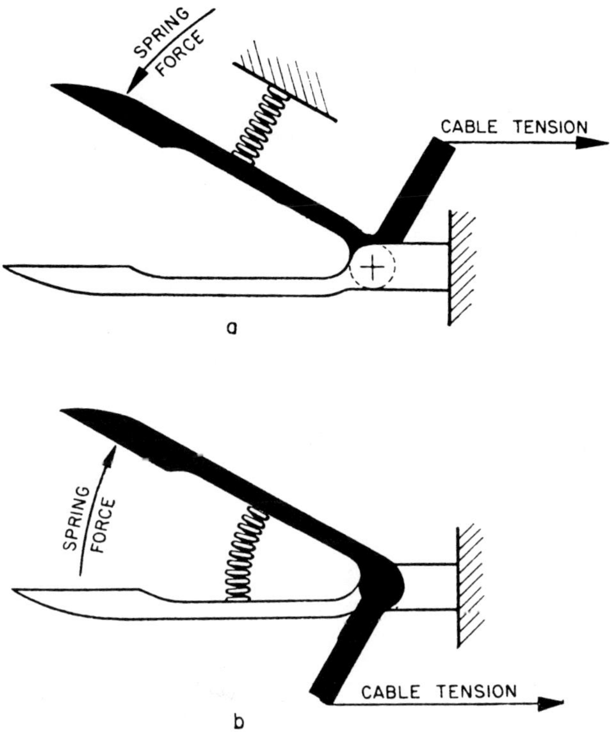

Fig. 5.7. Schematic drawing showing principles of *a*, voluntary opening and *b*, voluntary closing terminal devices (Reprinted with permission from M. J. Fletcher (22).)

to date is polyvinyl chloride which unfortunately stains easily and therefore requires frequent replacement (33).

Hands and hooks each have advantages and disadvantages. For most uses, hooks provide a greater variety of function but for some purposes the hand is superior. For patients who can benefit from use of both types of terminal devices it is possible to provide for quick interchangeability with very little added expense by use of the so-called quick-change wrist units (26).

WRIST UNITS

The primary purpose of wrist units is to provide attachment of the terminal device to the forearm portion of the artificial arm. Virtually all terminal devices for adults are provided with a stud with a $\frac{1}{2} \times 20$ thread and the wrist units are designed to accept this configuration. All wrist units in one way or another provide for pronation and supination of the terminal

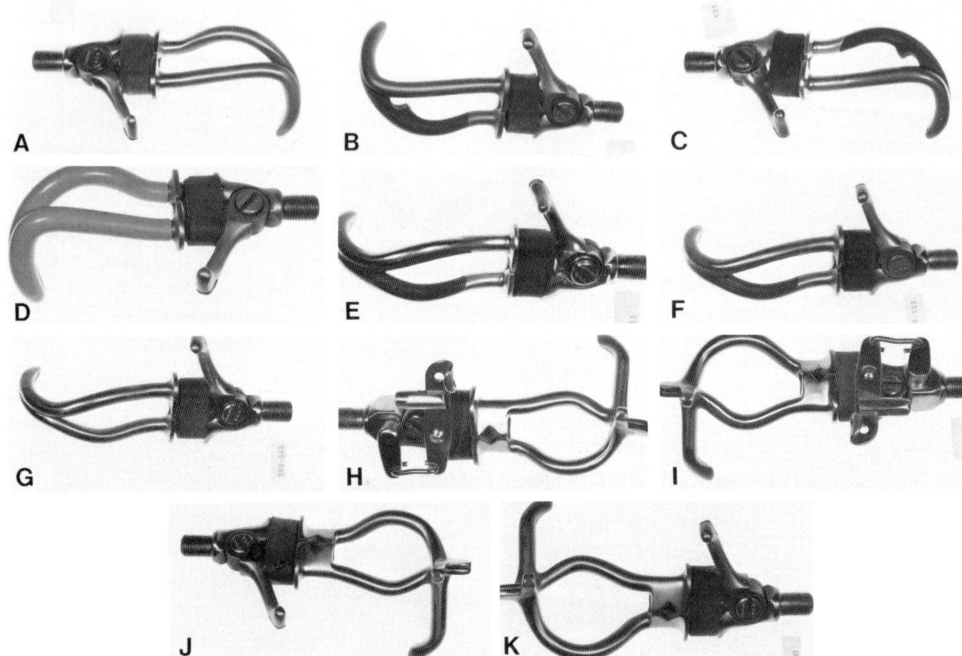

Fig. 5.8. *A–K*: Dorrance voluntary opening terminal devices. (Courtesy of the Hosmer-Dorrance Corp.) *A*, model 5—stainless steel; serrated holding surfaces; 4-⅞″ long; 7 oz weight. *B*, model 5X—stainless steel; neoprene-lined fingers; 4-⅞″ long; 7 oz weight. *C*, model 5XA—aluminum alloy; neoprene-lined fingers; 4-⅞″ long; 3 oz weight. *D*, model 5P—stainless steel; plastisol-coated fingers; 4-⅞″ long; 7-½ oz weight. *E*, model 555—aluminum alloy; neoprene-lined fingers; 5″ long, 3 oz weight. *F*, model SS-555—same design as model 555; stainless steel; neoprene-lined fingers; 5″ long; 7 oz weight. *G*, model SSS-555—stainless steel; serrated holding surfaces; 5″ long; 7-½ oz weight. *H*, model 6—heavy duty stainless steel; serrated holding surfaces; identical to model 7, but with valuable added feature of a lock to keep it closed on an object; 5-⅞″ long; 13 oz weight. *I*, model 6LO—heavy duty stainless steel; serrated holding surfaces; identical to model 7LO but with locking feature used on model 6; 5-⅞″ long; 13 oz weight. *J*, model 7—heavy duty stainless steel; serrated holding surfaces; specially designed for use with a variety of tools; 1-⅛″ handle opening, 5-¼″ long; 8-¾ oz weight. *K*, model 7LO—the same construction and features as model 7 except that the handle opening is wider (1-⅜″) for use with shovel handles; 5-¼″ long; 8-¾ oz weight

device. In the simpler units mechanical friction is used to provide resistance to turning forces after positioning by the other hand (or hook). A nylon plug forced against the threads of the terminal device stud by a setscrew is a common way of providing the friction needed.

For quick interchangeability of terminal devices plug-in or bayonnet-type designs are available (Fig. 5.15). An adaptor that is screwed onto the

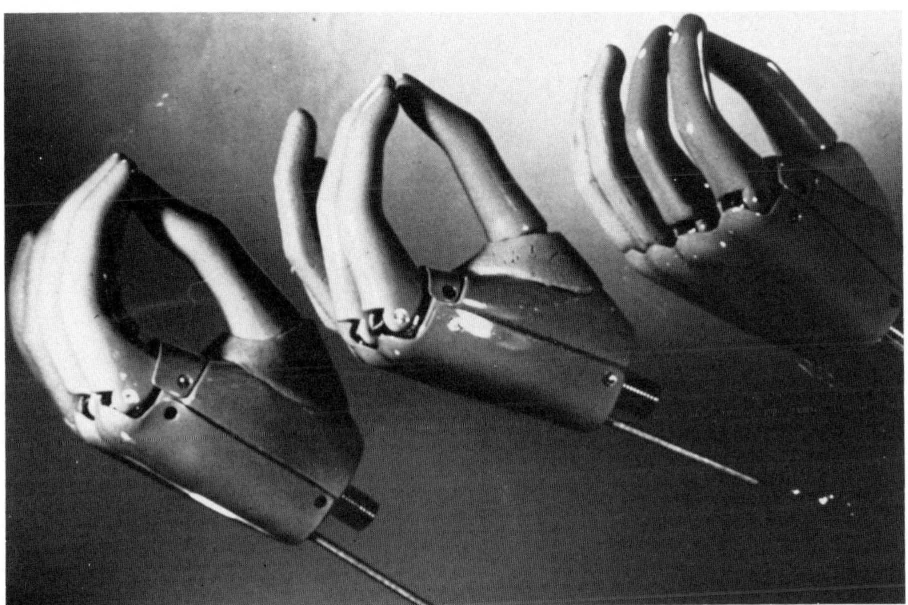

Fig. 5.11. Dorrance voluntary opening hands shown without cosmetic gloves (Courtesy of the Veterans Administration.)

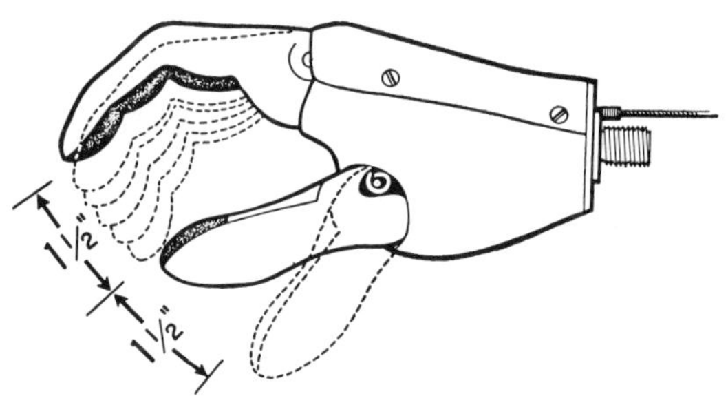

Fig. 5.12. Principles of the two-position thumb. In the closed position objects up to 1½" thick can be accommodated. In the open position objects between 1½" and 3" thick can be accommodated. An alternator-type lock holds the thumb in the closed position. A force in the direction toward the fingers releases the lock and a spring rotates the thumb into the open position. When the thumb is returned to the closed position, it is locked into place automatically. (Reprinted with permission from M. J. Fletcher (22).)

Flexion at the wrist can be provided by the interposition of a unit between the terminal device and the ordinary types of writs unit (Fig. 5.17) or the feature may be provided by a special type of wrist unit. Wrist flexion is appreciated most of all by bilateral arm amputees who have a need for terminal device function close to the body. Unilateral amputees who have a need to perform special tasks often find a wrist flexion unit very useful.

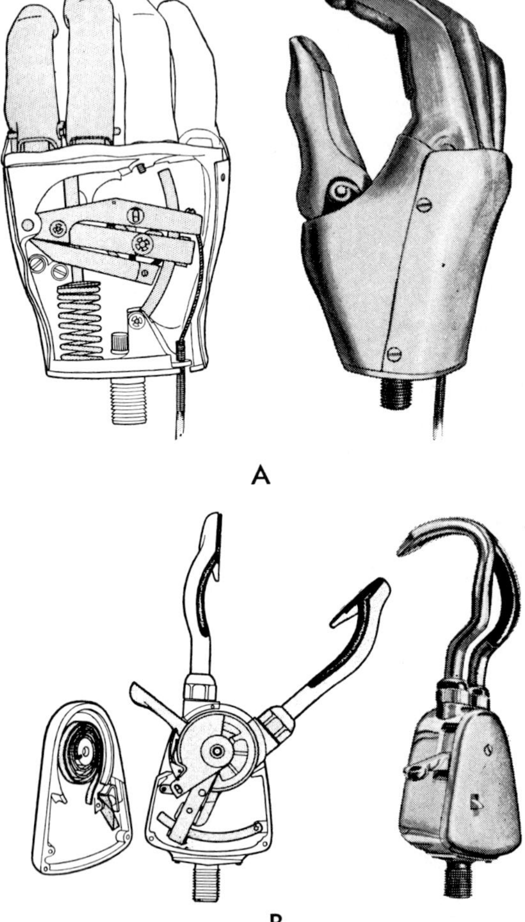

Fig. 5.13. Voluntary closing terminal devices. *A*, APRL-Sierra hand; left, cutaway view showing mechanism; right, assembled hand with cosmetic glove; *B*, APRL-Sierra hook. (Reprinted with permission from M. J. Fletcher (22).)

For both below-elbow and above-elbow amputees there is available a wrist unit that permits active control of pronation and supination by the relative motion between the arm and forearm (26).

ELBOW UNITS

Below-Elbow

At one time it was customary to provide below-elbow prostheses with metal hinges about the elbow to connect with a cuff about the humeral section to provide stability and suspension. With the advent of better socket designs, the need for rigid hinges has been reduced but they are needed often when heavy labor is required (Fig. 5.18). For those cases, where the stump is extremely short or where elbow flexion is weak there are available

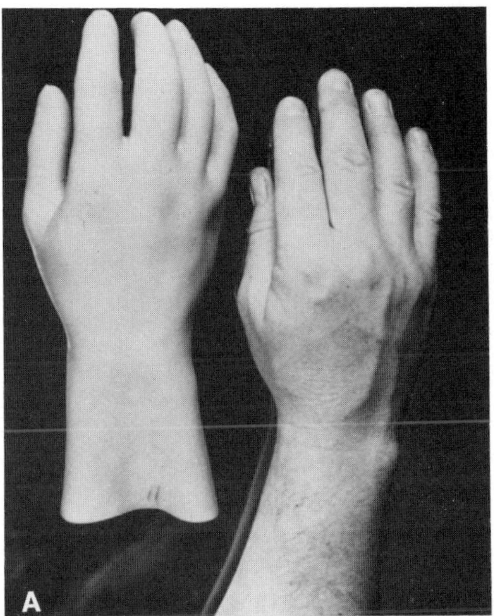

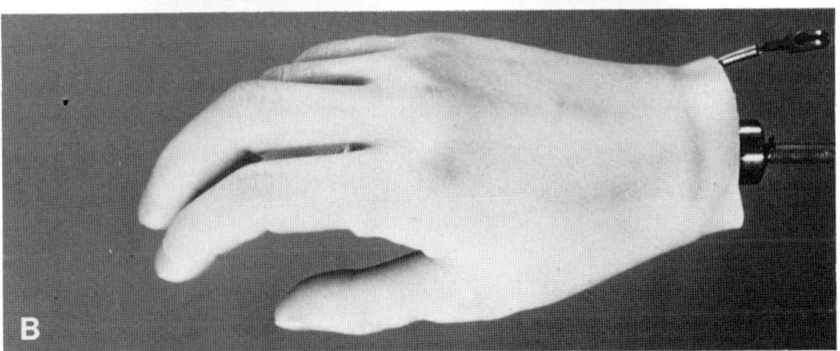

Fig. 5.14. Cosmetic gloves. Upper photograph, a glove shown along with a human hand. Lower photograph, a glove installed over a mechanical hand. In this instance, the gauntlet part of the glove has been cut away to make quick disconnect easier.

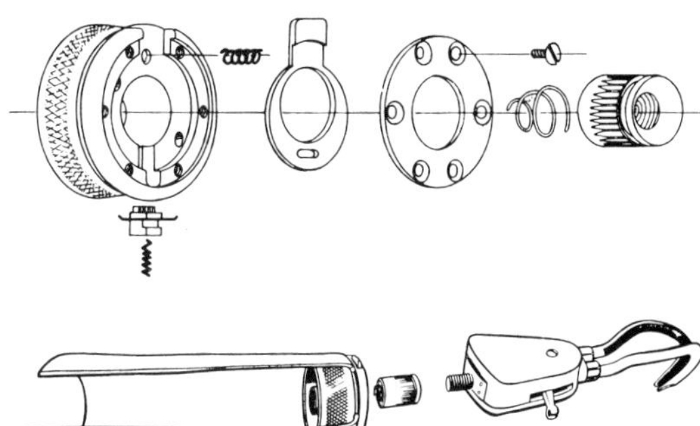

Fig. 5.15. Hosmer F-M wrist unit, with exploded view to show arrangement of parts and use in a prosthesis

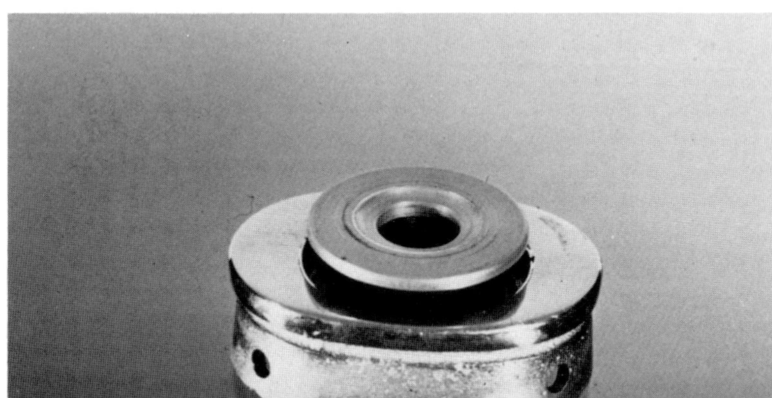

Fig. 5.16. Friction-type wrist unit. This model has an oval cross-section that is especially suitable for long below-elbow cases, and for use with Dorrance and Sierra mechanical hands. (Courtesy of the Veterans Administration.)

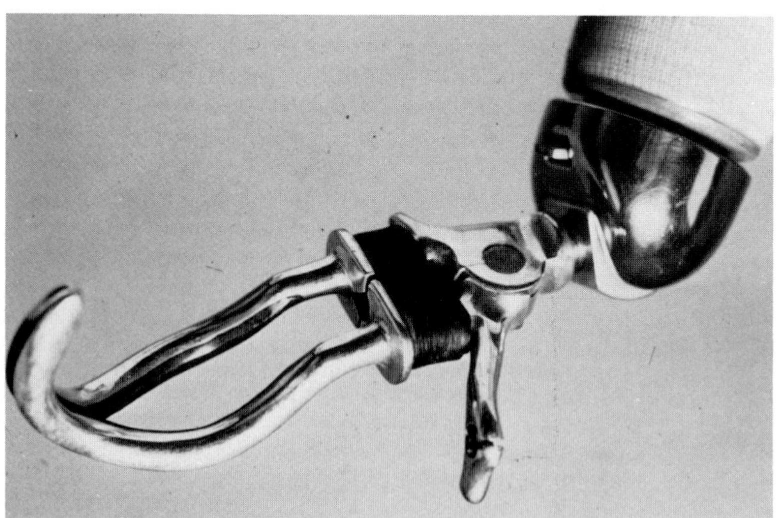

Fig. 5.17. Wrist flexion unit that is interposed between standard wrist units and terminal devices. Two positions of flexion are available. 22½° and 45° (Courtesy of the Veterans Administration.)

"step-up" hinges (Fig. 5.19), and stump-activated locking hinges to meet the needs of the individual (Fig. 5.20).

Above-Elbow

For the above-elbow amputee a single design using an alternator type of lock has become the unit of choice (Fig. 5.21). A short pull on a control

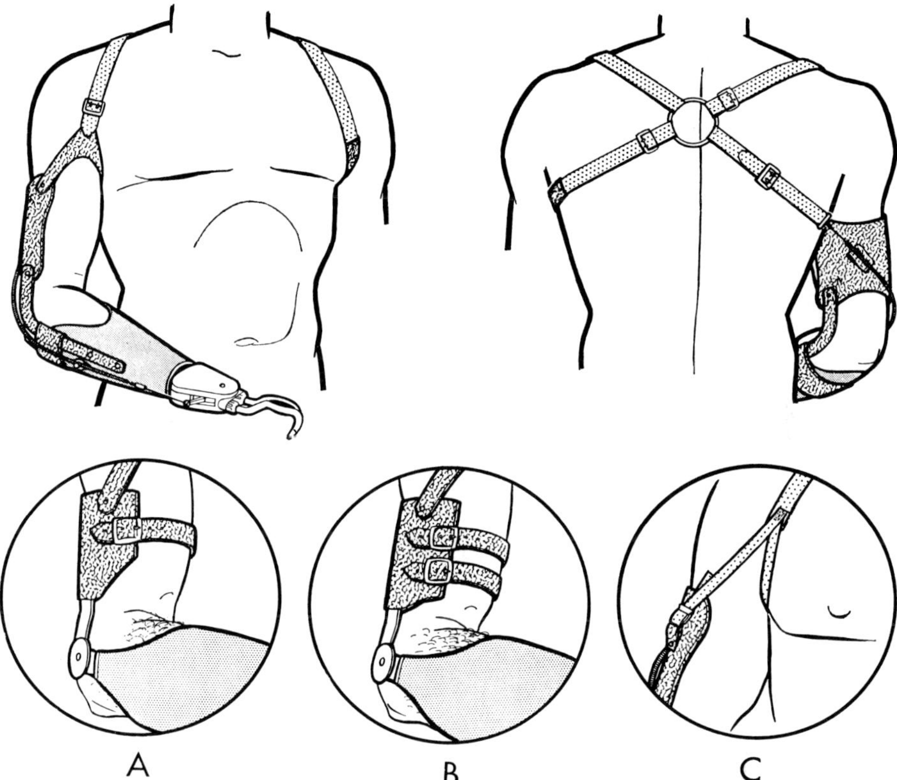

Fig. 5.18. Typical methods of fitting below-elbow amputees with medium-to-long stumps. *Above*, the figure 8 ring-type harness is most generally used. Where possible flexible leather hinges and open biceps cuff or pad are used. When more stability between socket and stump is required, rigid (metal) hinges and closed cuffs can be used (*inserts A* and *B*). In *insert C*, fabric straps are used for suspension in lieu of a leather billet (Reprinted with permission from A. B. Wilson, Jr. (60).)

cable alternately locks and unlocks the elbow unit in flexion. Eleven positions within the 0–135° range are generally provided. In the extended position the elbow is free, a feature much appreciated by the patients especially during walking and moving about generally. (This requirement often has been overlooked by designers of externally powered elbows and accounts for some of the resistance to acceptance of some of the externally powered units offered in the past (32).)

The connection to the humeral section of the prosthesis is through a single bolt along the long axis. A friction washer at this connection permits a certain amount of passive rotation, a feature that is necessary for proper function by bilateral arm amputees when one or both amputations are above the elbow. On occasion prosthetists have provided positive-type locks in the turntable to give active users the stability they need for heavy duty tasks.

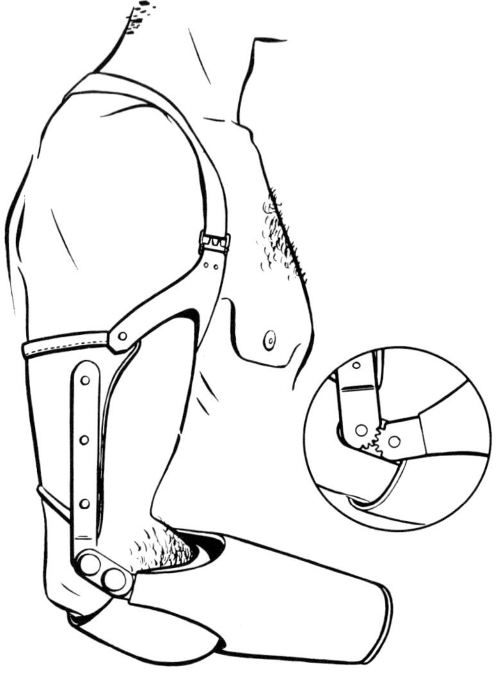

Fig. 5.19. Step-up hinges (*insert*) for short below-elbow amputations, especially for those cases where range of elbow flexion is limited.

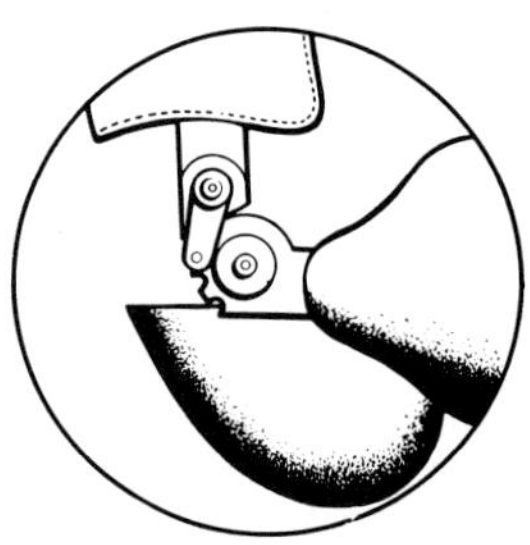

Fig. 5.20. Stump-actuated elbow lock for very short below-elbow amputations (Courtesy of Robin Aids).

SHOULDER UNITS

To date it has not been possible to design an actively controlled shoulder joint whether body powered or powered by external energy sources. Passively controlled units that offer three degrees of freedom are available and are used extensively in design and fabrication of prostheses for shoulder disarticulation and forequarter cases.

SOCKET DESIGNS

The configuration of the socket is as important as any other feature of an artificial limb. The optimum design provides the stability required yet is comfortable while permitting the musculature remaining in the stump to function adequately. Provision of the optimum design requires, on the part

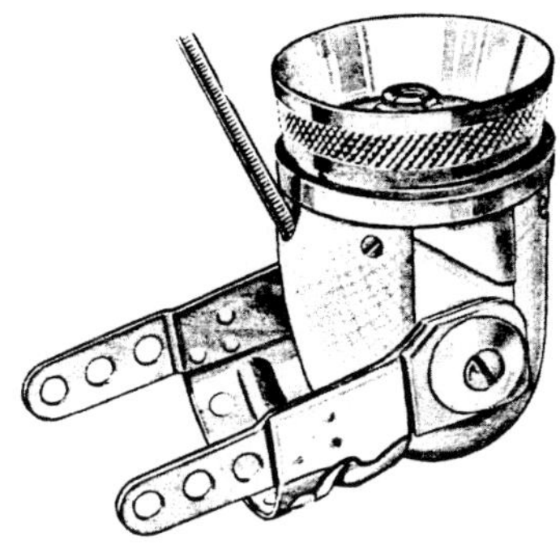

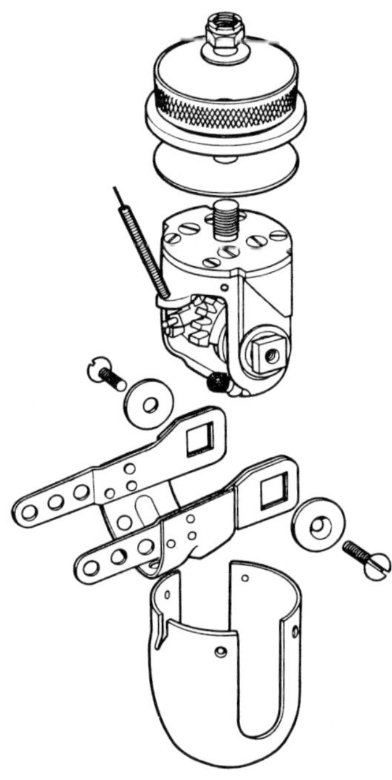

Fig. 5.21. Hosmer E-400 elbow unit (*top*) and an exploded view (*bottom*) showing the various components. The Hosmer E-200 is identical except that it is smaller.

of the prosthetist, a thorough knowledge of the anatomy and physiology of the upper limb, shoulder, and back. Guidelines for provision of satisfactory sockets have been provided in various texts (6, 11, 21, 39, 50, 52, 55, 56), and refined designs have been offered in the literature. Of especial note are the wrist disarticulation socket (59), the Hepp-Kuhn, or Münster, below-elbow socket (21) (Fig. 5.22), the suction socket of above-elbow cases by Pentland and Wasileff (39) (Fig. 5.23), and the air differential socket by Northwestern University (11), and the open-shoulder socket (34). All of these designs seem to have a place in the armamentarium but unfortunately the use of some

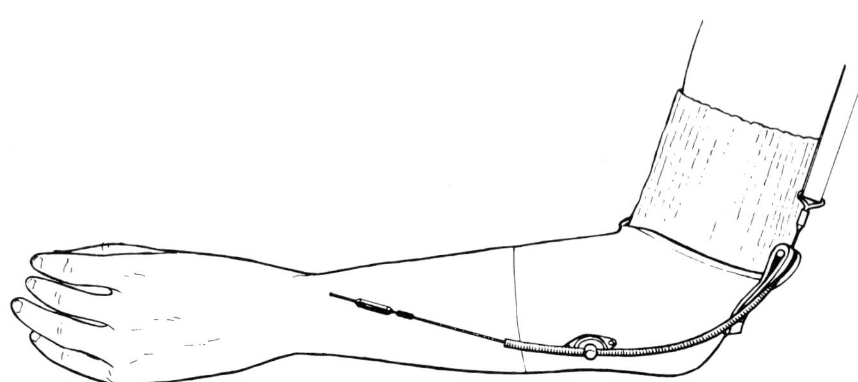

Fig. 5.22. Typical fitting of the Münster-type socket. Prosthetists usually provide some preflexion so as to give the amputee the optimum amount of flexion range. The preflexion is achieved by setting the long axis of the forearm at an angle to the long axis of the stump.

has not proliferated, no doubt owing to the absence of an evaluation program that could delineate the indications and contraindications for each of these variations.

Sockets for upper limb prostheses are made today almost universally of plastic laminates because they are easy to produce and easy to keep clean. However, this material in its present form leaves much to be desired since it is usually more rigid than is desirable for comfort and it does not "breathe."

HARNESS DESIGNS

One of the reasons that upper-limb prosthetics has seen little improvement during the last 20 years is probably owing to the exhaustion of ways to harness effectively body power for activation and control.

The present-day designs grew mainly from work carried out at Northrop Aviation shortly after World War II and refined later by UCLA and the Army Prosthetics Research Laboratory (37, 40, 56).

Power to actuate body-powered prostheses is derived from force and excursion generated by relative motion between two body parts. Tension is the type of force most easily harnessed.

Northrop Aviation introduced in 1944 the Bowden cable (Fig. 5.24) to prosthetics to replace the leather thongs and linen cords that had been used previously to transmit power. Northrop engineers also developed most of the hardware (retainers, clips, etc.) used today with the Bowden cable (37).

The major sources available for powering artificial arms are shown in Figure 5.25. In the typical below-elbow case the arrangement is quite simple (Fig. 5.26). An alternative sometimes used for partial hand cases and wrist-disarticulees is the butterfly harness (Fig. 5.27) which uses relative motion

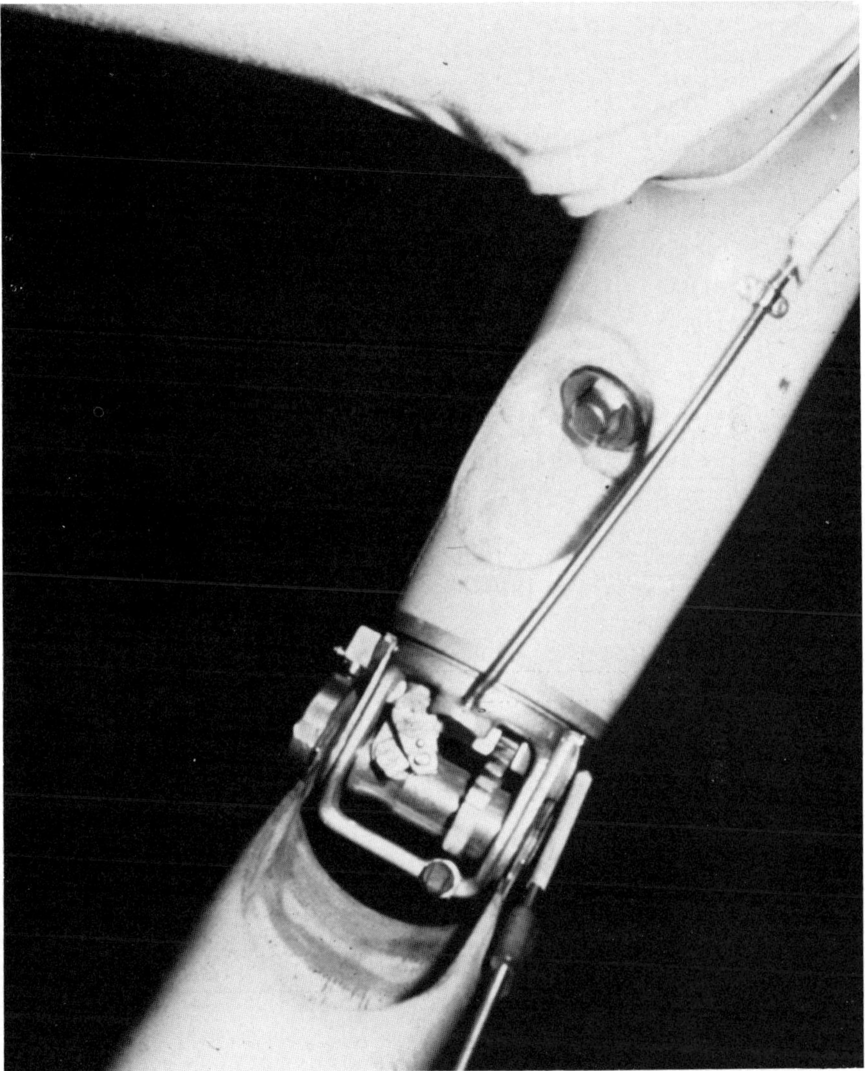

Fig. 5.23. Above-elbow suction socket showing location of the valve.

between the two scapulae to provide the force and excursion needed (40). The advantage of this arrangement is that power can be transmitted to the terminal device without movement of the terminal device relative to the upper arm, as is the case when humeral motion is used.

For the above-elbow and elbow-disarticulation cases the so-called dual control harness system (Fig. 5.28) is used almost universally in North America. In the dual control system the same motion and control cable is

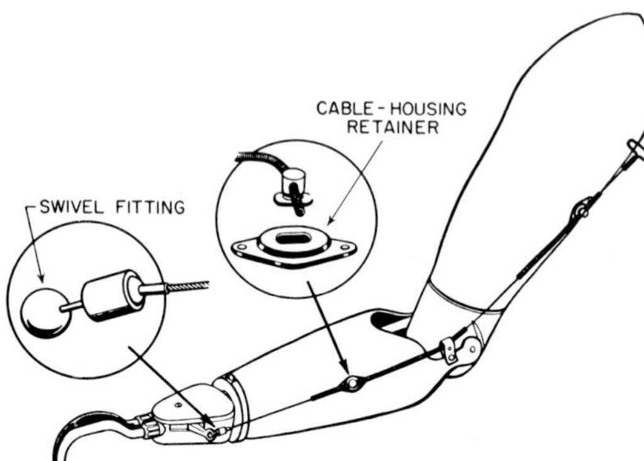

Fig. 5.24. Illustration of a typical above-elbow prosthesis with a dual-control system showing details of special hardware available for use with Bowden cable.

used to activate both elbow flexion and terminal device. When the elbow is unlocked and tension is imparted to the control cable, the elbow is flexed. When the elbow is locked, the tension is diverted to the terminal device. The disadvantages of this system are the need for a large amount of excursion and the need for the elbow to be locked for activation of the terminal device.

In Germany it seems to be rather common practice to provide the "triple-control" system (Fig. 5.29) in which separate control cables are used for elbow flexion and terminal device operation. This scheme has not been used widely in North America probably because the extra effort required by both prosthetist and patients has not seemed to have been worth the advantage accrued. An evaluation of the two systems carried out at the University of Poznan indicates that the triple control is preferred by laborers because of the greater stability afforded but other amputees preferred the dual control system because of the greater freedom of movement it permits (35, 53).

A disadvantage of the Bowden cable control system is the decrease in efficiency brought about as the radii of the bends in the cable are decreased during elbow and shoulder flexion. It has been proposed that hydraulic transmission systems be substituted for the cable system, and although some work in this area has been promising no sustained effort has been made to date to improve the efficiency of the power transmission system.

Typical Prosthetic Systems

PARTIAL HAND

Because loss of part of the hand invariably follows no patterns, there are no standard components readily available for application of a prosthesis, and it is a general practice for the prosthetist to design and fabricate a custom device to meet the individual needs of the patient. Hand surgery is quite specialized, and usually every attempt will be made to provide, through surgery, a functional extremity. Purely cosmetic prostheses usually will

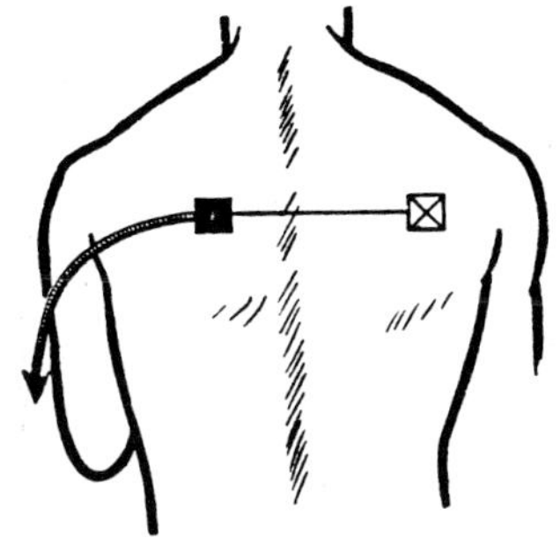

BISCAPULAR ABDUCTION (SHRUG)

APPLICATION: FOREQUARTER, PARTIAL SHOULDER DISARTICULATION, AND HUMERAL-NECK AMPUTEES

MUSCLES EMPLOYED: SCAPULAR ABDUCTORS

PROSTHESIS OPERATION: FOREARM FLEXION AND TERMINAL DEVICE

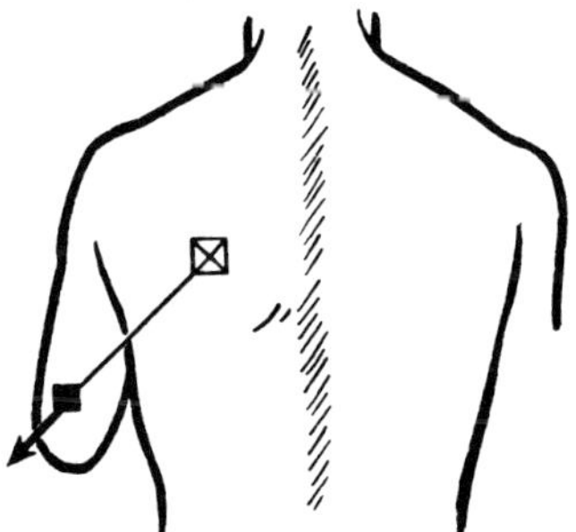

ARM FLEXION

APPLICATION: ABOVE- AND BELOW-ELBOW AMPUTEES

MUSCLES EMPLOYED: HUMERAL FLEXORS AND SECONDARILY THE SCAPULAR ABDUCTORS

PROSTHESIS OPERATION: FOREARM FLEXION AND TERMINAL DEVICE

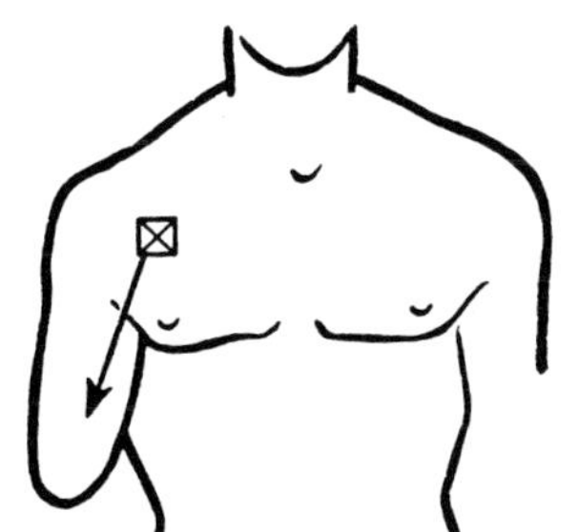

ARM EXTENSION

APPLICATION: ABOVE-ELBOW AMPUTEES

MUSCLES EMPLOYED: HUMERAL EXTENSORS

PROSTHESIS OPERATION: ELBOW LOCK

Fig. 5.25. Major harness controls. The points stabilized by harness (⊠) are beginning points for the control cable, which passes into a Bowden-type housing at movable points (■). The relative motion is transmitted *via* the Bowden cable (*top*) to distal points on the prosthesis. (Reprinted with permission from C. L. Taylor (52).)

result in less function because the sensation of touch is obscured by use of the cosmetic prosthesis. When additional function is required, the prosthetist must improvise.

Prosthetists have provided ingenious solutions for making many types of partial-hand amputees more functional (12, 8, 9). Several solutions are shown in Figures 5.30–5.32. The most comprehensive treatise on the subject of partial hand amputations and the provision of functional prostheses has been provided by Bunnell (12).

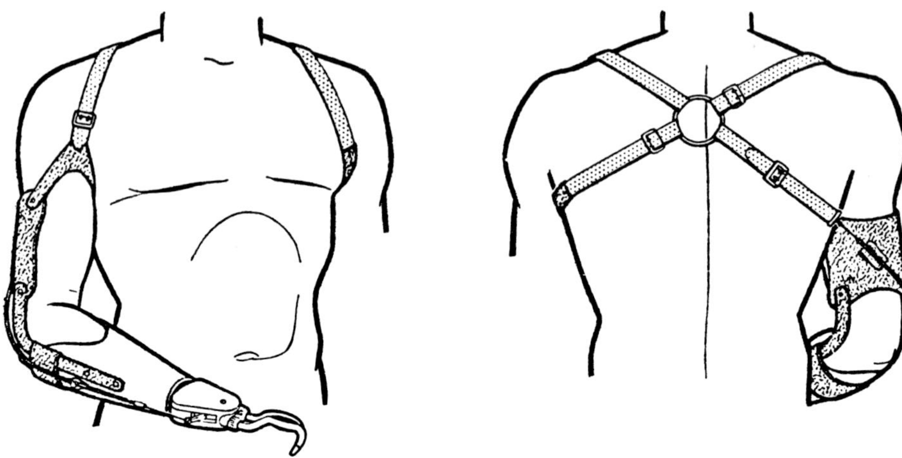

Fig. 5.26. Typical figure 8 harness for the unilateral below-elbow amputee.

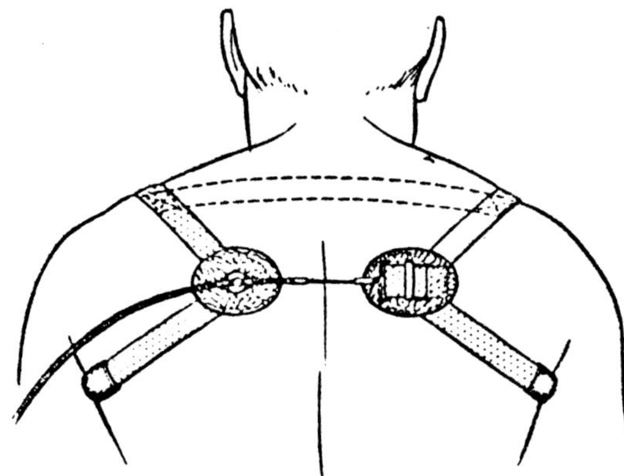

Fig. 5.27. The butterfly harness often used with wrist disarticulation and partial hand amputees where the only function needed is operation of the terminal device. The *dotted lines* represent an elastic strap that may be needed in some cases. (Reprinted with permission from R. J. Pursley (40).)

WRIST DISARTICULATION

One of the problems in fitting the wrist disarticulation in the past has been to keep the overall length of the prosthesis commensurate with the normal arm. The development of very short wrist units (26) especially for wrist disarticulation cases has materially reduced this problem. However, these units are available in only the screw, or thread, type and cannot be obtained in the bayonet type which lends itself to quick interchange of terminal devices.

The socket for the wrist-disarticulation case (Figs. 5.33 and 5.34) need not extend the full length of the forearm and is fitted somewhat loosely at the proximal end to permit wrist rotation. Either the "butterfly" harness or a simple figure 8 harness and Bowden cable are used to operate the terminal device.

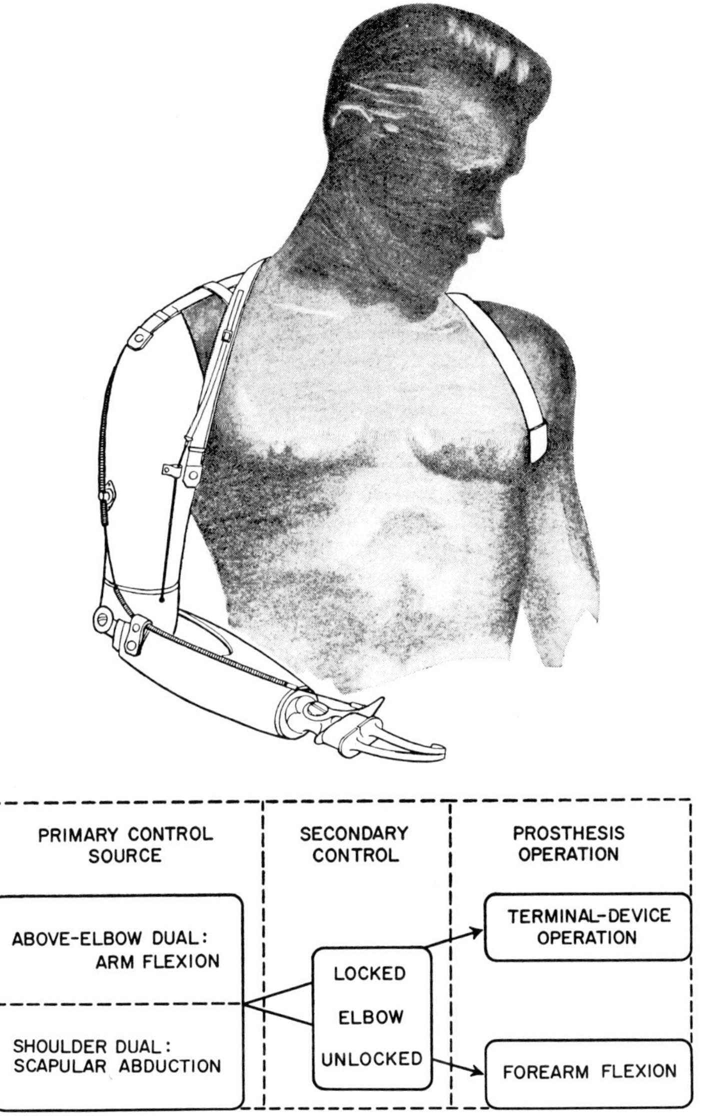

Fig. 5.28. Typical above-elbow prosthesis with the dual-control harness system (*top*). The diagram outlines the biomechanics of the system (*bottom*). (Reprinted with permission from R. J. Pursley (40).)

LONG BELOW ELBOW

The prosthesis for the long below-elbow case is essentially the same as that for the wrist-disarticulation patient except that the quick-disconnect wrist unit can be used when desired (Fig. 5.34).

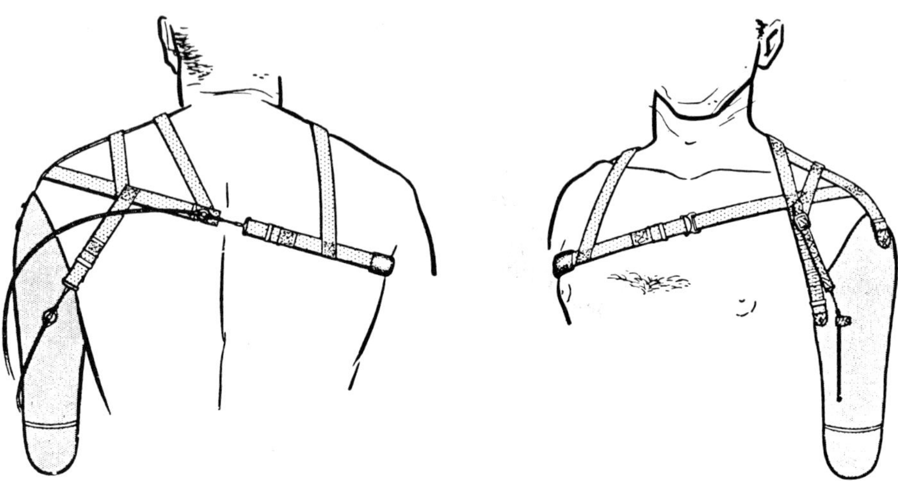

Fig. 5.29. The above-elbow triple-control harness. It differs from the dual-control pattern in that three body motions are required. The axilla loop uses shrug of the opposite shoulder to operate the terminal device, so that in this case the chest strap is separated at approximately the midspine position. Relative motion takes place between the axilla loop on the sound side and the reaction point located on the portion of the harness on the amputated side. A supporting shoulder saddle is constructed of a webbing network, and the control attachment strap for forearm flexion is attached to a point over the superior spine of the scapula on the amputated side. Arm flexion then lifts the forearm. Arm extension is harnessed as usual, a piece of elastic being used as the front suspensor strap to provide for the necessary relative motion (Reprinted with permission from R. J. Pursley (40).)

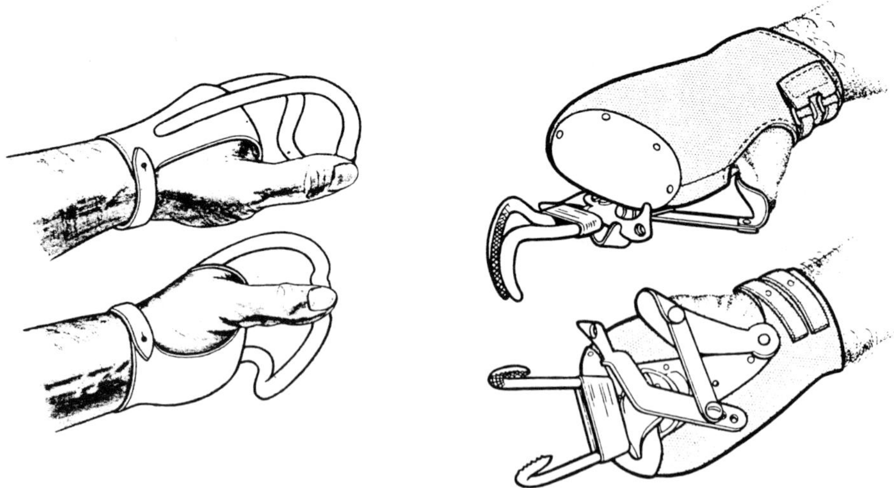

Fig. 5.30. Two examples of partial hand prostheses where a functional thumb is present (Reprinted with permission from S. Bunnell (2).)

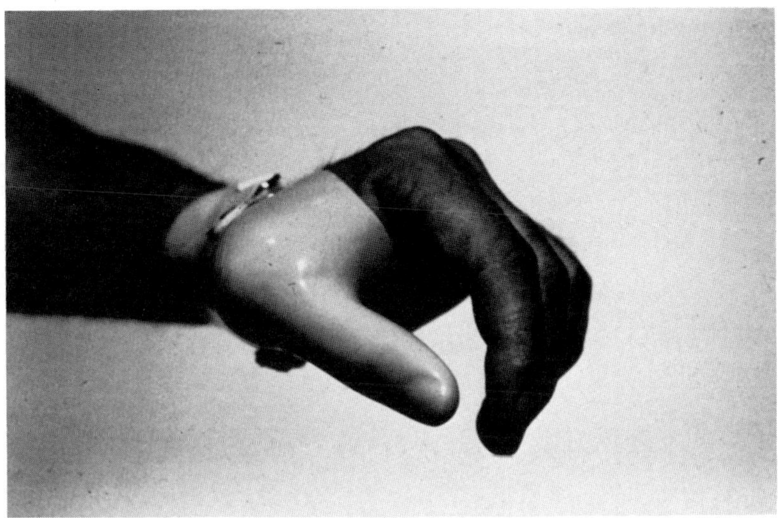

Fig. 5.31. A prosthetic thumb. (Courtesy of the Veterans Administration.)

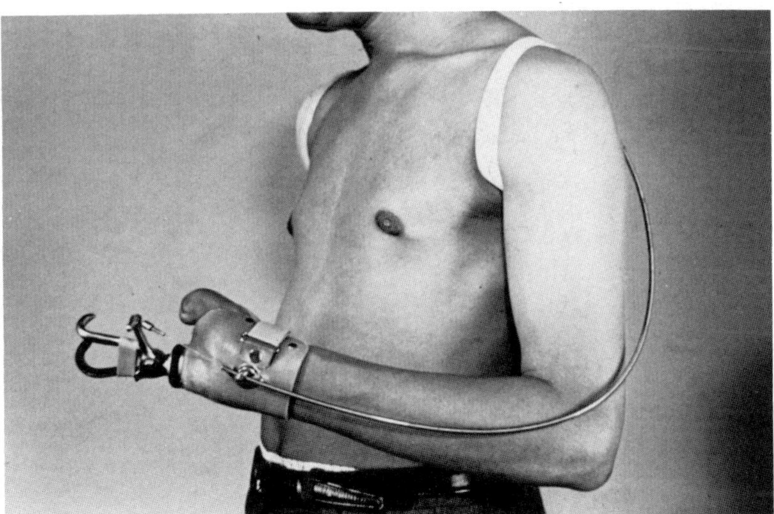

Fig. 5.32. Use of a voluntary opening hook by a partial hand amputee. (Courtesy of the Veterans Administration.)

SHORT BELOW-ELBOW

The socket for the short below-elbow stump, where there is no residual rotation of the forearm, is usually fitted snugly to the entire stump, and often rigid hinges connecting the socket to a cuff about the upper arm are used to provide additional stability. Either the figure 8 harness (Fig. 5.18) or

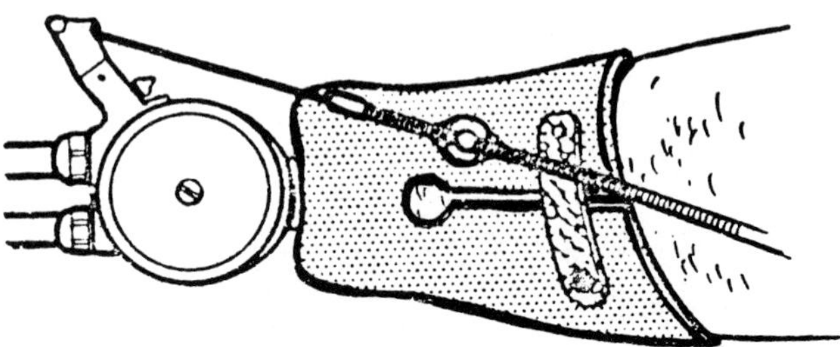

Fig. 5.33. One type of wrist disarticulation prosthesis. In this instance a special stud for the Northrup two-load hook is laminated into the socket in order to make the overall length of the prosthesis as small as possible. The butterfly harness (Fig. 5.27) is especially suitable for this type of socket. (Reprinted with permission from R. J. Pursley (40).)

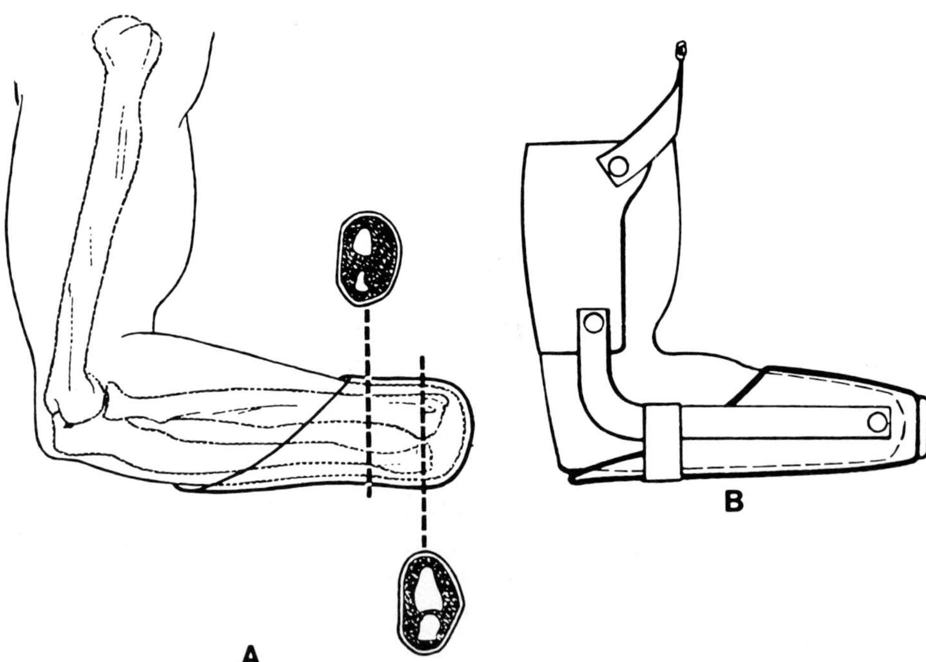

Fig. 5.34. *A*, relationship of the ulna and radius in a wrist disarticulation stump. Virtually no pronation-supination is lost when the gliding surfaces of the styloids are preserved. The socket may be a short cuff with an ulnar projection just long enough to provide comfort in lifting loads about the axis of the elbow. *B*, typical socket for a long-below-elbow stump. To protect the unpadded ulnar aspect and to provide stability, the socket may be extended to cover the olecranon without affecting the ability to pronate-supinate. (Reprinted with permission from C. L. Taylor (50).)

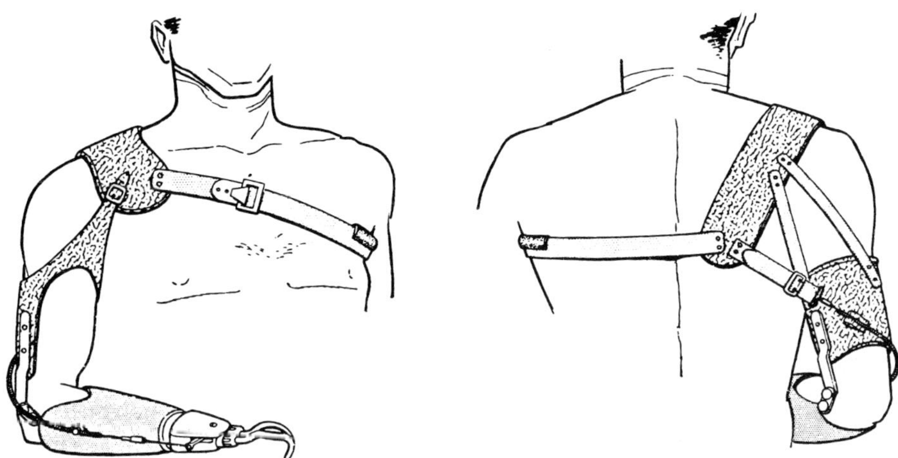

Fig. 5.35. The below-elbow chest-strap harness. Improved stability and reduced unit stresses over the shoulder offer greater ability to lift axial loads. Normally, the below-elbow chest-strap harness, used on amputees requiring heavy-duty service, is constructed in combination with a half-cuff and rigid elbow hinges. (Reprinted with permission from R. J. Pursley (40).)

the chest-strap harness may be used, the latter being preferred when heavy duty work is required since it tends to spread the loads involved in lifting over a broader area than is the case with the figure 8 design (Fig. 5.35).

A wrist flexion unit can be provided for the short below-elbow case but is seldom prescribed for unilateral cases.

VERY SHORT BELOW-ELBOW

Often the very short below-elbow case cannot control the prosthesis of the short below-elbow type through the full range of motion, either because of a muscle contracture or because the stump is too short to provide the necessary leverage.

When a contracture that limits the range of motion of the stump is present, a split-socket and step-up hinges may be used (Fig. 5.19). With this arrangement of levers and gears, rotation of the stump through 1° causes the prosthetic forearm to move through 2°; thus, a stump that has only about half the normal range of motion can drive the forearm through the desired 135°. However, when the step-up hinge is used, twice the normal force is required. When the stump is incapable of supplying the force required, it can be assisted by employing the dual-control harness wherein force in the terminal-device control cable is diverted to help lift the forearm. When the below-elbow stump is very short or has a very limited range of motion, an elbow lock operated by stump motion is employed to obtain elbow function (Fig. 5.20). When normal or nearly normal range of motion is available the Münster socket (Fig. 5.22) is usually used. Although full range of motion cannot be achieved, the other advantages usually outweigh this deficiency. Hinges and split socket are not needed, and sensory feedback is better. Furthermore, the harness is not needed for suspension of the prosthesis. The maximum forearm flexion may be limited to about 100°, but this does not appear to be a significant disadvantage to unilateral amputees.

ELBOW-DISARTICULATION

Because of the length of the elbow-disarticulation stump, the elbow-locking mechanism is installed on the outside of the socket. Otherwise the prosthesis and harnessing methods (Fig. 5.36) are identical to those applied to the above-elbow case. The function provided by the turntable in the conventional elbow unit is sacrificed, but the elbow disarticulation stump generally can provide sufficient humeral rotation.

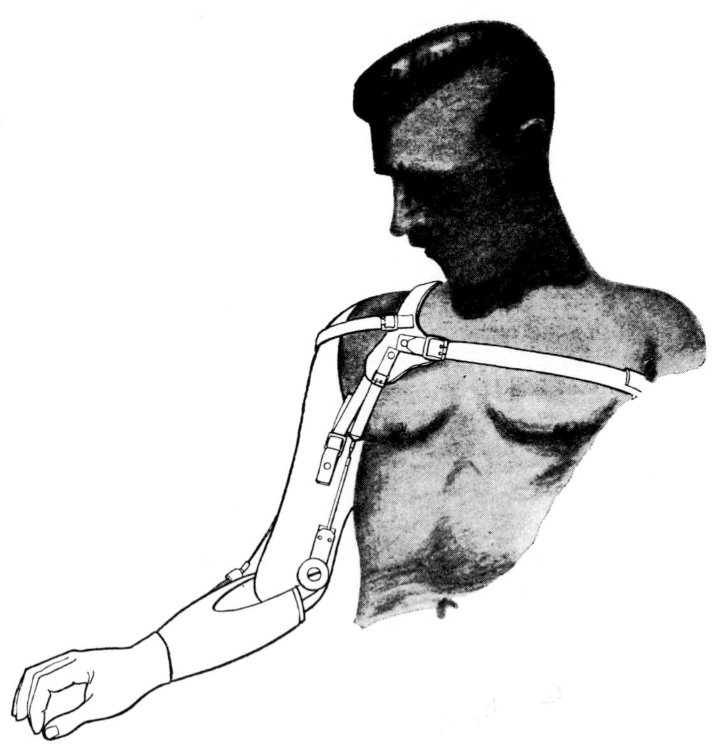

Fig. 5.36. Typical prosthesis for the elbow disarticulation case. The chest-strap harness with shoulder saddle is shown here, but the above-elbow figure 8 is also used. (Reprinted with permission from A. B. Wilson, Jr. (60).)

ABOVE-ELBOW

For the above-elbow prosthesis to operate efficiently, it is necessary that a lock be provided in the elbow joint, and it is, of course, preferable that the lock be engaged and disengaged without use of the other hand or pressing the locking actuator against an external object such as a table or chair.

Several elbow units that can be locked and unlocked alternately by the same motion are available. This action is usually accomplished by the relative motion between the prosthesis and the body when the shoulder is depressed slightly and the arm is extended somewhat. The motion required is so slight that with practice the amputee can accomplish the action without being noticed. These elbow units contain a turntable located above the elbow axis so as to permit the forearm to be positioned with respect to the humerus, supplementing the normal rotation remaining in the upper arm and thus allowing the prosthesis to be used more easily close to the midline of the body.

Elbow units are available with an adjustable coil spring to assist in flexing the elbow when this is desired. The flexion-assist device may be added or removed without affecting the other operating characteristics.

The plastic socket of the above-elbow prosthesis covers the entire surface of the stump. The most popular harness used is the figure 8 dual-control design (Fig. 5.28).

The chest-strap harness may also be used in the dual-control configuration.

SHOULDER DISARTICULATION AND FOREQUARTER AMPUTATION

Because of the loss of the upper arm motion as a source of energy for control and operation of the prosthesis, restoration of the more important functions in the shoulder disarticulation case presents a formidable problem; for many years a prosthesis was provided for this type of amputation only for the sake of appearance. In recent years, however, it has been possible to make available prostheses which provide a limited amount of function. To date it has not been possible to devise a shoulder joint that can be activated from a harness, but a number of manually operated joints are available. Socket configurations are shown in Figure 5.37. Various harness designs have been employed but, because of the wide variation in the individual cases and the marginal amount of energy available, no standard pattern has developed, each design being made to take full advantage of the remaining potential of the particular patient (Fig. 5.38). A device known as the nudge control has been found to be quite useful in providing control of the elbow lock by use of hand and chin motions (55, 56, 60).

BILATERAL UPPER LIMB AMPUTEES

Except for the bilateral, shoulder disarticulation case, fitting the bilateral case offers few problems not encountered with the unilateral case. The

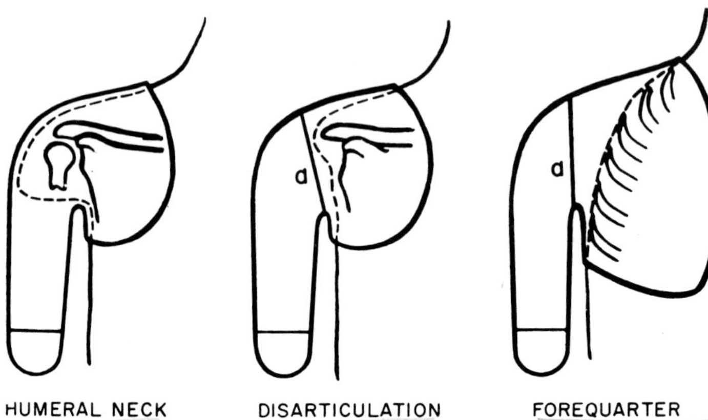

Fig. 5.37. Schematics of shoulder sockets. *Solid lines* show residual bony structure, *dashed lines* show the body contour and inner wall of the socket. Disarticulation and forequarter sockets may be two-piece with sectional plates at *a*. (Reprinted with permission from C. L. Taylor (50).)

prostheses provided are generally the same as those prescribed for corresponding levels in unilateral cases (49). Artificial hands are used rarely by bilateral amputees because hooks afford so much more function. Many bilateral cases find that the wrist flexion unit, at least on one side, is of value. The harness for each prosthesis may be separated, but it is the general practice to combine the two (Fig. 5.39). In addition to being neater, this arrangement makes the harness easier for the patient to don unassisted.

Some prosthetists have claimed success in fitting bilateral shoulder disarticulation cases with two prostheses. Because of the lack of sufficient sources of energy for control, most cases of this type are provided with a single, functional prosthesis and a plastic cap over the opposite shoulder which provides an anchor for the harness and also fills this area to present a better appearance (Fig. 5.40). Externally powered prostheses are certainly indicated in these cases.

Endoskeletal Prostheses

For those above-elbow, shoulder disarticulation and forequarter cases where, for either physiological or psychological reasons, a functional prosthesis is not indicated, consideration should be given to providing a cosmetic arm. At least one firm (38) offers the components for a limited function endoskeletal arm prosthesis (Fig. 5.41) that has proven to be useful to a significant segment of the upper limb amputee population.

The tubular arm and forearm components are covered with foam rubber so as to provide a somewhat natural response to touch while presenting a quite normal appearance because of its unbroken lines. The hand can be

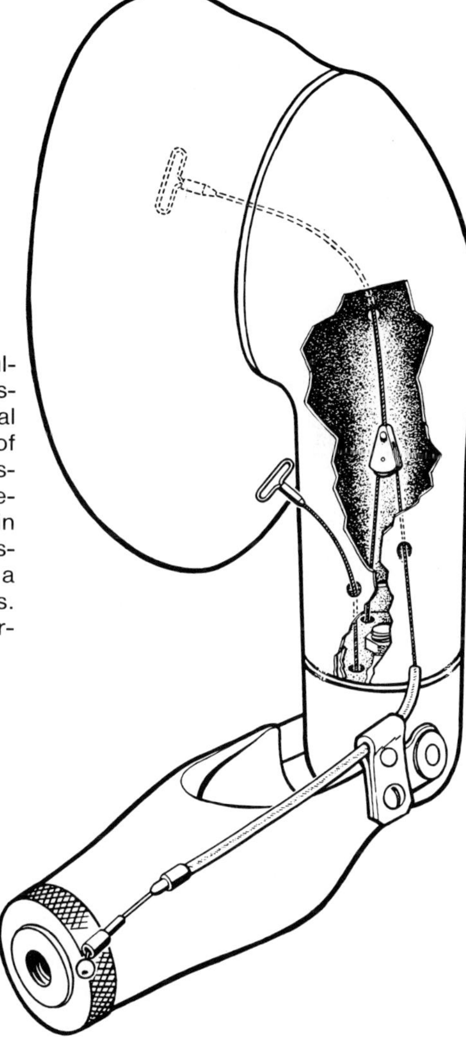

Fig. 5.38. One method of fitting a shoulder disarticulation case. The pulley system seen on the inside of the humeral section is used to reduce the amount of excursion needed in a dual control system. Obviously, gain in excursion requirement is offset by a 50% reduction in torque provided about the elbow. The system shown here might be applicable to a patient who has broad mobile shoulders. (Reprinted with permission from R. J. Pursley (40).)

controlled passively to provide holding of light objects, and the elbow can be locked in one of a number of positions by use of the contralateral hand.

Externally Powered Upper Limb Prosthesis

The earliest reference to externally powered upper limb prostheses seems to be in connection with experiments that took place in Germany about 1918 (45) in which electromagnets were used to close the fingers of an artificial hand. About the same time a design using compressed air as an energy source was reported (45). The next reported effort apparently is the

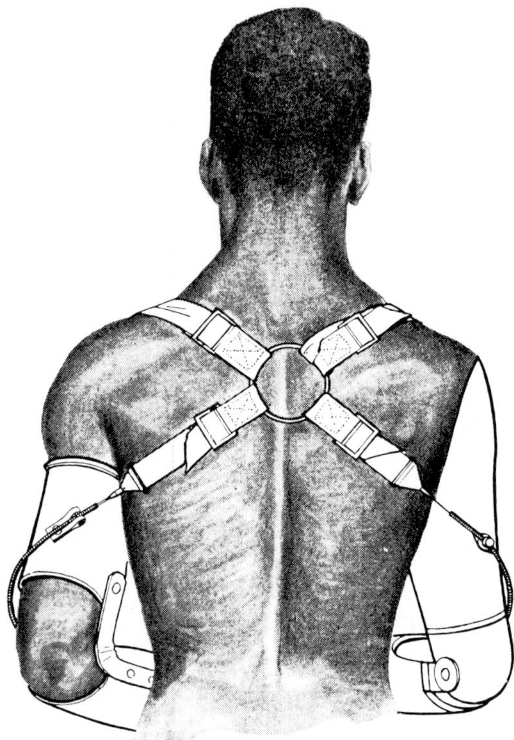

Fig. 5.39. Harness for the bilater
tee with below-elbow amputation on
above-elbow on the other. (Reprin
mission from A. B. Wilson, Jr. (69).)

research and development program proposed and carried out by Alderson (1) and Berger and Huppert (10) on electrically powered arm systems during 1946–1952 with support from International Business Machines, Inc. and the Veterans Administration.

Initial results of the Alderson-IBM project (1) (Fig. 5.42) were quite impressive with respect to operation, but an extensive evaluation at UCLA in 1951 revealed that a disproportionate amount of mental effort by the wearer was required for use of the various systems (17). As a result of the findings of the UCLA study, and because only a limited amount of money was available for work in artificial limbs, the Advisory Committee on Artificial Limbs (later the Committee on Prosthetics Research and Development) of the National Academy of Sciences recommended that development of actuators be delayed until sufficient research could be carried out concerning the control problem so as to provide means for control of the prosthesis without conscious thought by the wearer.

A project was initiated at UCLA about 1953 to explore various control methods. Among the various studies conducted at UCLA was an evaluation of the so-called Vaduz hand (16) (Fig. 5.43), a design that originated in Lichtenstein which used bulging of the residual muscles in a forearm stump

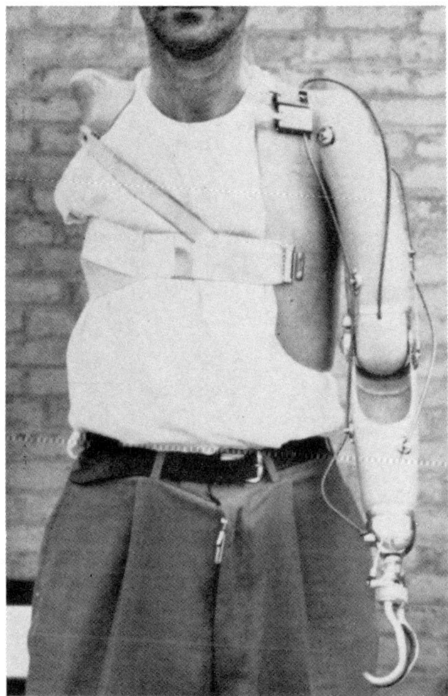
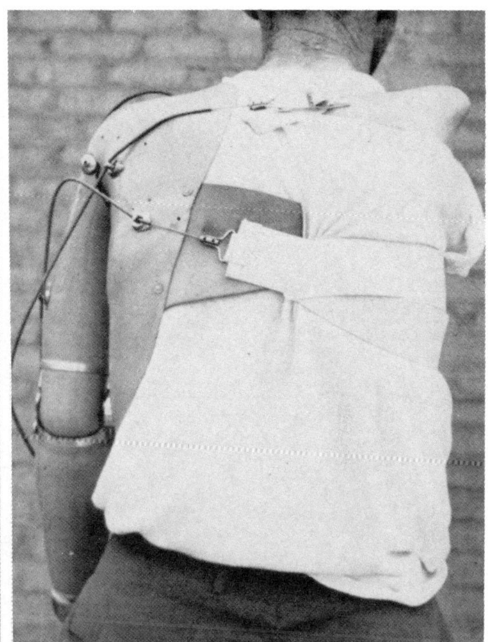

Fig. 5.40. Unilateral fitting of a bilateral shoulder-disarticulation case. Note use of the nudge control for the alternator type of elbow lock. (Reprinted with permission from A. B. Wilson, Jr. (60).)

to provide control of an electrically actuated artificial hand. Some rather positive findings were overshadowed by the poor quality of the one unit that was available for study at the time and, perhaps, by the introduction by Russia in 1958 of a "thought control" electric arm (31). The Russian device actually consisted of an electric hand controlled by myoelectric signals from the residual agonists and antagonists in the forearm stump of a below-elbow amputee.

The proposal by Reiter in 1948 (42) to use the EMG signals seems to have been overlooked.

The thalidomide tragedy (36) in 1958–1962 prompted England (4) and Canada to secure manufacturing rights to the Russian design, but fabrication and distribution was not successful in either country. The thalidomide tragedy also encouraged work at the University of Heidelberg in the development of pneumatically powered artificial arm systems (36), and an agreement was obtained by Kessler and Kiessling (29) for continuation of this work in the United States (Fig. 5.44). This project was carried out between 1960 and 1969. Again, the problem of control was the primary reason for discontinuing the work.

Because of the thalidomide tragedy, Sweden (25, 27) also launched a

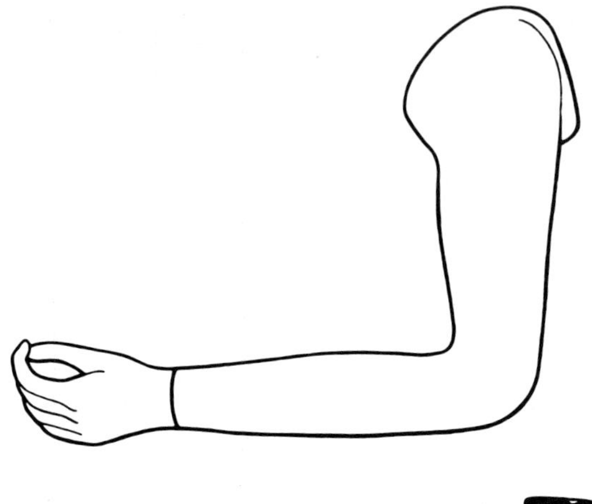

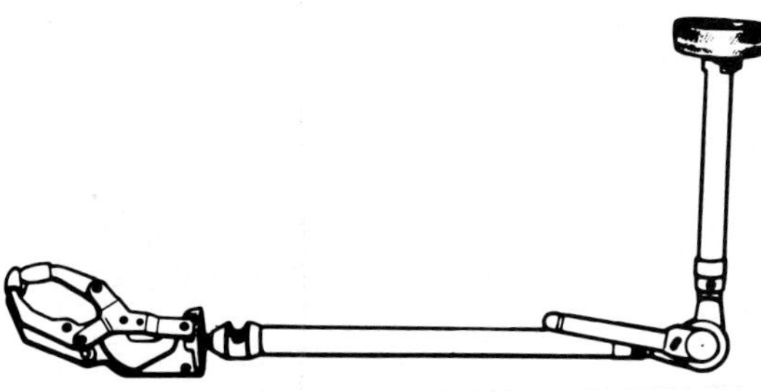

Fig. 5.41. The Otto Bock (38) endoskeletal system for above-elbow and shoulder disarticulation cases. Control of the elbow must be carried out by the hand on the contralateral side.

modest program in development of externally powered upper-limb prostheses about 1960. Work on this area has been carried out continuously since, and a child's hand is now commercially available.

The Russian design caused an Austrian group, Viennatone, and the Otto Bock Company in Germany, to develop and market similar devices beginning about 1962. A few years later Hannes Schmidl began fitting externally powered artificial arms on a relatively large scale at the INAIL (Instituto Nazionale per l'Assicurazione contro gli Infortuni sul Lavoro) Center, Budrio, Italy and continues to do so to the present time (47). Pneumatic models were used initially, but all designs used now are electric.

Simpson (48), at the Princess Margaret Rose Hospital, Edinburgh, Scotland, used routinely pneumatic prostheses for a group of thalidomide children, but his design is not widely available elsewhere.

In 1960, as a visiting professor at the University of Southern California, Tomović from the Institute Pupin, Belgrade, Yugoslavia, suggested the use of electromechanical pressure-sensitive devices to aid in solution to the control problem by introducing closed-loop feedback systems (41, 54). A number of prototypes (Fig. 5.45) were designed and fabricated upon the return of Tomović to Yugoslavia. Results of evaluation (28) also were overshadowed by poor workmanship and engineering, and work on this was abandoned about 1968.

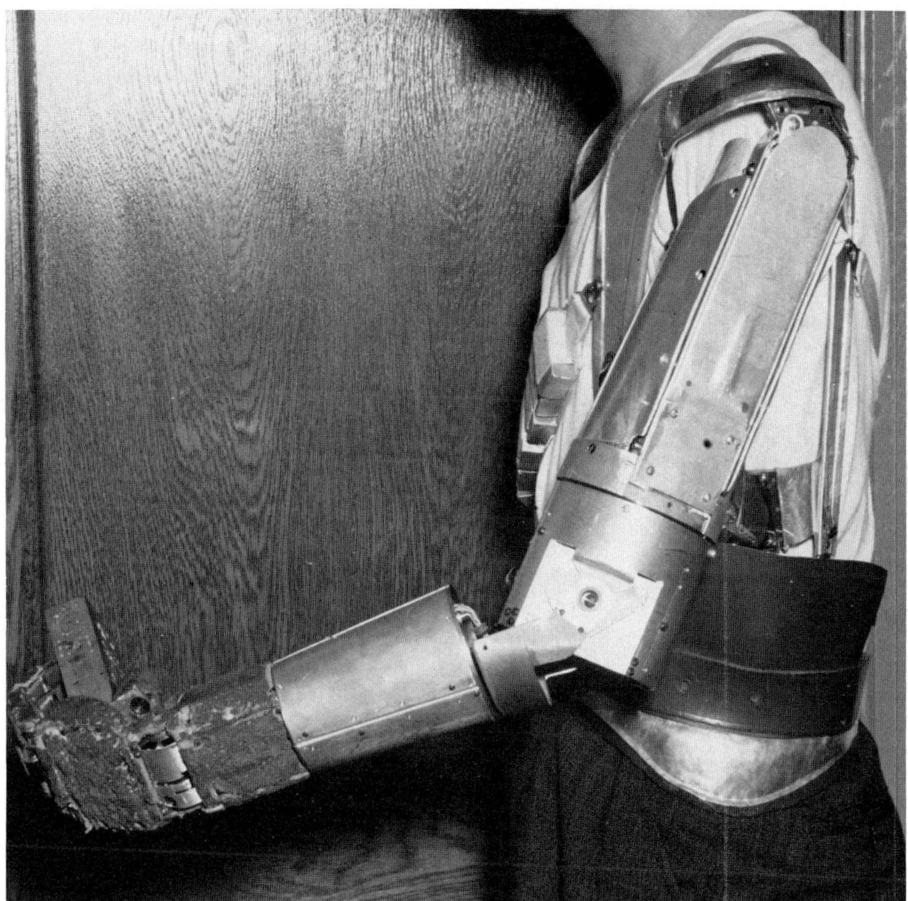

Fig. 5.42. An early model of the Alderson-IBM electric arm. (Courtesy of the Veterans Administration.)

McLaurin, while at Northwestern University, designed the so-called Michigan feeding arm about 1960 which used a linkage to coordinate motions about the elbow and the wrist to make it easier for young bilateral child amputees to feed themselves (23). This device met with considerable success in the hospital setting, but never became a commercial success.

McLaurin continued work on electrical arms for children at the Ontario Crippled Childrens Centre, Toronto, between 1963 and 1975. Although he was able to persuade the Variety Club to develop a facility for manufacturing, at cost, some of the products of research as a philanthropic endeavor, to date only an electric elbow has been made available; but because of the low volume, the cost is considered to be high for the benefits gained in spite of subsidization.

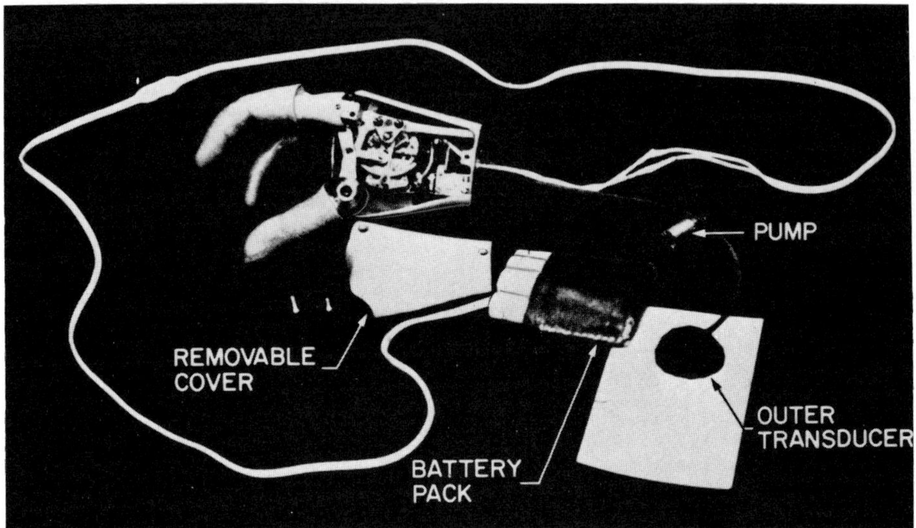

Fig. 5.43. The Vaduz hand and control system (Courtesy of the Veterans Administration.)

In the late 1960s a number of efforts in the United States were directed toward the development of electric elbows. By 1969 three designs were considered ready for clinical evaluation, the "Boston" elbow developed by the Massachusetts Institute of Technology and the Liberty Mutual Insurance Co., the AMBRL elbow, developed by the Army Medical Biomedical Research Laboratory, and a design by Rancho Los Amigos Hospital. The clinical evaluation program was organized and coordinated by the National Academy of Sciences in 1969–1970 (15).

Of 20 subjects in the study, only 3 elected to retain the electric device. Two of these subjects had physical problems that made operation of the body-powered prosthesis more difficult than would have been the case otherwise. Out of this experience came a revised set of design criteria and objectives (15).

In addition to all of these efforts, research and development programs in externally powered artificial arms have been carried out in North America at Temple University-Moss Rehabilitation Hospital (61), Northwestern University (14) (Fig. 5.46), Veterans Administration Prosthetic Center, Duke University, Rancho Los Amigos Hospital, University of California at Los Angeles, University of Colorado, Johns Hopkins University (18, 46), and the University of New Brunswick (43, 44). Sweden, Great Britain, Italy, Germany, Russia, and others have continued to support research and development in this field.

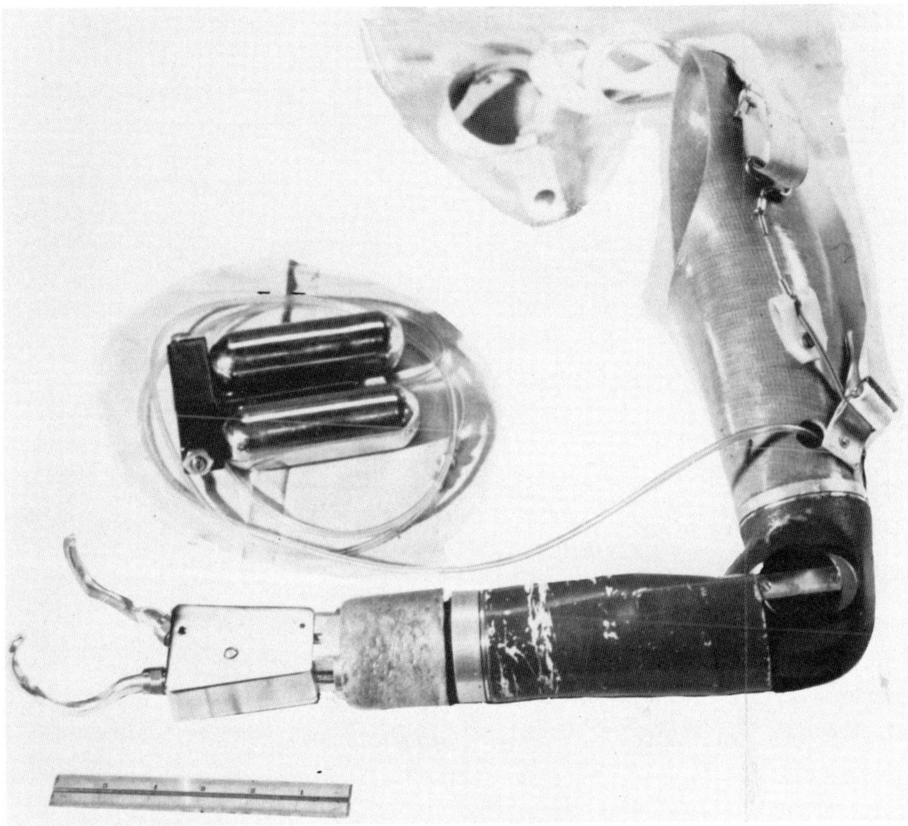

Fig. 5.44. One of the pneumatic above-elbow systems developed by Kessler and Kiessling at the American Institute for Prosthetic Research. (Courtesy of the Veterans Administration.)

In spite of the many efforts made in the development of externally powered prostheses, progress has been slow because it has been difficult to justify the expense of the individual fittings in view of the rather limited gains provided. Although some of the myoelectric below-elbow systems seem to provide control as good as the conventional systems, the above-elbow systems seem to be quite deficient and the patient has to be well motivated to continue using the devices generally available at this time.

Obviously, patients with bilateral upper-limb amputations resulting from trauma are apt to be motivated. However, unilateral upper-limb amputees, especially above-elbow cases, are not apt to be inspired to use a complicated piece of equipment that requires a great deal of maintenance.

The acceptance of externally powered artificial arms has not been enhanced by the lack of an externally powered hook.

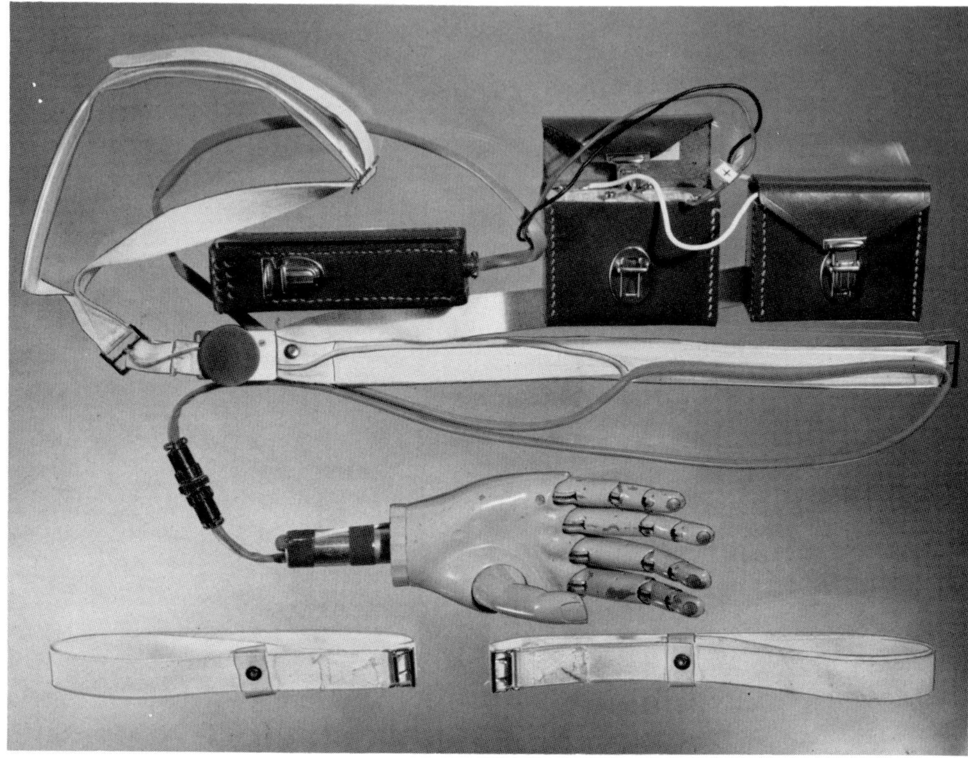

Fig. 5.45. The Belgrade hand and control system (Courtesy of the Veterans Administration.)

Part of the reason for a lack of widespread use of externally powered upper limb prostheses is owing to the high degree of sophistication needed by the prosthetist to obtain satisfactory results. Considerable experience is needed before most prosthetists can provide efficiently the service needed to fit and maintain externally powered prostheses. This suggests specialization. Several Canadian and United States centers offer this special service where various control systems and components can be used in combinations that best meet the individual needs of patients. No doubt, more centers will be formed to meet the demand that is expected.

However, until externally powered systems can provide sensory feedback superior to body powered prostheses, their application will be restricted to amputees who have special problems.

COMPONENTS AVAILABLE

Although a number of designers of externally powered upper-limb prostheses have offered more or less complete systems such as the pneumatic

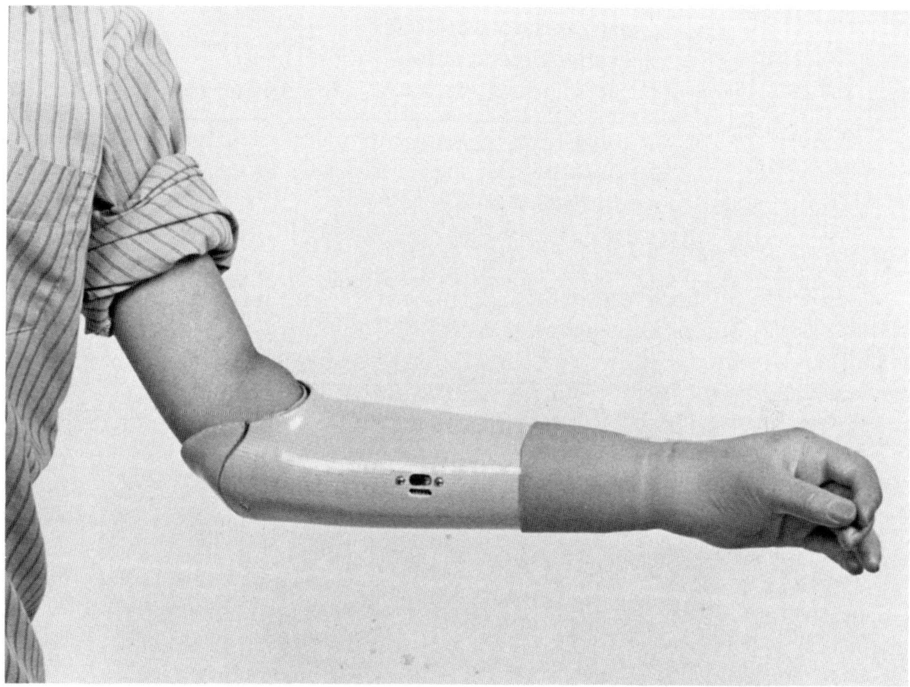

Fig. 5.46. The self-contained and self-suspended below-elbow system using myoelectric controls developed at Northwestern University. (Courtesy of the Veterans Administration.)

prostheses developed at Princess Margaret Rose Hospital in Edinburgh and the University of Heidelberg, and the electrically powered prostheses developed by IBM and Alderson, the present trend seems to be toward making available specific components, such as terminal devices and elbow units, that can be assembled by prosthetists to meet individual needs, just as is the case today with body-powered prostheses.

The components and control systems available for use with patients in North America today are described below.

TERMINAL DEVICES

Hands

A relatively large number of designs for externally powered hands for adults and children have at one time or another been developed for patient trials. Available in North America at the present time are:

Otto Bock electric hands in three sizes—adult male, adult female, children (38)

Electrolimb child size electric hand (child size)
Systems Teknik (Sweden) electric hand (child size)
VA-NU electric hand—United States Manufacturing Co. (58)

These hands can be controlled by either myoelectric signals or by excursion provided by body harness. All use a cosmetic glove, and the general appearance is as shown in Figure 5.46.

Hooks

The design of successful externally powered hooks has proven to be more difficult than hands for reasons that are not obvious.

Only one design is known to be available—the so-called Michigan external power system for Hosmer-Dorrance 10X and 10P hooks (Fig. 5.47). As the name implies, the design, which was initiated by the Michigan Crippled

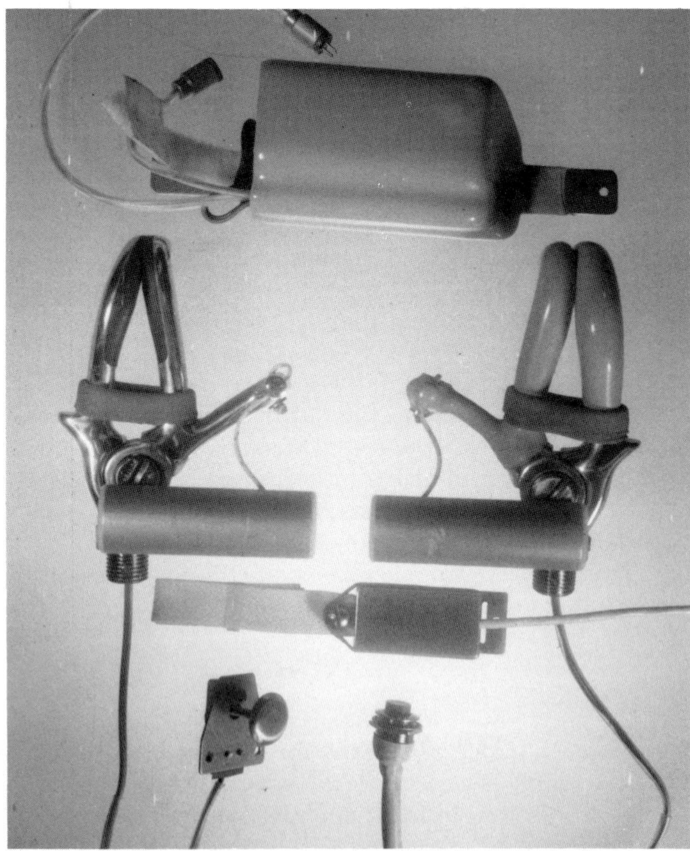

Fig. 5.47. The Michigan externally powered hooks for child amputees. Available are the 10P and 10X hook which can be operated by either compression (push) or tension (pull) switches. (Courtesy of the Hosmer-Dorrance Corp.)

Childrens Commission, consists of an externally powered actuator attached to the Number 10 series of Hosmer-Dorrance hooks. Two types of mechanical switches are available for control—a push button type for use with limb-deficient children who have a residual function available distally, and a pull-type designed for operation by a body harness.

Wrist Units

An electrically operated wrist rotation unit is available from Otto Bock.

Elbow Units

No externally powered elbow units seem to be generally acceptable at this time, although a number of designers hope to rectify this situation soon.

Cineplasty

At sporadic intervals throughout more than half a century, orthopaedic surgeons, sometimes urged by engineers, have experimented with surgical procedures that would permit direct coupling between a muscle and one or more components of an artificial arm in an effort to provide improved feedback of the forces involved and more efficient power transmission (7, 30). Experiments seem to have started with Ceci (7) who used knobs created in the ends of muscles for connection to the prosthesis. Sauerbruch (in Ref. 7), encouraged by an engineer, developed during World War I a procedure that resulted in a skin-lined tunnel installed through a muscle belly, the long axis of the tunnel being perpendicular to the long axis of the muscle (Fig. 5.48). Influenced by results obtained by German surgeons, United

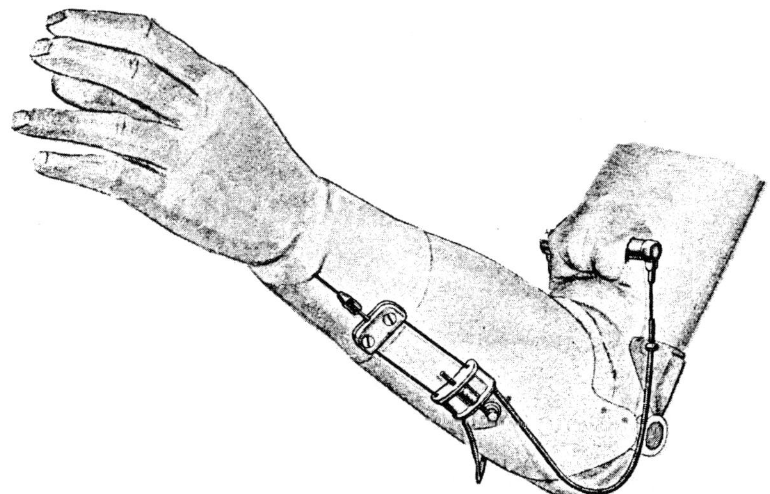

Fig. 5.48. One method of harnessing the biceps muscle provided with a cineplasty tunnel. (Reprinted with permission from C. O. Bechtol and G. T. Aitkens (7).)

States military surgeons, after World War II, engaged in a study to determine the benefits gained by cineplasty procedures. Evaluated were tunnels through the agonists and antagonists through forearm stumps, tunnels through the biceps for below-elbow and above-elbow patients, and tunnels through the pectoralis major for above-elbow and shoulder disarticulation cases (51).

Although some individual cases with tunnels through the biceps showed impressive results and some patients have been successful users for more than 30 years, the procedure has not been accepted as one that is appropriate for most amputees because of the need for keeping the tunnel clean and free of bacteria. Tunnels through other muscles, in general, are considered not to be worth the trouble for the advantages gained. Today, cineplasty tunnels are seldom indicated.

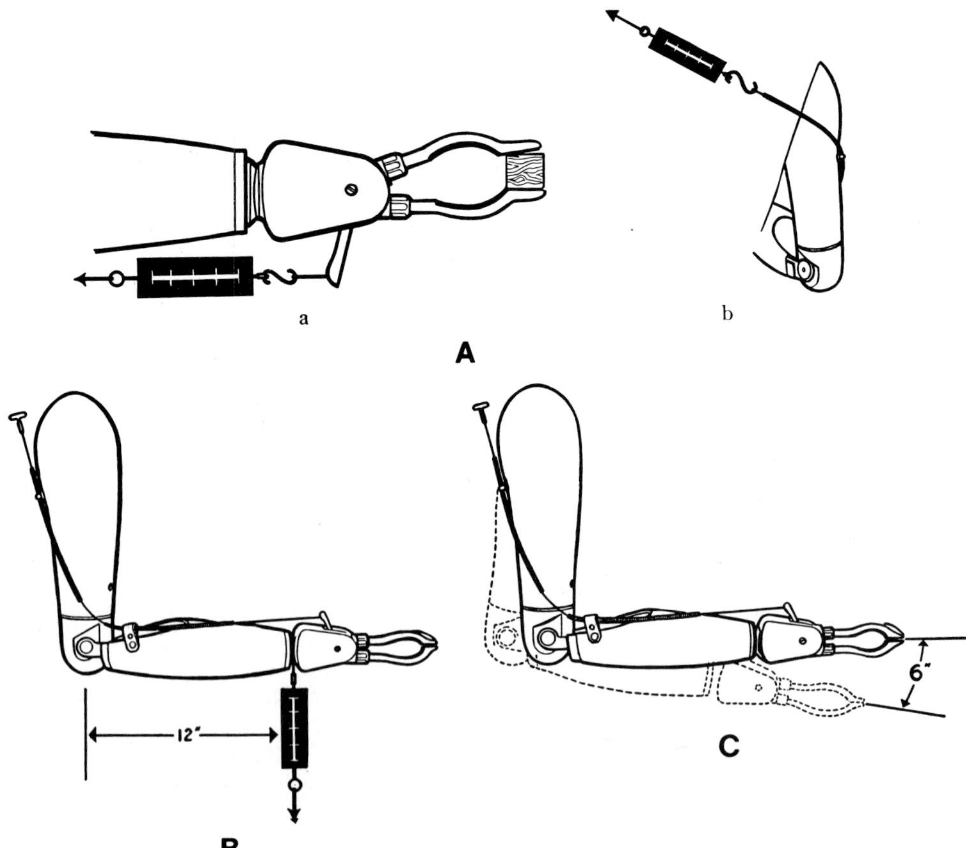

Fig. 5.49. Examples of the tests employed in checkout procedures. *A*, test for control-system efficiency. *B*, test for live-lift. *C*, test for motion of terminal device when locking elbow. (Reprinted with permission from L. Carlyle (13).)

Artificial Arm Checkout Procedures

The usefulness of well conceived, sensibly executed tests to determine the efficacy of the fitting of artificial arms seems obvious. To provide the standards for such tests, the Artificial Limbs Research Project and the University of California at Los Angeles conducted in 1952 a scientific study that led to the Artificial Limb Checkout Procedures (13, 55, 56) generally in use today (Fig. 5.49). The checkout procedures require the use of very simple, readily available tools, and should be used by every prosthetist to ensure that he has achieved an optimum set of conditions for each patient.

Most federal, state, and private organizations that pay for artificial arms use the checkout procedures described by Carlyle (13). Usually the checkout is carried out for the clinic team by the therapist. Most of the time, the checkout procedures have been beneficial to patient and prosthetist, but unfortunately there have been too many instances where rigidity in adherence to numbers, without taking into consideration other factors, has led to friction between the prosthetist and therapist, often to the detriment of the patient. It should be remembered by all that the checkout procedures were developed with the otherwise healthy upper limb amputee as the subject and, thus, allowance must be made for other problems, such as limited range of motion of joints, obesity, and muscle weakness.

Time of Fitting

There are no set rules about the management of upper limb amputees, except that every effort should be made to provide the devices and training that will best meet the needs of each individual patient.

Patients who are well coordinated and well motivated will solve many of their problems on their own. Other patients will require varying degrees of care.

It has been recognized that, in general, the earlier an artificial limb is fitted, the more apt an amputee is to accept and use the prosthesis, and ostensibly the more successful is the rehabilitation effort. A major reason for this probably is that during a long interval between amputation and fitting most unilateral patients discover the potential of the remaining hand, and are, therefore, reluctant to spend the time required to undergo the training necessary for them to make proper use of a prosthesis.

The principles involved in fitting lower limb amputees immediately after amputation surgery have been applied in a number of centers with very rewarding results (14, 19)—apparently partly because of the attitude of the patient resulting from the attention given, and because of the function provided so soon after the removal of the limb part. This conclusion is based on collective clinical judgment because the relatively small number of patients seen at any one hospital up to now has not made it easy to carry out a scientific study in this area. Nevertheless individual results are very impressive, whether body powered or externally powered systems are used. Good results have been obtained also with externally powered prostheses using either myoelectric or mechanical switches.

Considerations in Child Prosthetics

Children with amputations, especially infants and young children, obviously require special attention. In the case of congenital limb deficiencies, the parents need counseling beginning at the earliest possible moment after birth of the child. Proper counseling can save much time and trouble later for all concerned (57).

Whether the case is unilateral or bilateral, the general practice is to provide the child with a passive prosthesis about the time he or she is able to sit upright if this is practical. For this purpose the baby mitt (26, 57) is available. The mitt can, as the child progresses, be replaced with the child's wafer hook (Dorrance 10AW) (Fig. 5.50) or the newly available Child Amputee Prosthetic Program (CAPP) terminal device No. 1 (Fig. 5.51). The objective in fitting early, especially for the unilateral cases, is to provide the child with the capability of two-handed grasp at a normal distance from the eyes. This is achieved, of course, at the expense of some loss in sensation

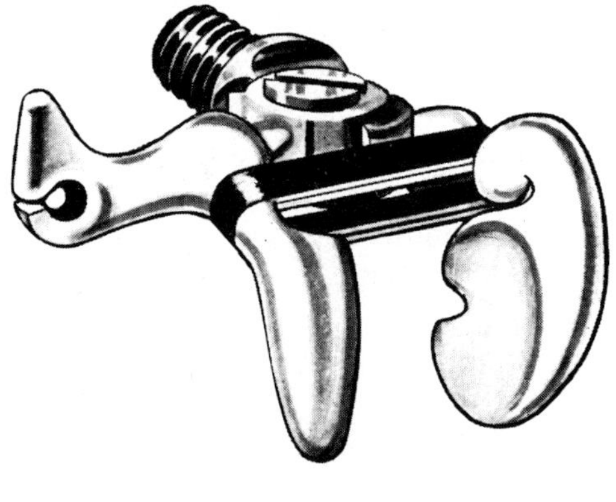

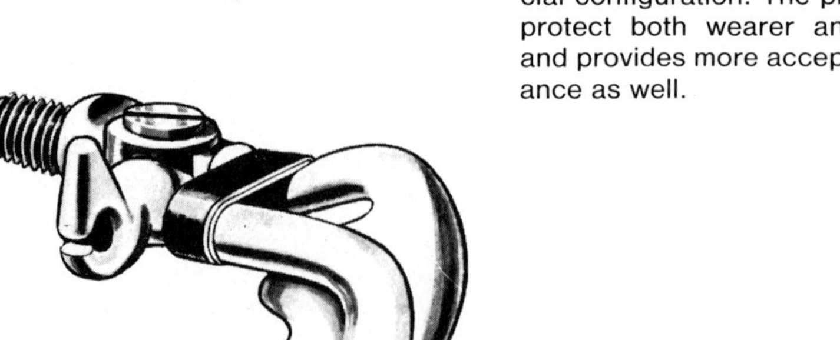

Fig. 5.50. The child's wafer hook, a Dorrance voluntary opening device. The hook fingers are covered with a flesh-colored plastic molded in a special configuration. The plastic helps to protect both wearer and associates and provides more acceptable appearance as well.

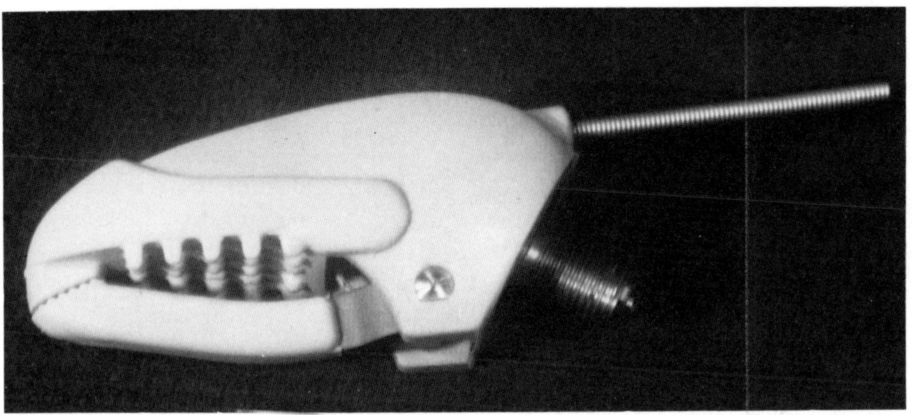

Fig. 5.51. The CAPP (Child Amputee Prosthetics Program, University of California, Los Angeles) terminal device No. 1. This terminal device, after many years of trials, is now available from the Hosmer Corporation. The objective of this rather revolutionary design which is based on many years of clinical experience is to provide a device that combines the best features of both artificial hands and hooks. (Courtesy of the Hosmer-Dorrance Corp.)

afforded by the stump. Most children seem to find benefit from early application of prostheses. However, each case is different and must be treated accordingly.

For the bilateral cases who have lower limbs, use of the feet should be encouraged. Even children with abnormal lower limbs can often use them surprisingly effectively as substitutes for missing upper limbs.

When children with high level amputations on both sides have been fitted with well designed functional prostheses, either body powered or externally powered, they will use them for a while apparently quite effectively, but usually will discard them after entering school, only to request a new set about or soon after puberty. Usually, the new set is well received for awhile but discarded later, because the energy cost is not worth the benefit.

This is not to say that children should not be fitted with artificial arms, nor should research be curtailed. The psychological benefit derived from the provision of artificial arms is almost always worth the cost even if they are abandoned before they are worn out (24). Research should continue to be supported, because, although progress is slow, it is quite probable that very useful prostheses can be made available.

Children with acquired amputations have somewhat different psychological problems but the biomechanical aspects of treatment are the same. The child should be fitted as soon as possible after the accident and surgery. Bilateral cases at high levels should be encouraged to use their feet.

Conclusions

Although the past 20 years have not seen the introduction of any great breakthroughs in upper limb prosthetics, a great many refinements have been introduced in body-powered systems and progress is being made in the control of externally powered systems.

Through experience, amputee clinic teams have become more realistic in management of upper limb amputees and the tendency to raise false hopes has abated.

Properly applied artificial arms, whether body-powered or externally powered, can be beneficial, but their value must not be oversold.

It is unfortunate that the work started at UCLA in the form of a case study, from which most of our present body of knowledge came, has not been continued there or elsewhere. Few of the innovations brought forth in the past 20 years such as the socket designs of Pentland and Wasileff (39), MaLaurin (34), and Childress (14), have been evaluated so that they can be accepted by the prosthetists and the agencies that provide upper limb prostheses.

Needed very badly throughout the world is an evaluation program that will provide an unbiased assessment of new devices and techniques as they emerge from research and development, whether from individual practitioners, component manufacturers, government laboratories, or groups supported by the government.

Prosthetists and other members of the amputee clinic team must remind themselves continuously that the guidelines provided by the standard texts generally deal with the uncomplicated cases who, except for amputation, are otherwise healthy individuals. Therefore when patients present with additional complicating problems, it is necessary to use all the information and originality available to provide solutions to unique problems that cannot be covered by texts (5).

REFERENCES

1. Alderson, S. W., The electric arm. In *Human Limbs and Their Substitutes*, edited by Klopsteg, P. E., and Wilson, P. D. Chapt. 13. McGraw-Hill, 1954, reprinted by Hafner Press, 1969.
2. American Academy of Orthopaedic Surgeons, Historical development of artificial limbs. In *Orthopaedic Appliances Atlas*, Vol. 2, Chapt. 1. J. W. Edwards, Ann Arbor, 1960.
3. Ballif, P., *Description d'une main et d'une jambe artificielles, inventées par Pierre Ballif*, Berlin, 1818, cited in Ref. 2 above.
4. Battye, C. K., Nightingale, A., and Whillis, J. The use of myoelectric currents in the operation of prostheses. *J. Bone J. Surg., 37B:* 506, 1955.
5. Batzdorff, J. A non-standard above-elbow prosthesis for a multiply handicapped patient. *Orthotics Prosthet., 30:* 1976.
6. Bechtol, C. O., Anatomical and physiological considerations in the clinical application of upper-extremity prosthetics. In *Orthopaedic Appliances Atlas*, Vol. 2, Chapt. 8. J. W. Edwards, Ann Arbor, 1960.

7. BECHTOL, C. O., AND AITKEN, G. T. Cineplasty. In *Orthopaedic Appliances Atlas*, Vol. 2, Chapt. 12. J. W. Edwards, Ann Arbor, 1960.
8. BENDER, L. F., Prostheses for partial hand amputations. *Prosthet Orthot. Int., 2:* 8–11, 1978.
9. BENDER, L. F., AND KOCH, R. D. Meeting the challenge of partial hand amputations. *Orthotics Prosthet., 30:* 3–11, 1976.
10. BERGER, N., AND HUPPERT, C. R. The use of electrical and mechanical muscular forces for the control of an electrical prosthesis. *Am. J. Occup. Ther., 6:* 110–14, 1952.
11. BILLOCK, J. N., The Northwestern University supracondylar suspension technique for below-elbow amputations. *Orthotics Prosthet., 26: 4*, 1972.
12. BUNNELL, S. The management of the nonfunctional hand—reconstruction vs. prosthesis. *Artif. Limbs, 4:* 16–23, 1957.
13. CARLYLE, L. Artificial arm checkout procedures. *Artif. Limbs*, 76–102, January 1954.
14. CHILDRESS, D. S., *et al.* Myoelectric immediate postsurgical procedure: a concept for fitting the upper-extremity amputee. *Artif. Limbs, 13:* 55–60, 1969.
15. COMMITTEE ON PROSTHETICS RESEARCH AND DEVELOPMENT. *Externally Powered Prosthetic Elbows—A Clinical Evaluation. Report E-4.* National Academy of Sciences, Washington, D.C., 1970.
16. COMMITTEE ON PROSTHETICS RESEARCH AND DEVELOPMENT. *The Application of External Power in Prosthetics and Orthotics, Publication 874.* National Academy of Sciences, Washington, D.C., 1961.
17. COMMITTEE ON PROSTHETICS RESEARCH AND DEVELOPMENT. *The Control of External Power in Upper Extremity Rehabilitation, Publication 1352. National Academy of Sciences, Washington, D.C., 1966.*
18. DANKMEYER, C. H., Sr., DANKMEYER, C. H., Jr., AND MASSEY, M. P. An externally powered modular system for upper-limb prostheses. *Orthotics Prosthet., 26:* 36–40, 1972.
19. DEPARTMENT OF VETERANS AFFAIRS OF AUSTRALIA. Child amputee prosthetic device. *J. Repatriation Artif. Limb Appl. Ser., 6:* 1977.
20. DORRANCE, D. W. U.S. Patent No. 1,042,413, issued October 29, 1912.
21. EPPS, C. H., AND HILE, J. H. Experience with the Münster-type below-elbow prosthesis, a preliminary report. *Artif. Limbs, 12:* 20–24, 1968.
22. FLETCHER, M. J. New developments in hands and hooks. In *Human Limbs and Their Substitutes*, edited by Klopsteg, P. E., and Wilson, P. D. Chapt. 8. McGraw Hill, 1954; reprinted by Hafner Press, 1969.
23. FRANTZ, C. H., An evolution in the care of the child amputee. *Artif. Limbs, 10:* 1–4, 1966.
24. FRIEDMANN, LIESL, Special equipment and aids for the young bilateral amputee. *Artif. Limbs, 9:* 26–33, 1965.
25. HEDSTRÖM, L., AND LYMARK, H. The SVEN-hand prosthesis. *Orthopädie Technik*, pp. 74–76, 1978.
26. HOSMER-DORRANCE CORP. *Catalog*, 9th ed., Rev., 1979.
27. KADEFORS, R., *et al.* Stryning Av Armprotes Med Myosignaler. *Electronik, 3:* 42–49, 1967.
28. KAY, H. W., KAJGANIĆ AND IVANCERVIĆ, N. Medical evaluation of the Belgrade electronic hand, advances in external control of human extremities. In *Proceedings of the Third International Symposium on External Control of Human Extremities*, Yugoslav Committee for Electronics and Automation, Belgrade, 1970.
29. KESSLER, H. H., AND KIESSLING, E. A. Pneumatic arm prosthesis. *Am. J. Nurs., 65:* 6, 1965.
30. KLOPSTEG, PAUL E., AND WILSON, P. D. The techniques of cineplasty. In *Human Limbs and Their Substitutes*, Chapt. 3, McGraw-Hill, 1954; Reprinted by Hafner Press, 1969.
31. KOBRINSKI, A. E., BOLKHOVITIN, S. V., VOSKOBOINIKOVA, L. M., IOFFE, D. M., POLYAN, E. P., PAPOV, B. P., SLAVUTSKI, Y. L., SYSIN, A. Y., AND YAKOBSON, Y. W. Problems of bioelectric control in automatic and remote control. In *Proceedings of the First Interna-*

tional Congress of the International Federation of Automatic Control, Vol. 2, p. 619. Moscow, 1960, Butterworth, London, 1961.
32. LeBlanc, M. A., Clinical evaluation of externally powered prosthetic elbows. *Artif. Limbs, 15:* 70–77, 1971.
33. Leonard, F., and Milton, C. L., Jr. Cosmetic gloves. In *Human limbs and their substitutes*, edited by Klopsteg, P. E., and Wilson, P. D. Chapt. 9, McGraw-Hill, 1954; reprinted by Hafner Press, 1969.
34. McLaurin, C. A., Fabrication procedures for the open-shoulder above-elbow socket. *Artif. Limbs, 13:* 46–54, 1969.
35. Miedzyblocki, W., and Suwalski, E. An evaluation of above-elbow prosthesis from the point of view of its mechanical performance. In *Rehabilitation of Unilateral Amputees*, edited by J. Tomaszewska. Polish Medical Publishers, Warsaw, 1976.
36. Marquardt, E. Heidelberg pneumatic arm prosthesis. *J. Bone Jt. Surg.*, *47B* 425–434, 1965.
37. Motis, G. M., *Contractors Final Report on Artificial Arm and Leg Research and Development Covering the Period January 2, 1945 to December 31, 1950.* Committee on Artificial Limbs, National Research Council, National Academy of Sciences, 1951.
38. Otto Bock Orthopedic Industry, Inc., U.S.A., 610 Indiana Ave. North, Minneapolis, Minn. 55422.
39. Pentland, J. A., and Wasileff, A. An above-elbow suction socket. *Orthotics Prosthet., 27:* 36–40, 1973.
40. Pursley, R. J. Harness patterns for upper-extremity prostheses. In *Orthopaedic Appliances Atlas*, Vol. 2, Chapt. 4. J. W. Edwards, Ann Arbor, 1960.
41. Rakic, M., Practical design of a hand prosthesis with sensory elements, *Proceedings of the International Symposium of the Application of Automatic Control in Prosthetics Design*, 103–119. Belgrade, Yugoslavia, August 27–31, 1962.
42. Reiter, R., Eine neue Electrokunsthand. *Grenzgeb. Med., 4:* 133, 1948.
43. Scott, R. N., Myoelectric control of prostheses and orthoses. *Bull. Prosthet. Res.*, BDR 10–7 93–114, 1967.
44. Scott, R. N., Myo-electric control. *Science*, pp. 2–7, 1966.
45. Schlesinger, G., Der mechanische Aufbau der kunstlichen Glieder. In Ersatzglieder und Arbeitshilfen, edited by M. Borchardt, *et al.* J. Springer, Berlin, 1919.
46. Schmeisser, G., Seamone, W. and Hoshall, C. H. Early clinical experience with the Johns Hopkins externally powered modular system for upper-limb prostheses. *Orthotics Prosthet. 26:* 41–52, 1972.
47. Schmidl, Hannes, The I.N.A.I.L. experience fitting upper-limb dysmelia patients with myoelectric control. *Bull. Prosthet Res. Spring:* 10–27, 17–42, 1977.
48. Simpson, D. C. An experimental design for a powered prosthesis for children. Health, Scottish Home and Health Department Bulletin, *22:* 75–78, 1964.
49. Sullivan, R. A., and Celikyol F. Post-hospital follow-up of three bilateral upper-limb amputees. *Orthotics Prosthet., 28:* 33–40, 1974.
50. Taylor, C. L. The biomechanics of the normal and of the amputated upper extremity, In *Human Limbs and Their Substitutes*, edited by Klopsteg, P. E. and Wilson, P. D. McGraw-Hill, 1954, reprinted by Hafner Press, 1969.
51. Taylor, C. L. Control design and prosthetic adaptations to biceps and pectoral cineplasty. In *Human Limbs and Their Substitutes*, edited by Klopsteg, P. E. and Wilson, P. D. Chapt. 12. McGraw-Hill, 1954; reprinted by Hafner Press, 1969.
52. Taylor, C. L. The biomechanics of control of upper-extremity prostheses. *Artif. Limbs., 2:* 4–25, 1955.
53. Tomaszewska, J., Rehabilitation problems of unilateral above-elbow amputees. In *Rehabilitation of Unilateral Above-Elbow Amputees*, edited by J. Tomaszewska, Polish Medical Publishers, Warsaw, 1976.

54. Tomović, R., and Boni, G. An Adaptive Artificial Hand, IRE Transactions on Automatic Control, pp. 3–10, April 1962.
55. University of California at Los Angeles, Artificial Limbs Project. *Manual of Upper Extremity Prosthetics,* R. D. Aylesworth, University of California Press, 1952.
56. University of California at Los Angeles, Artificial Limbs Research Project, *Manual of Upper Extremity Prosthetics,* 2nd ed., W. R. Santschi, (ed.), University of California Press, 1958.
57. University of California at Los Angeles, Child Amputee Prosthetics Project. *The Limb-deficient Child,* edited by B. Blakeslee. University of California Press, 1963.
58. United States Manufacturing Co., 180 North San Gabriel Blvd., Pasadena, Calif. 91107.
59. Wilson, A. B., Jr., and Purseley R. J. Fitting the wrist disarticulation case. *Orthop. Prosthet. Appl. J., September:* 17, 1952.
60. Wilson, A. B., Jr., *Limb Prosthetics,* 5th ed., Robert E. Krieger, Huntington, N.Y., 1976.
61. Wirta, R. W., Taylor, D. R., and Finley, F. R., Engineering principles in the control of external power by myoelectric signals. *Arch. Phys. Med., 49:* 294–296, 1968.

6

Rehabilitation Team

JOHN B. REDFORD, M.D.

The health care team—this expression is heard with ever increasing frequency in the corridors of hospitals and in the press. Seldom do those who speak or write this expression indicate the connotation intended. For example, much is said about the professional teamwork in rehabilitation settings such as in delivery of prosthetic services but the implications of this term is not always clearly defined. The purpose of this chapter is to define the amputee rehabilitation team and consider some of its functions.

The Webster dictionary defines team as "A group of people working or playing together, especially as one side in a contest" (4). Perhaps for the sportsminded, another definition of team is "A number of persons selected to contend on one side of a match (as in cricket, football and rowing or a debate)" (3). This comes closer to the usual association of the general public with the word, team.

Used in the general sense, the word "team" implies that there must be a captain or leader. Obviously no health care team without an acknowledged leader can function effectively. In any so-called team, one individual assumes responsibility for final decisions. Present day practices recognize that as the physician is legally responsible for the patient's well-being; he is the leader of the medical rehabilitation team and, in amputee care, the patient must ultimately rely on the physician's expertise. Although the final decision is made by the physician for the team, the basis for this decision does not mean physician "domination" nor does it mean a dictator, as the physician must heed opinions and respect the expertise of other members of the team. Without this, the patient becomes confused, delays in treatment occur and, ultimately, the patient suffers from inadequate treatment.

Although the physician has legal responsibility for team action, the moral responsibility of carrying out treatment with fullest dedication in each case lies with each team member. In a well run team, all personnel have their respective roles; failure of any individual to play his part results in poor treatment, often a weakness in service provision by rehabilitation teams. Furthermore, the patient's role must not be overlooked as he or she is the only reason for the team's existence. Unless he/she is mentally incompetent, the patient has the final say in any team decision and in whether or not any of the expert advice is taken.

In amputee care, effective communication and teamwork are best established through a prosthetic clinic. This should meet regularly to ensure an effective working relationship between team members. If the members of the team see and report the patient's problems serially, without regard to others, interprofessional and interdepartmental conflicts are sure to arise. Therefore, a time should be set aside for all to meet together and discuss each case in a clinical setting. As in team sports, when the amputee team assembles, each participant must not only know the rules of the game and the capabilities of the other players, but especially know the score.

Historical Perspective

The team concept of amputee management was developed as a result of military experiences in World War II. The Surgeon-General of the United States Army established a number of amputee centers in Army hospitals to upgrade management of these patients. Before the war, a small number of institutions such as industrial clinics were using the prosthetic team approach but, in general, a surgeon referred a patient to a prosthetist. Only occasionally did the prosthetist have communication with the surgeon prior to definitive limb fitting. Few physical and occupational therapists were really involved in training patients with prosthetic limbs. Patients were left to learn on their own, consulting the prosthetist when problems developed. As a result, amputee care had changed little since the preceding century. Now, 40 years later, the situation is entirely different. Not only have the quality and the functions of artificial limbs been completely revolutionized but systems of delivery and training amputees have improved immeasurably. Nearly all the amputees in the Veterans Administration (VA) hospital system and the majority of the civilian amputees in the United States receive services through a coordinated team approach. Rehabilitation teams for amputees which were pioneered in the United States by VA medical services have expanded to include hundreds of amputee teams throughout this country and the world (1).

It generally has been accepted that a multidisciplinary team functioning in a coordinated effort is the only way to identify and resolve the complex problems of the amputee—especially those of the very young and the very old.

Amputee Team

The minimal number of persons on an amputee team consists of the physician, prosthetist and therapist. In the early stages of developing amputee clinics, these were the only disciplines on the amputee clinic team.

Nowadays, however, a wide variety of persons with related disciplines may enter or leave the team setting as their services are needed. Amputee team clinics also may have a different emphasis depending on whether they are dealing with child amputees, geriatric amputees or adults whose injuries are work-related.

There are usually two settings in which an amputee team functions. One is during the acute phase prior to, and immediately after, surgery. The other is at a later phase, usually when the amputee is an outpatient or housed in a rehabilitation facility.

ACUTE PHASE

During the acute phase the amputee team involves primarily the surgeon, nursing staff and therapists—rarely the prosthetist unless he/she is employed by the hospital or working in a very close relationship with the surgeon. Ideally, prior to the amputation, members of the rehabilitation department will advise the patient about preoperative exercises and the stages of rehabilitation which will follow the operation.

The nursing staff is with the patient 24 hours a day and they obviously have a significant role in supporting a patient emotionally through the ordeal of amputation. Preoperatively, the nurse may be involved in patient care while the underlying pathology is being evaluated and treated. At this stage, a perceptive nurse may be helpful in gathering information about the patient's desire for prosthetic fitting and encouraging a positive attitude toward rehabilitation. Postoperatively, the nurse takes care of the dressing changes and early stump exercises and patient mobilization. She instructs the patient regarding stump hygiene, skin inspection and, when indicated, stump wrapping. The nurse, usually the patient's advocate in the hospital setting, is in the best position to provide continuous psychological support through this early phase. In settings where immediate postoperative prosthetic fittings are performed, the nurse should be thoroughly familiar with the stages of cast changes, application of the walking pylon or temporary prosthesis, and exercises. She may be the main team coordinator during this phase of care and may continue in this role in an outpatient clinic setting.

The surgeon makes the decisions about the general medical status of the patient, wound care and advice to the patient's family. Depending on the particular situation, the surgeon may continue to direct patient care throughout the entire rehabilitation process. However, if he does not have the time or knowledge to fully participate in prosthetic management, he should consult with another physician who specializes in amputee rehabilitation. Generally, this is a physiatrist or an orthopaedic surgeon. Decisions regarding the care of the patient and follow-up of the amputee in the amputee clinic during the rehabilitation phase then become the responsibility of the rehabilitation consultant.

The physical therapist, in an acute setting, should help prepare the patient psychologically and physically for the amputation, using exercises and other modalities preoperatively. Postoperatively, the physical therapist assumes daily patient contact and responsibility for the patient's exercises, standing and protective weight bearing. In the immediate postoperative prosthetic fitting case, she/he should pay precise attention to details and phases of management. Catastrophic complications with this procedure have occurred when the surgeons, nurses, physical therapists and prosthetists do not work as a well coordinated team. In fact, unless a well established coordinated working team participates in patient care with immediate postoperative prosthetic fitting, the procedure has not been practical or particularly helpful (1).

The occupational therapist in an acute hospital setting will play a similar role to the physical therapist for patients with upper limb amputations. However, in many settings where there may not be occupational therapy program, the physical therapist may have to assist in a similar manner for both upper and lower limb amputees.

REHABILITATION PHASE

The acute phase of amputee care generally can be considered complete when the wound is healed sufficiently for suture removal and no other postoperative medical complications persist. At this point, the patient is generally discharged from the hospital or transferred to another facility specializing in rehabilitation. Ideally, this early phase should be followed by a preparatory prosthesis with supervision in training and care by the amputee team. In other words, there should be no gaps in time between suture removal and prosthetic fitting. The patient should walk out of the hospital with the temporary prosthesis or leave wearing a temporary upper limb. In reality, for medical, financial and social reasons, there is usually a time lapse before the amputee actually receives the prosthesis or even has an assessment for the possibility of using one.

Under ideal conditions, the amputee team involved in rehabilitation should work with the patient prior to discharge from the hospital. However, this is only possible where organized rehabilitation services are closely associated with acute care. Many patients who have amputations in an acute-care hospital will require a complete follow-up at a different facility. If, ultimately, training with a prosthesis is a feasible goal, at the very least, amputees should have a well established exercise and wrapping program for the amputation stump prior to leaving the acute hospital.

AMPUTEE CLINIC

Amputee clinic teams have been founded on the premise that the most effective delivery in prosthetic services require a specialized team familiar with prosthetics and amputations who meet together regularly to review cases. An amputee clinic (or prosthetic clinic—the two terms are interchangeable) can operate in a number of ways and in many different settings. The team involved may be very extensive or rather small. For convenience, clinics usually are located in a physical therapy department.

Scientific study into the effectiveness of the prosthetic clinic team as compared to an unorganized approach to amputee care has not been done. In fact, there are only a few good solid studies on the effectivenss of team care in chronic illness (5). There is certainly a universal agreement by the regular readers of the *Amputee Clinic Newsletter* that amputee clinics in the United States and Canadian institutions serve a very important function. We personally are acquainted with one center where the number of amputees successfully rehabilitated was very limited prior to the development of an amputee clinic. After its development, the number of patients successfully fitted with prostheses reached 80–90%.

The amputee clinic team approach has definite advantages.

1. The various disciplines represented offer the best means of arriving at a good prosthetic prescription or, in some cases, based on knowledge of physical and pyschosocial factors, no prescription at all.
2. The patient is assured of proper fitting, training and follow-up. Thus, he is unlikely to become disgusted and develop the "limb-stored-in-the-closet" syndrome.
3. Financial, social and psychological problems can be discussed and managed. Experience suggests that lack of success in prosthetic fitting is more often due to psychological, social or vocational factors than unsuitable stumps or prostheses.
4. Clinics usually are conducted in educational institutions, thus leading to exchange of new ideas concerning medical care, prosthetic prescription and training. Critical analysis of prosthetic problems in relation to alignment, gait, suspension, etc. are lost unless students can benefit by the interchange between the prosthetist, physical therapist and nurse.
5. Clinical research in fitting and trial of new prosthetic devices is almost impossible without an organized clinic team approach. Clinical experiences reported through the journal of the interdisciplinary child amputee clinics are excellent examples of joint cooperations in research by various clinics throughout North America. Progress in child amputee care might have been nearly non existent without the availability of these clinics.

Establishing an Amputee Clinic

In developing an amputee clinic, some of the considerations in organization are as follows:

1. There should be a simple method for referral and criterion for admission. Really, the only criterion needed should be that the patient has a limb amputation.

2. Comprehensive medical care should be easily available, for example, cardiology opinion or pulmonary function testing should be easily accessible.
3. The service should be open to all from the community even though the clinic may be located at a particular institution. Lack of this has been a real drawback of the excellent clinics at the VA Medical Centers.
4. The team should have full representation of various disciplines including social and vocational services. All should attend regularly when their cases are discussed and participate in the disscussions concerning treatment.
5. A secretary or other person must be available for scheduling patients, maintaining records and billing third-party payers when necessary. In large clinics, an additional staff person such as an amputee clinic coordinator may be required. Not only should such a person have responsibility to oversee communication between members of the amputee clinic team, outside limb companies and third-party payers, but this person also can provide a vital link between the patient and the many parties involved in his/her care (6).
6. A complete medical record should be kept so that progress can be checked and accurately assessed. Use of preprinted prescription and check-out forms such as those used in prosthetic training courses can be very helpful in this regard.
7. Clinics should establish a regular time and place to hold meetings and they should start on time whether there are 2 or 20 patients to be seen. Actually, the number of amputees at each clinic will be set by the clinic chief depending on the scope of the particular program. There is disagreement as to whether all patients should come at the same time and wait or whether they should be given separate times. The former system, although regarded by some as wasteful of the patient's time, has the advantage of creating a small-group discussion opportunity for those who are waiting and are perhaps, unfamiliar with the various options.
8. Amputees complain of the impersonal character of clinic and that the first visit can be emotionally traumatic. A perceptive amputee has made the following suggestions:
    a. Always have some reading matter. There is always a period of waiting—and the longer the wait, the easier for psychic withdrawal.
    b. Assign someone to the first-time patient, prior to the patient entering the clinic, to explain the physical layout and describe functions of those with whom he will be involved.
    c. When the patient comes into the room for observation by the team, introduce him to the staff so he knows who the clericals

are, who are his therapists, and who the possible substitutes may be (2).

PHYSICIAN

The amputee clinic chief should be a physician with special interest and expertise in amputees and their prostheses. He or she is usually either a general surgeon, an orthopaedic surgeon or a physiatrist. The clinic chief makes a complete diagnosis of the patient's medical problems by a review of the chart, physical examination and help from medical consultants when necessary. He/she also prescribes various services needed to meet the goals including prescription of drugs, X-rays, laboratory studies and other services. The physician in charge also sets limits and outlines precautions so that all persons will work toward the same goal. The clinic chief must be responsive to suggestions of others and make changes accordingly. If the prescription and treatment are not conducted satisfactorily, he/she is ultimately legally responsible for the action of the clinic.

Controversy has existed over which particular medical specialist should be in charge of the amputee clinic. The key to successful clinic operation appears to be not which brand of specialist is used but whether his or her training in all aspects of amputee care is adequate and, perhaps more importantly, whether he or she has the attitude and interest to work in a rehabilitation team environment.

PHYSICAL THERAPIST

The physical therapist evaluates the patient's strength and range of motion and general functional ability, reporting findings both in progress notes and at the team meeting. On the basis of findings and guidance from the clinic chief, the therapist plans and executes a program designed to improve patient's strength and functional ability.

Any physical therapy program for the lower extremity amputee will include establishing independence in use of crutches and/or wheelchairs and training the lower limb amputee in the use of the prosthesis. The physical therapist will be responsible for bandaging or otherwise treating the stump to reduce edema and if necessary applying various physical modalities to speed healing or to control stump pain. After completion of training with the prosthesis, the physical therapist may be responsible for the final "check-out". In some cases, the therapist may be responsible for dressing changes or even cast changes if this is an immediate postoperative fitting program where therapists are specially assigned duties of this type.

To function optimally in a clinic, the physical therapist must keep abreast of the latest prosthetic developments and training procedures. It follows that he/she must maintain a continuing interest in the prosthetics literature, attend courses to learn new material and work closely with the prosthetist(s) members of the clinic. As the therapist is in almost daily contact with the patient during preprosthetic and prosthetic training, he/she gets to know the patient perhaps better than any other member of the team. As patients often confide their family and economic problems to the therapist, he/she learns of patient's motivations and psychological hang-ups and may have to undertake the role of psychologist or social worker, particularly if none is associated with the amputee clinic. Therefore, therapists often have more to contribute to the amputee rehabilitation team than simply supervising exercises and teaching the use of prostheses (7).

OCCUPATIONAL THERAPIST

The occupational therapist, like the physical therapist, will evaluate the patient's strength, range of motion and functional abilities, particularly in view of activites of daily living. She/he also plans and develops a program to teach the patient independence in daily living without the artificial limb. The occupational therapist trains the upper extremity amputee in the use of the prosthesis and, depending on the circumstances, may be involved in improving the strength and ability to don and doff the prosthesis in the lower extremity amputee. Once the prosthesis is accepted and the patient trained, the occupational therapist may be responsible along with the prosthetist for the final check-out. All comments made concerning a more general role for the physical therapist apply equally well to that of the occupational therapist.

PROSTHETIST

The prosthetist advises on the prothesis and its component parts based on the individual needs of the patient. It is his responsibility to build the prosthesis and keep the clinic informed of any construction or other problems that occur. Obviously the prosthetist is a key person in the operation of a prosthetic clinic and must work in close collaboration with the clinic chief to prevent any misunderstanding by the patient concerning his expectations for the device. For the most part, prosthetists today are highly skilled persons with a rapidly broadening educational base as defined by the American Board of Certification for Prosthetists. Today when prosthetics include such factors as hydraulics and pneumatics, endoskeletal or exoskeletal prostheses and external power, it is vital that prosthetists be regularly consulted by the clinic chief in the best interests of the patient and the team. Thus, the prosthetist should share the responsibility for prescription writing; he should be able to design innovative prosthetic systems for difficult and ususual cases. Ron Snell (12), a well known prosthetist, has commented, "Unless a clinic is willing to create a situation where their prosthetists are required to think and participate, their team will have to settle for mediocrity in prosthetic service."

SOCIAL WORKER

The social worker associated with the amputee clinic interviews the patient's family members and others in the patient's social environment to help assess the patient's psychosocial functioning since the onset of disability. The social worker may make recommendations about family problems and other problems such as housing, finances, social isolation and psychological disturbances in the patient. The psychosocial information she/he brings to the clinic may be vital in influencing the overall rehabilitation program and goals. She/he also may be involved with third-party payers and other forms of finance for the patient's care. Educational and vocational counseling for the amputee also may be assigned to the social worker if no rehabilitation counselor is available.

REHABILITATION COUNSELOR

The function of the rehabilitation counselor is to evaluate employment status of the patient prior to his amputation and assess his present vocational potential and interests including, if necessary, recommending further aptitude testing, training and placement. He or she may advise the team that further psychological testing is necessary for proper vocational placement.

In many clinics, a rehabilitation counselor is assigned to the clinic through the State Department of Rehabilitation Services. This is an excellent arrangement as it helps ensure early re-employment or training of the amputee who may otherwise be lost to vocational follow-up were there no clinic team visits.

NURSE

In a clinic setting where hospitalized patients attend, the nurse may continue to have an important role beyond the acute phase advising the various team members of the day-to-day functioning of the patient. Along with the physical and occupational therapist, she/he can help to carry out the activities of daily living in the hospital setting and determine how well the patient can learn to use the prosthesis. Thus, the nurse may have a particularly helpful role in dealing with elderly or multiply handicapped amputees who are often found on rehabilitation wards. From the time of admission, the nurse works with the clinic team in developing a comprehensive discharge plan. She may be responsible for informing the team where further assistance from a visiting nurse or physical therapist may be obtained after discharge or whether there may be problems in the home.

It also has been proposed that a nurse may serve as a casefinder; suggesting patient referrals to the amputee clinic team for evaluation and follow-up. Furthermore, if a patient known to the team is admitted for problems other than the amputation, the nurse should be quick to inform other nursing staff involved about the specifics of this patient's amputation status and methods necessary to prevent regression during this hospitalization (13).

PATIENT

The most important member of the amputee clinic team is the patient. He or she must evaluate the recommendations of the rest of the team in terms of his or her own life-style and personal goal and decide whether or not to play an active role in his or her rehabilitation. The patient should accept the advice of the clinic chief and must work to achieve the goals that have been recommended by the team. Only he or she can make a success out of the whole approach outlined as follows.

Amputee Clinic Operation

For new patients, in the usual amputee clinic operation, the chief of the clinic reviews the medical record, examines the patient and his/her stump and orders further investigation, if needed. The chief usually will order treatment by the therapist and a further medical consultation if there are unresolved medical problems. The amputee then has further assessment and treatment by the physical therapist, prosthetist or other members of the team.

Usually at this initial assessment other team members schedule individual visits with the patient. A return appointment is then made for a more complete conference to be held with the team members at a succeeding clinic. Rehabilitation goals are set out at this time. At the end of the conference, the physician writes a treatment prescription acting on advice from all members of the team and advises the patient about the program. Plans are made to resolve any nonprosthetic problems and provide maintenance therapy to keep the patient in good condition while his prosthesis is being made. When the artificial limb is ready, the patient returns to the clinic for a limb check-out and a prescription of a training program.

A different style of operation than the above method is to have the preliminary evaluation by all team members on an individual basis prior to the first visit to the clinic. This can be arranged, for example, during the morning of the clinic day, then the patient is seen by the whole team and discussed in the afternoon clinic. This method saves time and is particularly helpful if patients must travel long distances. However, this method may rush the patient somewhat and not permit him the relaxed atmosphere and familiar settings available in a system where his physical therapist and occupational therapist and others see him for longer periods prior to his return clinical appointment for full team assessment.

Not all patients, particularly those who wear old prostheses, need undergo such elaborate assessment. However, we feel that a perfunctory clinic operation where the clinic chief examines the stump accompanied by the physical therapist and the prosthetist and then prescribes the whole program from start to finish is not a good procedure. The setting is uncomfortable for the patient and no opportunity occurs to derive relevant information at a personal level or make other clinic members feel a part of the team approach. This type of evaluation, therefore, has to be gross and possibly incomplete. It also lacks opportunity to demonstrate teaching points to students and visitors.

After the limb has had a preliminary check-out, the patient undertakes a period of training. This is usually as an outpatient but may have to be as an inpatient if he lives far from a rehabilitation facility. As mentioned earlier, the physical therapist trains a lower limb amputee and the occupational therapist trains the upper limb amputee. Length of time for training will vary depending on the type of amputation and the individual. During this training period, the social worker or rehabilitation counselor may maintain contact with the patient to assist with any problems arising in their areas of interest.

When the therapist believes the patient has obtained optimal benefit from training, a recheck is scheduled at the clinic. Patient is then asked to demonstrate his skill at handling and using the prosthesis and further check-out is made of comfort, fit and alignment. The patient will then be discharged from the clinic and then perhaps return in a month or 6 months depending on the period prescribed. He or she should be followed up on a long-term basis to be assured that the prosthesis is being used correctly. In addition, once patients leave the clinic they may continue to have contact with the social worker or rehabilitation counselor to be sure they have made a smooth transition to their new life situation or that they are able to adapt to their changing labor market.

Problems with Amputee Clinic Approach

As in any multidisciplinary medical team, the disadvantages of operating an amputee clinic are obvious and continue to receive attention and discussion in prosthetic literature. Some of the disadvantages that have been listed are the following:

1. Amputee clinics are expensive in time for the professional staff. The cost of such a large team meeting really can not be met through the patient or the insurance carrier payments.
2. Clinics are inconvenient and expensive for patients. Amputees often have to come long distances and there may be wasted periods of up to 1 or 2 hours of waiting. Furthermore, clinics only meet at certain times so delays may occur in prescriptions and check-outs.
3. The impersonal nature of the approach where the patient is introduced and displayed to a group of professionals may be intimidating and, for sensitive people, embarrassing.
4. The prosthetist may resent criticism created by a clinic system,

particularly if younger therapists are given the authority to make check-outs and strictly stick to the rules.

In answer to the first two points, the costliness and the delays in treatment, McCullough (10) has some notable comments. When in his amputee rehabilitation program some team members meet without the physician clinic chief, and others, present (the meetings are mostly for routine follow-ups and training in prosthetic problems), he found that many medical, social and vocational problems were not identified. Therefore, these problems became expensive later in terms of time and money wasted and delays in full rehabilitation. Furthermore, the value of the interchange between the physicians, therapists and prosthetists for teaching and ideas in research was lost to students and others who had formerly attended the clinic. He believes that although other systems of amputee care may seem less expensive and more convenient, multidisciplinary team approach with all participants attending is sound and has no equal in educational sphere. Efficiency of the system may be less than ideal but benefits are greater in the long run (10).

To meet the complaints that limited-number amputee teams with set times for clinic operation may inhibit early amputee rehabilitation, it has been proposed to have traveling clinic teams who would consult and assist in postoperative amputee care in different hospitals. Such a team, comprised of a physician-coordinator, a prosthetic assistant and a consulting board of physicians, was active in immediate postoperative prosthetic fitting in Boston for 3½ years, 1969 through 1972 (14). The results were moderately successful but not ideal. The real needs seemed to be for better training and cooperation of the operating surgeons toward their understanding of the total approach to postamputation care and the provision of some type of practical "going-home" prosthesis that could be supplied in each hospital where the patients had their amputations. Instead of a roving clinic team, there seems to be no good substitute for early referral in the community to one or several clinics where a full range of services are available. These clinics may create some inconvenience for patients but many of the problems can be solved with a flexible system of operation as outlined in this chapter.

It is difficult to answer the third question that lack of privacy and embarrassing personal situations created by the theatrical atmosphere of the multidisciplinary team offends some patients. Suitable precautions must be taken to avoid "depersonalization" of the amputee in this multidisciplinary environment. There is probably no better way to help in establishing a warm, friendly atmosphere than by personal introductions to the team members prior to the assembling of the group. If the clinic chief can be warned in advance by his/her staff of a particularly concerned patient, the chief should contact patient personally and discuss his/her fears frankly.

Earlier in this chapter we suggested that by meeting other patients waiting in an anteroom prior to meeting time, the new amputee's fears can be allayed. Personal contact with other amputees who have been through the clinic process can be very helpful and should be encouraged. A model program, using rehabilitated amputee visitors to counsel cancer amputee patients, has been in operation at the Mayo Clinic for several years (9). This could have wider application in other programs, particularly for geriatric amputees.

In answer to the final problem raised, the resentment by the prosthetist to the clinic system, Marschall (8), a prosthetist, recently spoke out against the traditional check-out sheet. He would like to see the check-out sheets scrapped and replaced by one consisting of only three questions: is the prosthesis/orthosis as prescribed?; is the patient comfortable?; and is the prosthesis/orthosis functional?

Marshcall (8) believes that the decision as to cosmetic apperance should be left to the patient and the decision on whether or not accepted standards and principles have been met in fitting, alignment and fabrication of the device should be entirely that of the prosthetist-orthotist. Perhaps a number of clinics where the standards have been rather rigid should consider this advice as it might make programs run more smoothly.

Conclusions

The amputee team approach has proven of great value both in assuring a high rate of success in new patients and in determining the reason for past prosthetic failures. The number of persons involved in the amputee team may vary at times but, ideally, there should be more people involved than simply the physician, therapist and prosthetist. Sarno (11) emphasizes that the psychosocial and vocational services should not be grafted onto the process of providing a prosthesis but should be an integral part of that process for optimal results. To quote his conclusion "The acceptance and efficient use of a prosthesis goes beyond the technical factors. If the patient is depressed or fearful, ashamed or discouraged, overwhelmed by circumstance or unconsciously tired of trying, the very best prosthetic prescription will be a failure. Herein lies the strength of the clinic team approach" (11).

REFERENCES

1. Burgess, E. M., and Alexander, A. G. The expanding role of the physical therapist on the amputee rehabilitation team. *Phys. Ther., 53:* 141–143, 1973.
2. Fogel, H. H. Role of patient in the amputee clinic. *Newsletter—Amputee Clin., 6:* 1, 1974.
3. Gove, P. B. (ed.) *Webster's Third New International Dictionary of the English Language.* Merriam, Sprinfield, 1971.
4. Guralnik, D. B., and Friend, J. H. (ed.) *Webster's New World Dictionary.* World Publishing Company, Cleveland, 1962.
5. Halstead, L. S. Team care in chronic illness: critical review of the literature of the past 25 years. *Arch. Phys. Med. Rehabil., 57:* 507–511, 1976.
6. Hodges, M. T. The role of the coordinator of amputation services. *Newsletter—Amputee Clin., 6:* 2, 1974.

7. Lisle, Jamie L. Role of physical therapist in the amputee clinic. *Newsletter—Amputee Clin., 6:* 1, 1974.
8. Marschall, K. To check-out or not to? *Newsletter—Prosthet. Orthot. Clin., 3:* 1, 1979.
9. May, C. H., McPhee, M. C., and Pritchard, D. J. An amputee visitor program as an adjunct to rehabilitation of the lower limb amputee. *Mayo Clin. Proc., 54:* 774–778, 1979.
10. McCullough, N. C. Thoughts on the amputee clinic team. *Newsletter—Prosthet. Orthot. Clin., 3:* 2, 1979.
11. Sarno, J. E. Amputee clinic or clinic team. *Newsletter—Prosthet. Orthot. Clin., 3:* 7, 1979.
12. Snell, R. Role of prosthetist in amputee clinic. *Newsletter—Amputee Clin., 6:* 1, 1974.
13. Thomas, E. L. The nurse on the amputee clinic team in the inpatient setting. *Newsletter—Amputee Clin., 6:* 1, 1974.
14. Warren, R., James, R. C., Banks, H. H., Barr, J. S., Bonner, C. D., and Mooney, H. V. The Boston interhospital amputation study. *Arch. Surg., 107:* 861–865, 1973.

7

Physical Therapeutic Management for Lower Extremity Amputees

G. MENSCH, M.C.P.A.
P. ELLIS, M.C.P.A.

The standard and quality of health care which is provided in today's developed societies lengthens the lives of our citizens. Consequently, a trend toward a greater number of geriatric amputees is evident (28, 33). Also, the success of vascular surgery often postpones the need for amputation and when patients eventually come to amputation they are generally more debilitated, making careful treatment planning and realistic goal setting necessary. This chapter covers all phases of physical therapeutic measures in amputation rehabilitation for lower extremity amputees.

The treatment plan, based on sound rehabilitation principles, is unique for each patient and varies considerably with the individual.

The rehabilitation process for the amputee patient begins as early as the preoperative phase where a development of good lines of communication and rapport between patient and therapist can create a sound base for future rehabilitation treatment.

Preoperative Procedures

Preferably, the therapist visits the patient prior to amputation surgery to prepare him for all postoperative treatment activities and to answer as many questions as possible that the patient and his family may have (10).

A preoperative assessment may include examination of the patient's

1. Chest condition,
2. Arm strength,
3. Remaining leg strength,
4. Sensation in the lower extremities,
5. Trunk strength,
6. Ability to transfer.

The therapist should use discretion in performing the assessment. In some cases toxicity due to gangrenous changes or the patient's psychological condition due to pain or anticipation of amputation may hinder completion of a full assessment.

Following assessment, if possible a light-weight walker is adjusted to the patient's height, labeled with the patient's name and left on the ward away from the patient, not at the bedside, because supervised walking is necessary initially. The patient is taught transfers from bed to chair. He also is instructed in active range-of-motion exercises for the uninvolved leg. Quadriceps and gluteus muscle contractions are practiced in preparation for postoperative activities. The patient's shoes are checked for comfort and support and labeled with his name and ward.

Reassurance should be given that amputation surgery is not the end result of treatment but only the beginning of a process which may enable the amputee patient to walk in a modified way. It also should be stressed that the patient and his family are an integral part of the rehabilitation team and will have an input into the decision making regarding the treatment plan. At this time strong family support is necessary for the emotional well-being of the patient.

Whenever possible the physical therapist should be present during amputation surgery (10). In this way, the therapist can observe the stump condition at the time of surgery and will have a better base for judgement during the following treatment sessions (*see* Chapt. 2).

Postoperative Activities

INITIAL TREATMENT FOLLOWING SURGERY

Prior to visiting the patient for the first time following amputation surgery, the physical therapist has to investigate the patient's condition from the chart. Information regarding sleep patterns, pain, blood pressure, temperature, mental status, amount of bleeding, medication, and pulse rate will indicate to the therapist the amputee's ability to cope with early activities. The first postoperative treatment contact is psychologically and physically most important (*see* Chapt. 2).

Following reevaluation of the patient's condition, treatment procedures include:

Deep Breathing and Coughing. This is a postoperative preventive measure to avoid static pneumonia. The increased oxygen intake also assists in overcoming the possibility of postural hypotension when the patient changes position from lying to standing.

Isometric Gluteus Muscle Contractions. Muscle contractions of the hip extensors prepare the amputee for standing in the upright position. Since hip extension controls the locking of the artificial knee in above-knee (AK) amputees, early muscle reeducation is necessary in order to provide the patient with strong hip extensor muscle control. When teaching gluteal contractions, one can get the patient to place his hands over the buttock area so that he feels his muscles contract. In this way the patient controls and feels the correct muscle action. Request repeated muscle contractions every hour on the hour during the day.

Isometric Quadriceps Contractions. In below-knee (BK) amputees the quadriceps muscle is two-thirds covered by the postoperative plaster cast. The therapist's hands should rest on the upper third of the anterior portion of the thigh, the patient then contracts the muscle against the therapist's hand, and learns the correct muscle action by placing his own hands over the area. He also can feel the muscle contracting against the cast wall. Bilateral contractions aid muscle activity on the amputated side. If phantom sensation is present, encourage the patient to use this sensation and incorporate the feelings into his exercises. The quadriceps muscle stabilizes the knee during weight bearing and functions as a knee extensor.

In cases of Gritti-Stokes amputation, one has to avoid early quadriceps contractions. Bone has to heal to bone and contractions too soon after surgery may detach the patella from the femur.

Abdominal Exercises. Modified sit-up exercises with the postoperative cast supported are used to strengthen the rectus abdominis as well as the internal and external obliques. The degree of difficulty of these exercises are graded according to the patient's ability and tolerance. This muscle group provides counterbalance to the back extensor muscle group. Together these trunk muscles will aid in controlling the patient's sitting and standing balance.

Hip Abductor and Adductor Muscle Groups. These muscles are contracted and exercised isometrically by pushing against manual resistance. The therapist uses both hands placed against the hip abductors on the lateral thigh of both legs. This bilateral muscle action assures contraction of the appropriate muscle group. By switching the hands to the medial side of the thigh, the same technique is used for the adductors. These muscles are used to control the pelvis and thus aid mediolateral stability in stance.

Exercises for Remaining Leg. Range of motion to all joints is indicated. Weight-bearing can be simulated while the patient is still in bed by stepping into a towel. The patient holds both ends of a long bath towel and steps into the sling, controlling his own stepping force. This activity exercises the complete leg which must assume a dominant role in ambulation. Emphasis should be placed on total body extension because this will encourage an upright posture when standing later on.

Early initiation of bed activities will facilitate nursing care as well as prevent venous thrombosis and development of pneumonia.

Sitting Balance. Before attempting to stand, sitting balance should be assessed. The sitting position provides a wide base which enables the patient to feel secure performing balance exercises. Good sitting balance will increase the patient's confidence about the first attempt at standing. Also, exercises for a period in sitting before standing may reduce the possibility of postural hypotension.

Standing with Walker. Check cast position and cast suspension, then support and guide the cast until the patient has stability in the standing position. If the patient shows signs of postural hypotension, return him to the sitting position and encourage deep breathing.

When standing up the first few times, the dependent position of the residual limb may cause throbbing. This is normal. Some patients describe this feeling as pulsating or pumping; it gradually diminishes with increased muscle activity and later weight bearing.

Standing Balance. Standing balance also is assessed and practiced prior to ambulation, again to improve the patient's confidence.

The therapist also can assess for the presence and severity of claudication pain during these early standing and ambulating activities.

Permitting the amputee to proceed with the walker to the bathroom is the first step toward independence in activities of daily living. The length of treatment time and frequency of treatment of all postoperative activities is geared to the patient's tolerance.

EARLY AMBULATION

Rigid Dressing. The nonremovable rigid dressing which is applied following amputation surgery is primarily used for BK amputees but rigid dressing also is possible for other levels of amputation. The rigid dressing has several advantages: to protect the stump and the surgical wound from impact and allow it to heal with support; to provide a quiet wound environment; and to prevent edema because the plaster cast walls will maintain the shape of the stump and can permit early ambulation (9, 10, 33).

For several reasons, the practice of initiating ambulation immediately following amputation surgery is not now favored. If a patient, following amputation surgery, transmits too much weight through the stump, there is the possibility of stump breakdown or splitting of the suture line (1, 9). Even if a patient is able to control the amount of weight passed through the rigid dressing, they may have problems balancing on one leg following surgery and, at intervals, may put too much body weight through the cast which would interfere with wound healing. Analgesics administered to patients following major surgery reduce the amount of pain felt to such an extent that the patient easily can misjudge the amount of weight being passed through the cast to the stump.

The first cast change is usually carried out approximately 10 days following amputation surgery. The surgeon checks the wound, observes the stump, and asks the patient to bend the knee a few times to prevent knee stiffness. The feasibility of progression to early weight bearing is assessed and some sutures may be removed at this time. The physical therapist should be present to observe the following:

1. Amount of healing at the suture line,
2. Presence of any cast pressure areas,
3. Color of the skin,
4. Temperature of the skin,
5. Patellar mobility,
6. Range of motion at the knee,
7. Presence of a popliteal pulse,
8. Stump edema.

Recognition of these conditions will permit better judgment in treatment planning and progression (10). For example, the amount of healing at the suture line will determine the amount of weight bearing.

A nonremovable cast has to be reapplied immediately because recent stumps without the protection of a cast will quickly become edematous. When a gait attachment unit is indicated, the patient then can stand on both legs, taking a few steps using partial weight bearing on the amputated side (*see* "Cast Care and Cast Changes").

Patient Transfer with Nonremovable Cast. The attachment for the gait unit is incorporated into the cast by metal prongs (*see* Fig. 7.3) (9). The bottom part of this attachment, the cast base plate, has a receptacle which enables the foot unit to be detached when the patient is in bed and which allows the unit to be securely fixed to the socket by either a wedge system or a screw attachment when the patient is ambulatory. The foot unit is attached in the proper position while the patient is still lying. The shoe is placed on the sound foot at the same time. Then the patient is assisted to the standing position.

The gait attachment unit is aligned to provide the patient with full foot support during midstance. If the foot unit is poorly attached initially, the prosthetic foot could invert or evert excessively. Either deviation causes stance and alignment errors and transmits incorrect weight-bearing pressures to the stump onto areas where it is not desirable, anatomically, for the stump to bear body weight. Stump complications could result from this. It is therefore imperative that the connection between the cast base plate and foot unit is securely set before attempting to transfer the patient out of bed.

When assisting the patient during transfers, the physical therapist has to support the weight of the prosthetic unit (Fig. 7.1). The foot attachment is heavy and if a patient attempts to hold the temporary prosthesis by raising his stump, the weight, combined with the added leverage, causes pressure over the distal end of the stump which could produce pain and pressure over the distal tibia.

The therapist carries and guides the unit while the patient changes

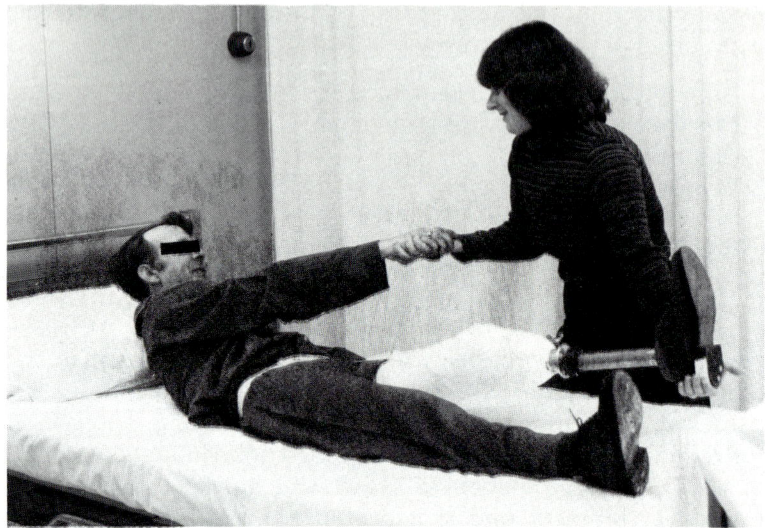

Fig. 7.1. The physical therapist supports the weight of the prosthesis to avoid pain and pressure over distal tibia of the patient.

position from lying to sitting at the side of the bed until the patient's remaining leg touches the floor and until the prosthetic foot reaches the floor (Fig. 7.2).

Walking with Walker. The first rule prior to taking steps is to check the alignment and cast suspension. Both feet should be on the ground 6–10 cm apart, in a parallel position; the body centered over the legs; a firm grip on the walker; the patient looking up.

If, in this stance position, the artificial foot deviates from a foot flat position, alignment adjustments are indicated to prevent development of gait deviations. Correct leg length also may have to be adjusted at this time. Gentle weight-transfer exercises are guided by the patient's tolerance and precede taking steps. Patients usually walk according to what they sense. Therefore, any alignment adjustment presents a proprioceptive change to them.

The nonremovable cast in the B/K amputee immobilizes knee motion. This permits the surgical wound to heal without friction by motion. Therefore, concentrate on small steps. Too long a step with a fixed knee increases weight bearing, distorts the gait cycle, and can lead to gait adaptations. Gait adaptations are usually demonstrated in the form of gait deviations. All gait deviations, if not detected and corrected early, become fixed habits and can, in some instances, lead to complications.

Weight-Bearing Control. The amount of weight bearing transmitted through the amputated side is difficult to judge. Weight bearing is guided by sensation, coordination, proprioception and by the ability of the muscles to contract. Any analgesics will diminish the patient's judgement of the amount of weight being placed through the prosthetic device, and a possible balance disturbance can accidently increase the amount of weight distribution to full weight bearing. This is undesirable at this time, as excess weight bearing may cause suture line separation.

To provide some feedback to the patient, one can use a scale or a set of double scales allowing the patient to exert from 0–25 kg of pressure on his training unit (1, 2). However, these scales are in a stationary position and many patients cannot accurately transfer the feeling of static scale compression into the gait cycle. It is, therefore, only a partial guide.

If the ability to bear weight adequately remains a problem, the limb load monitor may be used in later stages of rehabilitation (*see* "Physical Therapeutic Modalities").

In another weight-bearing test, the therapist's hands are placed between the patient's hands and the parallel bars or walker. In this way, one can judge the amount of weight being passed through the patient's hands to the gait aid.

Most patients walk by what they feel. This is particularly evident in the early stages following amputation surgery when the patient tries to adapt his locomotor control after loss of physical function. It is, therefore, essential

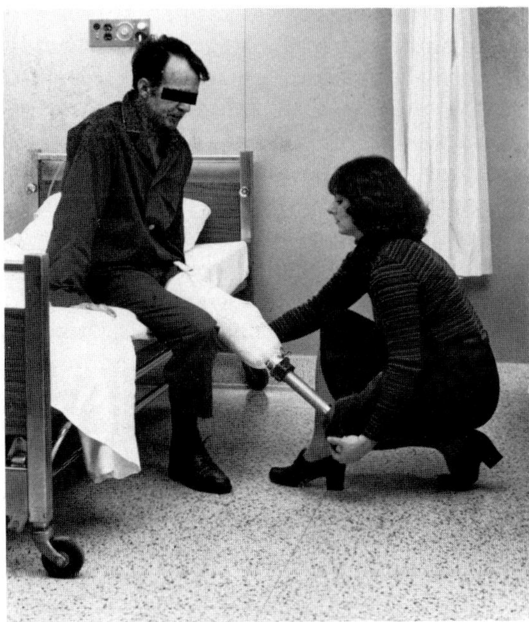

Fig. 7.2. The physical therapist supports and guides the prosthetic unit while the patient moves from a lying to a sitting position.

that therapists provide precise unit alignment. This ensures that the patient gets accurate proprioceptive feedback when trying to walk.

This first awareness of gait will help him/her to adapt and regain confidence in coordinated body motions, which will assist him/her in later stages of gait training. The longer the patient is without the proprioceptive feedback of weight bearing, the more difficult it will be to relearn the gait pattern.

Cast Care and Cast Changes

To provide expert care, physical therapists have to be equipped with:

1. Detailed knowledge of the techniques of plaster socket fabrication,
2. Understanding of the surgical procedure,
3. Reasons for various socket shapes,
4. Knowledge of the correct areas of weight distribution (9, 31).

The plaster sockets can be economically and easily constructed. They always provide a perfect fit during the postoperative treatment period when stump shapes alter.

BELOW-KNEE POSTOPERATIVE CAST POSITION

Postoperative BK plaster casts extend well above the knee to past the midthigh level in order to restrict all knee motion. This immobilization of the stump provides a total postsurgical rest for the stump and therefore aids in healing of the wound (9, 10, 33). A circular cast window directly over the patella avoids a possible pressure area over the knee if the patient tries to move or contract the muscles of the stump within the cast.

If the cast was brought only just above the knee and not extended past midthigh level, increased stump mobility within the cast would then contribute to cast slippage and possibly irritation of the wound.

Careful stump cast care at this early phase in the amputee's recovery is imperative. Emphasis should be placed on contouring the plaster cast above the condyles as this compression will reduce the possibility of cast slippage. In this way, distal cast contact can be maintained. This distal cast contact is necessary at all times to prevent stump edema, and to support the healing surgical wound (9).

Suspension straps are incorporated into the cast to prevent the plaster from either sliding down and/or from rotating. In a very few instances, contouring of the plaster above the condyles may be satisfactory for cast suspension, however, in most situations suspension straps are definitely necessary. Both cast position and cast suspension have to be checked frequently by all of the staff following surgery. A pelvic belt suspension has to be worn at all times and the suspension straps have to be connected to the belt. Casts are contoured to the anatomical landmarks of the stump and if the cast position is lost, the resulting cast malalignment can cause edema, pressure areas, blisters and discomfort. Therefore, if a cast slips or loses its position, it must *never* be pushed back on. It must be reapplied.

ABOVE-KNEE POSTOPERATIVE CAST POSITION

An AK quadrilateral postoperative cast is the most difficult one for rehabilitation personnel to control. It is held in position with suspension cables and a waist belt (9). A cast position check includes observations of the following landmarks:

1. The adductor longus tendon shall be in the anteromedial cast groove,
2. The femoral triangle (Scarpa's Triangle) has to be in place,
3. The medial cast rim has to be in contact with the pubic ramus.

Cast slippage usually occurs when the patient tries to master the bedpan. If this cast slippage is then combined with cast rotation, usually medial rotation, the cast position is lost and the immediate postoperative wound support is not maintained.

Although, postsurgically, a hip spica would be a more secure way to control AK cast alignment, it is not recommended because proper sitting posture cannot be attained with the hip spica. Since a hip spica inhibits stump motion, the AK amputee would be unable to activate a gait unit during early ambulation.

INDICATIONS FOR POSTOPERATIVE CAST CHANGES

1. For regular postoperative wound inspection,
2. When cast slippage occurs,
3. When the cast appears to have rotated,
4. When a patient reports severe tightness and pain,
5. When the patient is febrile with no systemic cause evident,
6. When the patient complains of pressure points,
7. When piston action is observed,
8. When a patient says that the cast feels too loose,
9. When a cast is visibly loose. (Not every patient can tell if the cast is loose.)

FABRICATION OF PLASTER CAST SOCKETS

Removable Below-Knee Plaster Sockets

Positioning and Testing. Weight-bearing and end-bearing considerations are vital for BK socket fabrication. The severed distal end of the tibia is not designed, by nature, to carry body weight, therefore, body weight must be distributed to other areas, for example the patellar tendon (31).

Before casting, one should examine the stump, the skin, the healing of the wound, and range of motion of the knee joint.

The patient should be placed in a supine or sitting position. Weight-bearing potential can be tested by applying thumb pressure with both hands over the patellar tendon or by placing both thumbs laterally and medially to the patellar tendon while, at the same time, pressing with the fingers against the popliteal area. While applying pressure, the patient flexes and extends his knee. The therapist should feel the muscle and skin mobility of the stump.

Increased knee flexion increases the amount of weight bearing in a kneeling position away from the end of the stump. This is one of the features of weight-bearing distribution in BK sockets. Even pressure in the popliteal area holds the patient's stump against the patellar tendon bar which is built into the socket.

BK sockets can accommodate a certain amount of built-in flexion, approximately 3–5°, in order to fully use the patellar tendon weight-bearing area on stance.

Casting.

1. The surgical wound is protected with a dressing and a Spandex stump sock.
2. The stump is wrapped in 2 or 3 layers of Webril to provide a smooth, perspiration absorbing, socket wall.
3. Cut felt pads are placed in appropriate areas to protect the patella, tibial crest and fibular head. Principle: to relieve hard areas; and to compress soft areas.
4. Using elasticized plaster, which permits a mild increase or decrease of tension, the suture line is approximated, bringing firm plaster support from posterior to anterior. This minimizes the possibility of suture line separation during weight bearing and helps to reduce the sometimes present throbbing sensation.
5. The socket is reinforced using regular plaster.
6. The socket is moulded by compressing the patellar tendon and applying slight pressure over the popliteal area. In a supracondylar removable socket, the cast border extends anteriorly above the knee but posteriorly the hamstring tendons remain free. This type of plaster socket shape allows knee motion but needs a well-functioning suspension system in order to avoid piston action and to provide stance stability, particularly for the short BK stump. The Sarmiento block can be used to assist in shaping the posterior socket rim.
7. The suspension straps are incorporated into the anterior and posterior walls of the socket.

Gait Attachment Unit. The prosthetic attachment unit is composed of two separate parts. The metal strips of the upper part are bent to conform to the cast shape and are incorporated into the socket wall with plaster. The base receptacle of the foot and pipe unit must fit exactly because this base will determine, to a large extent, the foot position and this, in turn, will reflect pressure from the ground back to the cast and hence to the stump.

The adjoining pipe and foot piece are attached to the base plate either with a push-button device similar to adjustable metal crutches or with a wedged groove which slides back and forth and fastens with a screw.

Correct leg length is roughly determined by placing the patient supine with shoulders and hips 90° to the spine in order to avoid a pelvic drop. The artificial foot can be held against the physical therapist so that the patient experiences the feeling of stance (Fig. 7.3). In this way the patient is sometimes able to tell whether the foot position is comfortable. Final alignment adjustments are carried out with the patient standing between the parallel bars.

Above-Knee Plaster Sockets

Positioning and Testing. Above-knee quadrilateral sockets can be fabricated with a casting device, or all four walls of the socket can be duplicated with the aid of wooden or metal angles if a prosthetic casting device is not available.

The patient is in a side-lying position with the amputated side up, leaning against a pillow with the remaining leg in a flexed position at hip and knee level. This permits the patient to balance and hold the stump position during casting. This position also avoids an increased lumbar lordosis so that the elderly patient fighting a hip flexion contracture can extend the stump sufficiently to the neutral position.

Hip flexion at this point has to be avoided, otherwise the cast would gape in front and does not give enough pressure in the femoral triangle area, which must fit snugly in order to allow adequate ischial seat weight bearing.

Also, abduction of the stump must be avoided. This would force the

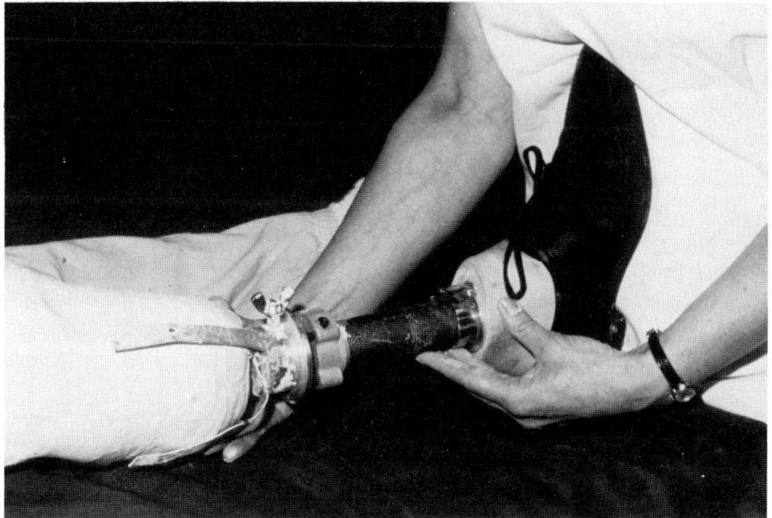

Fig. 7.3. The recent amputee can experience the feeling of stance by pressing the artificial foot against the therapist.

medial wall out of socket alignment and flesh could slip out at the adductor area, where prevention of an adductor roll is of major concern. Also, the patient loses the intimate contact of the lateral wall which is so necessary for support during stance phase.

Hip joint range of motion is tested prior to casting and the patient is made aware of the stump position he has to hold during plaster cast application.

Casting.

1. The stockinette is pulled over the stump extending it generously proximally and distally.
2. The stockinette is cut at the level of the adductor tendon to permit socket fit high into the groin.
3. Webril is used sparingly except under the ischial seat. If taped with adhesive, it will stay in place.
4. Plaster is applied in circular turns from distal to proximal with the physical therapist standing behind the patient while an assistant standing in front keeps tension on the stockinette.
5. The anterior and lateral socket walls are constructed higher than the medial and posterior walls. The function of the anterior wall is to force the tissue onto the ischial shelf. The lateral high wall aids in medial lateral stability during stance.
6. As the plaster sets, wooden or metal angles, which provide the groove for the adductor longus tendon, are pressed against the adductor area. At the same time, the other hand provides pressure under the buttock area. In this way, one is able to provide the ischial shelf which most closely duplicates the final quadrilateral socket shape.
7. When the open-ended cast is carefully removed, shape adjustments can still be made.
8. Straps are incorporated into the anterior and posterior socket walls and suspended with a pelvic belt.

Gait Attachment Unit. The temporary AK gait unit consists of:

1. Metal prongs which are incorporated into the plaster socket,
2. A single axis knee which has a manual lock to permit selective knee motion,
3. Pipe and SACH foot.

Alignment is achieved by observing the pelvic level in a supine or standing position depending on the tolerance of the patient.

The supine position has advantages for geriatric patients as they often have problems remaining stable on one leg and they are inclined to hike or drop the hip which makes it difficult to determine the correct leg length.

Windowed Rigid Dressing

This technique, as practiced by Dr. A. H. MacMillan (27), Amputation Clinic Chief at the Henderson General Hospital, Hamilton, Canada, maintains the stump in a protected environment while providing easy access for wound inspection and debridement.

Indications.

1. Delayed healing.
2. When medicated dressings are necessary and the patient is uncomfortable with a stump bandage over the dressing.
3. For restless patients who would possibly disturb the dressing.
4. Visible edema around wound areas.
5. Prevention of potential contracture.

Procedure.

1. Dressings are applied as prescribed to the affected area, and one extra layer of Curity gauze sponge is added.
2. A Spandex stump sock is applied to cover the dressing.
3. One even layer of Webril is applied over the Spandex sock. This serves to absorb perspiration and permits cutting of the cast window without cutting the stump sock.
4. One roll of elasticized plaster of Paris is applied initially. This permits tension control and wrinkle-free, smooth application. The cast is completed with ordinary plaster and incorporates cast suspension straps.
5. The area to be windowed is marked immediately on the cast.
6. The cast is allowed to dry for 24 hours. A dry cast permits a smooth cutting of the window. Tape does not stick to wet plaster.
7. Following the outline for the window, one can feel when the cutter touches the Webril. The window is cut in a fashion that permits the sock to remain intact. The window is then carefully lifted.
8. The Spandex stump sock is cut in the center and then extended towards the corners as if making a tailor's buttonhole, and the sock edges are bent after pulling slightly to prevent wrinkles over the cast rim. The sock is taped to the outside cast wall. Some Webril will bend over the sock. This will protect the patient's stump from a sharp window border. This also ensures that no plaster dust enters the area to be dressed.
9. The extra layer of gauze is removed but the dressing is left in place.
10. The window edges are taped and the fit of the window is retested.
11. Velcro closure is attached and landmarks are indicated (this is important to ensure that the window is not attached upside down following subsequent dressing changes).

After window completion, daily wound care can be attempted (Fig. 7.4). The physician may prescribe Varidase jelly, consisting of fibrinolytic enzymes which digest purulent material, or Hygeol which is a surface cleaner and a mild astringent. Cicatrin powder which is an amino acid and an

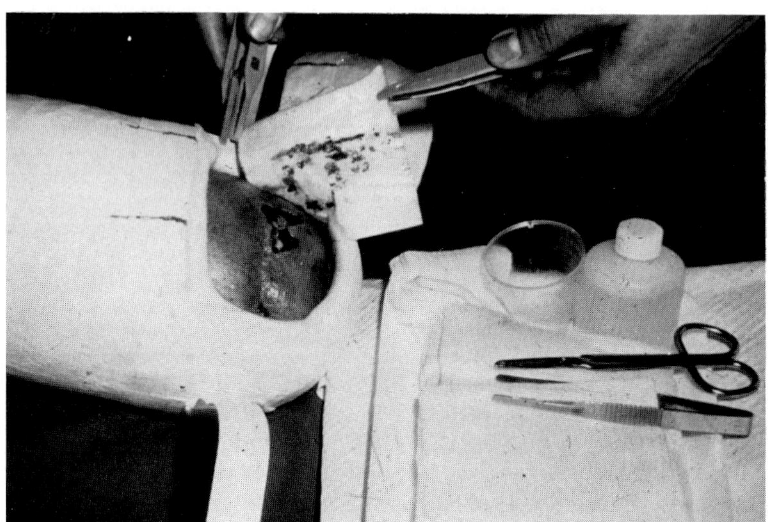

Fig. 7.4. Daily wound care through a windowed rigid dressing.

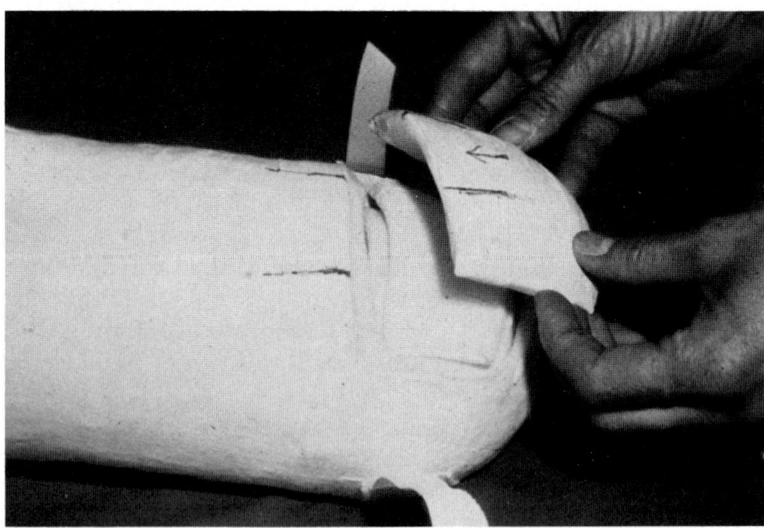

Fig. 7.5. After wound care, the window in a rigid dressing is carefully reapplied.

antibiotic mixture also may be used. Debrisan powder, a dextrose polymer which absorbs serosanguinous drainage, may be prescribed.

Physical therapeutic treatments such as ultraviolet also can be given through this windowed opening of the rigid dressing.

Note: after each dressing change or treatment, it is imperative that the window be reapplied with equal firmness in order to avoid window edema (Fig. 7.5).

Referral and Initial Contact with the Amputation Clinic Team

Recent amputee patients referred by their physicians to the amputation clinic have undergone major surgery. They are generally debilitated regardless of the reason or reasons for amputation. In addition, patients are usually experiencing one of the mourning stages (25). The stage could be typified by behavior such as anger or hostility. Thoughts of adjusting physically, emotionally and socially after amputation surgery raise many questions in their minds. The clinic assessment team must be prepared to deal with as many of the patient's concerns as possible. All health care workers in contact with these patients must be aware that these problems do exist and be able to cope with them as they may arise at any time during the rehabilitation process.

The amputation clinic core team consisting of a physician, a physical therapist, a prosthetist and a social worker is often the first contact between the patient and the rehabilitation team following amputation surgery. The core team should conduct a thorough initial assessment of the patient's specific needs, and the outcome of their findings will determine the structure of the total rehabilitation program.

Many factors, such as the patient's general health, the level or levels of amputation, the age, the types of activity which the amputee expects to perform with a prosthesis, as well as the individual's motivation and attitude towards amputation rehabilitation, determine the selection of the treatment approaches.

The results of the assessment made by the team are discussed with the patient and preferably with at least one of his family members. The treatment program, the necessity of the patient's active participation during treatment sessions, and the progression to fitting with a prosthesis are presented at this time. The decision whether or not to accept this treatment proposal must be made by the patient for without his cooperation the possibility of maintaining achieved goals is often remote. The aims of treatment are:

1. To help the patient understand and adjust to his condition,
2. To restore physical function,
3. To assist the patient in learning to live as independently as possible with an irreversable handicap.
4. To reinforce that rehabilitation is the beginning of an adapted way of locomotion not the end of physical function.

The team's ultimate reward will be in seeing a physically rehabilitated, emotionally adjusted, amputee return to the community as a respected contributing member of society.

COMMUNICATION

One major factor in establishing a good rapport is communication. To set up this communicative bond between the amputee and the rehabilitation team members, early positive contact through exchange of information is essential.

Initially the patient should receive, together with a notice of his first amputation clinic appointment, an amputation rehabilitation sheet containing basic and practical information. This can ease the recent amputee's fears of the unknown and help him to understand what the amputation clinic team plans to do. Early communication establishes a firm base for mutual exchange of information in the months to come. Any communication with patients or their relatives should avoid complicated medical terminology and state clearly the intent of the program.

Assessment

Amputation rehabilitation is both a physical and psychological challenge for the physical therapist, who holds a key position on the rehabilitation team. Communication and close liaison with other health care professionals such as physicians, prosthetists, nurses, social workers, occupational therapists and psychologists are essential (35).

The physical therapist's knowledge of anatomy, human physiology, locomotion, biomechanics and pathology help to provide a sound basis for physical treatment, but equally important is the need to understand the patient as a human being and to support him psychologically during his rehabilitation (13, 15). The attitude and manner of the physical therapist greatly influence the amputee's cooperation and emotional well-being. The patient's social and emotional adjustments are just as important as his physical performance during this complex rehabilitation program. Physical therapy sessions tend to be methodical and repetitive, therefore, precise explanations will help the amputee to understand the reasoning behind treatment. One should not forget that the patient is the most important member of the team.

The assessment procedure is detailed and includes general and specific information. All assessment observations have to be recorded for future reference, for comparison, to evaluate treatment progression, and to permit research studies to be carried out at a future date. The following headings will serve as practical guidelines for evaluating the amputee patient's physical rehabilitation potential. The outline is structured and discusses the assessment procedure under five major headings, and concludes with a treatment plan.

1. Personal data,
2. Medical history,

3. Physical therapy assessment,
4. Social history,
5. Vocational and avocational interests.

A printed assessment form will ensure a standard collection of all data.

PERSONAL DATA

The patient's name, address and telephone number, marital status, sex, age, insurance coverage, etc., will be listed. These identifying records usually comply with the institutional or medical record procedures and will vary, accordingly from center to center.

MEDICAL HISTORY

A summary of the patient's general medical condition should be provided to the amputation assessment clinic by the referring physician prior to the patient's arrival. The following pertinent information should be included:

1. A brief past medical history,
2. Date and level of the amputation,
3. The reason or reasons leading to amputation (trauma, peripheral vascular insufficiency, malignancy, congenital defects, etc.),
4. Amputation-associated diseases (diabetes mellitus, Buerger's disease, cardiopulmonary, and cardiovascular difficulties),
5. Amputation-associated symptoms,
6. The range of vital signs,
7. Any known preexisting social or behavioral problems,
8. List of present medications,
9. Any other pertinent information which could be of value to the amputation assessment team during this initial visit.

The amputation clinic physician will do a complete medical assessment at the time of the clinic visit. A medical history from the referring physician as well as a resume of patient's present status and prognosis will determine his ability to actively and successfully participate in an intensive rehabilitation program.

Energy consumption required for the performance of any physical task is, for an amputee, greater than for a healthy individual of the same sex, age and build (18, 46). For this reason, more energy is expended during all phases of training as well as for activities of daily living (ADL). Any underlying disease process will further tire the patient. Therefore, one must know the specifics of the patient's medical condition in order to judge factually the patient's rehabilitation potential (35). The clinic physician has to consider medications and the control of nutritional intake required. The physical therapist must provide a careful balance of activity and rest.

PHYSICAL THERAPY ASSESSMENT

Assessment of Residual Limb

Every amputation stump will undergo considerable change from surgery to the final prosthetic fitting. It matures and toughens with wound healing, stump shrinkage, and mobility. The duration of stump maturation will depend on several factors, therefore precise observation during the initial stump examination must be made and recorded.

Rigid Dressing in Place. Most recent BK stumps are protected by a cast. It is of major importance to check during the assessment the position and condition of the cast as well as the effectiveness of cast suspension (*see* "Rigid Dressing" under "Early Ambulation").

If a cast change is indicated, it is important to inspect the wound and immediately reapply the next cast. This will avoid the quickly developing stump edema (9) and support and protect the recent surgical wound (*see* "Cast Care and Cast Changes").

Shape. If the recent amputation stump is not covered by a rigid dressing, the stump shape should be noted. Stumps can be conical, bulbous, cylindrical or edematous. Some stump shapes lend themselves to a better prosthetic socket fit than others. The stump must, therefore, in the very early stages be bandaged to encourage proper shrinkage and shaping before stump stabilization occurs (*see* "Bandaging Techniques" under "Shrinkage and Shaping Techniques").

Scar and Skin Condition. It is important to record the condition and size of the surgical incision, any scar tissue, adhesions, the presence of sutures, or tissue flaps, the presence of other scars (previous bypass surgeries) and appearance of the skin, any open areas and their size, and areas of tenderness.

Ideally, in later stages, the skin has to be intact and toughened in order to take stress from socket friction and weight bearing during ambulation.

Circulation. The temperature, the texture and, in particular, the color of the distal end of the stump as well as palpable pulses will indicate to some degree that adequate circulation is present. Ischemic stump conditions will tend to prolong the duration of the amputee's rehabilitation.

Range of Motion. Although it is desirable that all joints are free of contractures, one usually detects mobility restrictions in geriatric patients. It is necessary to record all range limitations and any pain within joint range. Particular attention should be given to the level of free hip extension in AK amputees and knee extension in BK amputees.

Some geriatric amputees have experienced prolonged illness and inactivity prior to amputation surgery, in which case consideration must be made for preexisting joint restrictions and decreased strength.

All joint range limitations must be documented. Measurement comparisons at a later date during treatment will indicate contracture fixation or joint range improvement. Measurements can be recorded in goniometer readings by degrees or in centimeters with the tape measurement technique (*see* "Contractures").

Muscle Strength. The stump muscles must be strong in order to carry body weight and to accelerate and decelerate the prosthesis during ambulation. Muscle strength is one indicator of the amount of weight bearing that will be possible.

Individual muscle strength is recorded on a scale from 0–5 and tested manually (12). The levels are:

0: The inability to move;
1: A muscle flicker is apparent;
2: Full movement with gravity eliminated.
3: Independent full motion against gravity.
4: Strength against some resistance;
5: Strength against strong resistance.

In testing muscle strength and control in a recently amputated limb, one has to repeat the isolated motion frequently until the amputee can perform the range in a smooth fashion. Lack of stump control at this early stage is often a sign that the patient has not yet adjusted to the weight loss of his amputated leg and that proprioception is somewhat impaired. Proprioception returns more readily if the physical therapist's hands initially guide the expected movement.

Sensation. Skin sensation tests include assessment of pinprick, light touch and temperature. Intact sensory perception provides the amputee with stump awareness. The patient who can feel and distinguish stump sensation has a better chance for establishing stump proprioception, which will assist him/her during gait training.

Proprioception. Proprioception, or the awareness of the position of the limb in space, also must be assessed. The presence of proprioception will, in later stages of the ambulation, assist the patient in the placement of his prosthesis during gait training.

Stump Pain. The description of pain in the stump by the patient is often vague. The type of pain experienced must be investigated to rule out possible future complications. The nature of pain can be expressed by its character as throbbing, biting, burning, sharp, etc.

A patient presenting with a painful stump is unable to walk. He will compensate during the gait cycle with gait deviations if stump pain is present.

Phantom Pain and Sensation. Phantom pain relates to the body part which has been amputated and is most puzzling to patients (24, 30). It can be present in varying degrees. Phantom pain is real discomfort and its presence interferes with rehabilitation. For recording of this phenomenon the patient can be asked to describe the nature of the pain and to rate phantom pain on a scale of 1 to 10, with the upper margin of the scale being the most severe pain.

However, initial phantom pain, which is not experienced by all amputees, will in most cases subside and change gradually into phantom sensation.

Phantom sensation is an awareness which gives the patient the feeling of being complete, and it is expected to be present. Phantom sensation is helpful during rehabilitation as it can help the patient in the placing of the prosthesis during the gait cycle (39). During assessment, one must establish the difference between the two phantom feelings. The patient can expect phantom sensation while severe phantom pain is not the rule.

The recording of fading phantom pain will be helpful in modifying the patient's rehabilitation program. Documentation also will help to establish a comparison of this still little understood phenomenon.

Measurement. Stump measurements taken during the assessment and later during treatment at regular intervals, indicate when stump shrinkage has reached a plateau. Length measurements are taken from a fixed point.

Below-knee (BK) amputees are measured from the tibial plateau to the bone end with girth measurements at approximately 3 cm apart. If measurements are taken in any other way, for instance in congenital deformities or unusual stump shapes, the measurement landmarks then have to be recorded on the patient's chart.

In above-knee (AK) stumps, one can measure from either the greater trochanter, if palpable, or the anterosuperior iliac spine to the end of the bone. Care must be taken if measuring from the anteriosuperior iliac spine to eliminate the possibility of a hip flexion as a flexed joint shortens the actual distance. Bone length within the stump is the true length of the stump because the bone acts as a lever. Redundant tissues have no leverage value, therefore existing redundant tissue has to be compressed against the bone when the length measurements are taken.

Circumferential measurements are repeated at selected intervals along the stump. Following the initial assessment, all these measurements are recorded on a weekly basis.

Condition of Remaining Leg

The remaining leg, in geriatric patients often not a sturdy leg, has to be examined with care using the same principles as for stump examination (8). Assessment investigation must include the following observations.

Shape. Is edema present? Excessive edema has to be controlled before more strenuous activities for this leg are planned.

Skin Condition. Special attention has to be given to the skin of the remaining foot (42). Areas of skin breakdown can occur between and around toes. Toenails in geriatric patients, often overgrown and brittle, can irritate preexisting skin lesions. Abrasions or tender areas have to be protected prior to ambulation.

Circulation. The recording of pulses (femoral, popliteal and pedal) are specified as strong, weak, faint, absent, or unable to palpate. Also noted is whether the patient experiences rest pain or claudication pain with activity. The color of the skin is observed as this can indicate the viability of the circulation.

Range of Motion and Muscle Strength. The range of motion of all major joints and muscle strength have to be tested and recorded. The remaining leg must now function as the dominant leg until the patient is able to master the prosthesis. The additional strain of standing on one leg can often initially cause leg fatigue and can lead to instability in standing.

Pain and Sensation. Pain and sensation in the remaining leg are assessed in the same fashion as previously discussed under stump assessment.

Upper Extremity, Trunk and Balance

Locomotion involves total body movement. All body parts are subject to a gait acceleration and deceleration pattern during locomotion. Since body weight is only initially transmitted through the remaining leg, other body parts must assist in compensating for the loss of the limb. The trunk partially controls standing and sitting balance. Arm strength, specifically the triceps and wrist extensors, will assist during crutch walking. Strength and ability to carry this extra load have to be assessed.

Ambulation

The patient's preamputation method of ambulation and walking endurance will partially determine the postamputation level of ambulation which may be achieved. An ambulation prediction during assessment will guide realistic treatment goals.

Previous Prosthetic History

Not all patients referred are recent amputees. Assessments should therefore include a section discussing the previous amputation(s). Such information as distance of pain-free walking with the prosthesis, endurance, the prosthetic-wearing tolerance, and the number of stump socks worn within the prosthesis or training unit should be recorded. Also, the name of the prosthetist should be obtained in order to facilitate the continuity of contact while in hospital.

Motivation

The patient's attitude toward amputation rehabilitation is of utmost importance. Does the patient wish to have a prosthesis? Are the patient's goals realistic? Does the prosthesis serve only as a cosmetic appendage? Is the family advising the amputee to give it a try? Is the amputee overenthusiastic? Does he understand the level to which he will be required to participate during the rehabilitation program? Does he understand that he will walk with his prosthesis, the prosthesis will not walk for him? Recognition of the patient's emotional status and his desires, his understanding of his physical capabilities, and the support of his family all contribute to the patient's motivation (13, 15, 25).

SOCIAL HISTORY

The social history should include the availability of family support, the layout of the home (number of stairs, the situation of the bathroom, etc.), as well as the avocational interests of the patient. Availability for financing of the prosthesis and any other ambulation aids should be determined also at this time. This information will help the team formulate more realistic goals.

Worry over such things as "How will I pay for the leg?" or "Who will manage things at home while I am unable to work?" can often hinder a patient's total concentration on his physical program. Reassurance at this point can often allay these concerns.

VOCATIONAL AND AVOCATIONAL INTERESTS

Physical mobility is a basic requirement for every job performed, be it sitting, standing, walking or driving. The amputee's educational skills, his previous activity level and the extent of his loss of physical function often will be a determining influence in the type of prosthesis ordered. The nature of the job to which the amputee hopes to return also is taken into consideration.

The patient's avocational interests also are investigated. The prescription for the prosthesis may include an ankle rotator if the patient is interested in playing golf. He also may want to know about the advisability of a swimming prosthesis. If he hunts or fishes and he is an AK amputee, a safety knee or a manual lock knee may be used to provide stability on rough ground. These are some of the things which should be considered before writing the prosthetic prescription.

TREATMENT PLAN

The treatment outcome depends to a large extent on how well the individual patient's multiple problems have been diagnosed and analyzed and how well the team integrates all assessment findings into a precise treatment plan. During the patient's first amputation clinic visit, each core team member meets individually with the amputee and, following their independent assessments, they meet to discuss problems, the potential for prosthetic fitting and, finally, to formulate immediate goals. This team interaction is the basis for establishing an individual and realistic treatment program which may include necessity of cast changes, pylon fabrication, the prescription of a gait training unit, wound care, stump shrinkage and shaping, general and specific exercises, positioning such as prone lying, ambulation, ADL, the patient's attendance at amputee discussion groups and any other physical modalities which may be indicated. Medical treatment, medications and advice regarding nutrition also are included in the total treatment plan.

During rehabilitation the patient's status may change, therefore treatment progression and treatment goals have to be reassessed frequently in order to provide the best of care, with the final goal being to arrive at a practical prosthetic prescription which will enable the patient to function within his capabilities.

At this point it should be mentioned that not all amputees are prosthetic candidates (28, 39). Considering the increased energy consumption required to use a prosthesis, preexisting medical conditions such as severe respiratory or cardiac disease, neurological problems, the presence of a previous amputation (which now makes the patient a bilateral amputee) and the inability of tissues to heal adequately enough to allow weight bearing, may make prosthetic fitting an unrealistic goal.

The treatment plan in this case would focus on wheelchair independence with extensive input by the occupational therapy staff.

Previously, these patients often have been looked upon as "failures" because no amount of conditioning or prosthetic input by the team would allow them to walk. Quite the contrary is so. Many patients are able to manage at home in a wheelchair and maintain a quality of life which may not have been possible with the effort required for them to use a prosthesis(es).

"Ideal" Residual Limb

A so-called "ideal" stump, which rarely exists, consists of adequate length, sufficient strength, adequate proprioception, full joint range of motion, sufficient nerve supply, intact circulation, presence of phantom sensation, and sufficient skin sensation.

LENGTH

Enough stump length allows for adequate leverage of the stump within the socket. It also ensures a more intimate socket fit during ambulation and sitting because the stump will maintain its socket position. Very short stumps have a tendency, particularly during sitting, to partially slip out of the socket which then causes stump replacement problems when the patient stands and attempts to walk. Enough length, therefore, assures a better socket contact fit and permits the amputee better control of his prosthesis during ambulation.

STRENGTH

Sufficient muscle strength within the stump enables the patient to achieve a stable and efficient gait. Not only is the forward motion of the socket controlled, the patient is able to carry the weight of the prosthesis more efficiently.

PROPRIOCEPTION

Proprioceptive awareness can, to some extent, be assisted by muscle fixation and early ambulation. The ability to receive stimuli within stump muscles, tendons and joints varies greatly in patients and seems to decline with age. Proprioception is necessary in providing the patient with joint position sense. Directional motion awareness, another component of proprioception (11), allows the patient to know where the stump is in space, thus permitting a patient with intact proprioception to achieve a more controlled and automatic gait pattern.

RANGE OF MOTION

A full range of motion of the joint next to the level of amputation will allow normal mobility. If contractures develop, two complications will arise: restricted step length, and displacement of weight bearing, both of which result in gait deviations.

NERVE SUPPLY

If the nerve supply to all muscle fibers remains intact following amputation surgery, the patient has a better opportunity to build up muscle strength and to recognize proprioception through joint position sense.

CIRCULATION

Adequate circulation and the forming of a collateral circulation in the amputated limb is essential in maintaining a healthy stump and healthy skin. Intermittent claudication in a stump can present problems by limiting gait endurance.

PHANTOM SENSATION

Phantom sensation is an awareness of the missing part which makes the amputee feel physically complete. It is not an unusual sensation. It aids in proprioception and is useful during gait training (24). Phantom sensation will usually not subside completely, but it can telescope. If it telescopes after a long period of time following amputation surgery, then a patient may describe phantom sensation as follows, "I feel my foot, but it's not where it's supposed to be. It is higher up, underneath my knee." Explanations for these telescoping sensations are not complete at this time (30).

SKIN SENSATION

Intact skin sensation will alert the patient to any area of excess stump pressure during ambulation and will act as a warning system indicating when tissue stress should be reduced.

SUMMARY

The presence of all of these qualities will enable the stump to take the stress from friction and weight bearing and will provide the patient with a functional stump. Physical therapists must be able to understand and recognize stump conditions and stump problems during rehabilitation and deal with them effectively.

Care of Residual Limb

HYGIENE

Stump

Stump hygiene is important because only a healthy, cared-for stump can function as an activator and lever for the prosthesis. The stump has to carry body weight on anatomical areas which have not been designed by nature to do so. Care has to be meticulous to permit the stump, following surgery and in later stages, to take on these extra functions.

Basic principles of hygiene have to be followed and the amputee has to learn to care for these stump needs independently (2, 20).

1. The stump has to be washed daily with warm water and mild soap. This avoids a build-up of salt deposits on the skin.
2. Rinsing the stump well and towel drying is essential. A soap residue will leave a film over the skin, thus reducing the ability of the skin to breathe. Complete towel drying leaves the skin smooth.
3. Skin folds have to be cleansed with an applicator or cotton swabs, to eliminate bacterial growth in dark, moist, stump fold areas.
4. Abrasions, open areas, scratches, bruises, etc., have to be observed and reported for appropriate treatment.
5. The amputee has to learn to examine his own stump with a hand mirror and to be taught to report any skin condition which he may observe. Areas to watch for in BK amputees are the tibial crest, the distal end of the tibia, the area around the fibular head and the distal end of the fibula. AK amputees have to inspect the distal end of the femur, the skin condition in the groin area and the skin around the ischial seat.
6. Stump bathing is recommended in the evening. Following a bath, an increase in circulation, may cause the skin to "puff." If this happens in the morning, it may cause problems in donning the prosthesis.

Skin care has to be taught in a repetitive manner as the procedure now has to become part of the amputee's daily routine. After careful supervision, the patient will achieve independence. Close adherence to these procedures will enable the stump to take on the stress of weight and friction from the socket wall without complications.

Bandages and Stump Socks

An increase in perspiration due to the loss of skin surface and the increased effort required for activities, necessitates that socks and bandages be washed frequently.

All stump covering materials have to be washed by hand (bandages, shrinker socks, stump socks) in warm water using mild soap. They must be rinsed thoroughly to eliminate any soap residue. The items are not to be wrung because this twisting motion destroys the elastic fiber which is necessary to maintain stump support during bandaging. Excessive heat and hanging to dry have to be avoided for the same reason.

The shape of the stump sock end can be preserved to some extent by placing a ball (the diameter of which is comparable to the width of the stump sock) into the stump end during the drying period. Each amputee should be supplied with several stump socks and bandages to allow for daily change. Any stump socks or bandages which have lost their fiber elasticity will not support stump end tissue and should be discarded.

Hygiene is ultimately the amputee's responsibility but it is up to the physical therapist and the nursing staff to explain and establish these daily hygiene procedures.

SHRINKAGE AND SHAPING TECHNIQUES

Bandaging

Correct bandaging is a reliable, effective and economical method of achieving maximum shrinkage, shaping and toughening of the residual limb. It should be fully understood by nurses, physical therapists, occupational therapists and prosthetists. It is the physical therapist's responsibility to teach the amputee the exact bandaging technique and to explain the purpose and goals of the procedure. The patient should learn how to bandage for himself and should be instructed to wear the bandage at all times except when the prosthesis is worn. This is particularly important for the amputee who has lost his limb due to circulatory disorders because his stump will not stabilize as quickly as that of the patient who has lost his limb due to trauma. The bandage should be removed every 2–3 hours and the stump should be checked for excess bandage pressure. Range-of-motion exercises also can be performed at this time.

Various bandaging techniques can be used as long as they achieve the desired results. It is easier for rehabilitation staff and patients alike to practice one specific method because this is less confusing, especially for the geriatric patient. It is therefore advisable for the institution management to decide upon one specific method which is to be used by all staff members. This basic method, however, *must* be adapted to the patient's specific needs when the use of a routine bandaging procedure is not indicated.

Therapist's Position. The physical therapist, if right-handed, stands on the right hand side of the patient when applying the bandage; if left-handed, on the left side. However, when teaching the patient to bandage, the therapist should sit or stand beside the patient to demonstrate the technique in such a way as to closely approximate the patient's visual perspective. This is less confusing to the patient because he is not trying to follow the "mirror image" effect which occurs if the therapist is facing him.

Materials Used.

1. Two elastic bandages are sewn together so that tension is not lost during bandage applications. In cases of large stumps, three bandages should be sewn together. The bandage can be either 10 or 12 cm in width, depending on stump size.
2. An emollient such as Nivea Cream or Vaseline also can be used. It is applied over the stump to help lubricate the skin, except for areas which will later be weight bearing, because these areas need toughening. Open areas are not covered with the emollient. The application of the emollient prevents the bandage from slipping off, reducing the necessity of frequent rebandaging.
3. A safety pin is necessary for fastening the bandage at its completion.
4. Retelast, an elasticized net, can be applied to help maintain the bandage in position.

Below-Knee Bandaging Procedure. The aims of BK bandaging are:

1. Shrinkage and shaping of the stump,
2. Prevention of knee flexion contracture.

Distal pressure is important in order to achieve shrinkage and shaping of the stump. The tension should be firm but not tight. A bandage wrapped too tightly can cause irritation over the patella and tibial crest where skin viability is marginal.

The bandage is anchored distally over the stump and led in a figure-8 fashion toward the proximal end of the stump, and continues to proceed above the femoral condyles to include the tissues behind the knee. The coverage of the posterior section of the knee is necessary to achieve total shrinkage, for later the supracondylar strap has to hold the prosthesis suspended.

A different BK bandaging method sometimes leads the bandage above the knee, in front of the knee, to aid knee extension. In this instance, the popliteal area is kept uncovered to permit free range of motion of the knee joint (Fig. 7.6). This technique is advisable for stumps which are not too edematous initially. This bandaging technique permits more knee mobility.

A lubricant over the end of the stump, except on weight-bearing or open areas, is advised to help the bandage from slipping. However, in BK amputees, slipping of the bandage is not quite as common as in AK amputees. The reason may be that it is easier for an amputee with a BK

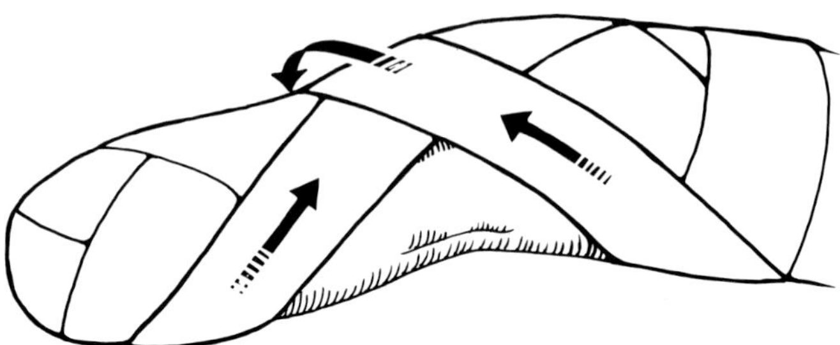

Fig. 7.6. A below-knee (BK) amputation bandaging method. To permit free range of motion of the knee joint, the popliteal area is kept uncovered.

amputation to learn to bandage while an AK patient, who has less mobility compared to the BK patient, finds it cumbersome coping with the pelvic turn which anchors the bandage. The prominence of the femoral condyles also may aid in the anchoring of the BK bandage.

Above-Knee Bandaging Procedure. The aims of AK bandaging are:

1. Shrinkage and shaping of the stump,
2. Prevention of an abduction contracture,
3. Prevention of an adductor roll.

The stump is examined; the bandage is anchored diagonally over the stump with the first bandage turn directed medially. This is of major importance for this medial turn will later determine the direction of the bandage pull, which has to be toward body midline, when the pelvic turn suspends the bandage. This also is useful in preventing an abduction contracture of the hip.

The bandage is initially anchored without applying tension and it is led in a figure-8 fashion over the distal end of the stump where most of the pressure has to be applied. Bandaging should always be firm, never tight. The patient is often the best guide to judge the amount of tension of the bandage. Distal pressure applied to the stump results in rapid and uniform shrinkage.

The bandage is continued towards the proximal end of the stump in figure-8 turns. As the bandage is applied from distal to proximal, it is essential to decrease the amount of bandage tension in order to obtain the desired stump shaping.

When the bandage is led across the front of the pelvis towards the nonamputated side, the stump is kept in a relaxed extended position (Fig. 7.7). In this way, hip flexion is not encouraged, the bandage is merely pulling the stump toward body midline and thus preventing it from abducting. The bandage is then placed over the iliac crest, around the pelvis and brought to the front again. It is then continued high into the groin in a diagonal fashion, covering the adductor region (Fig. 7.8). This helps to prevent an adductor roll.

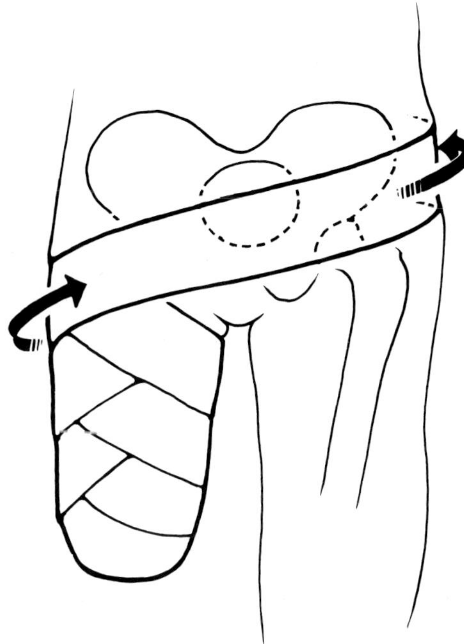

Fig. 7.7. Above-knee (AK) amputation bandaging procedure showing the wrap across the front of the pelvis.

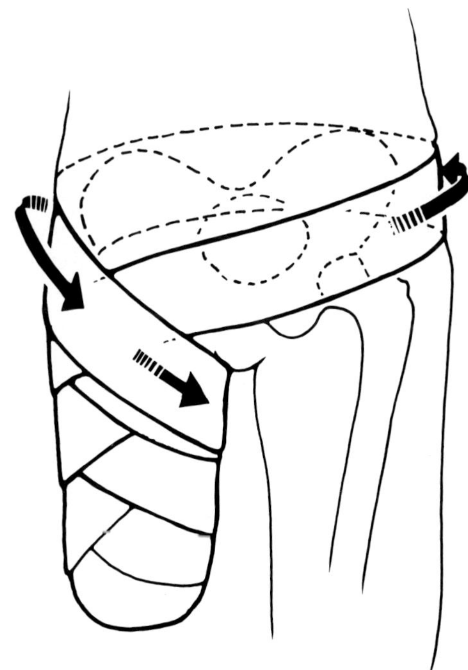

Fig. 7.8. A continuation of the above-knee (AK) amputation bandaging shown in Figure 7.7 after the bandage is brought forward again and continued, diagonally, high in the groin.

The pelvic turn is repeated before securing the bandage. This diagonal approach into the adductor area helps to prevent the bandage from rolling down and cutting into the flesh.

The bandage is completed by being securely pinned. The therapist's fingers are placed under the bandage so that the patient is not injured during application of the pin. Retelast can be used to secure the bandage.

Advantages. Each bandage turn permits precise moulding of the stump and tension control. The application of distal pressure and reduction of bandage tension towards the proximal end of the stump encourages venous return and lymphatic drainage. A firm bandage gives the patient the feeling of comfort and support. Bandaging is the most precise method of stump shrinkage and shaping because every bandage turn can be contoured to each stump size.

Disadvantages. It is at times cumbersome, particularly for geriatric patients and rehabilitation staff alike, to rebandage whenever the bandage becomes loose or tends to "pop off" during activity periods. When this happens, the distal pressure of the bandage is lost and the bandage becomes ineffective. A bandage improperly done is worse than no bandage at all.

Shrinker Socks

Shrinker socks are like stump socks but they are made of an elasticized material with a straight and diagonal stretch. They come in three sizes and are tapered from bottom to top.

Advantages. Shrinker socks are easy to pull on and they give a feeling of support to the stump. If correctly worn, they apply distal and lateral pressure to the stump and encourage venous return (19). They are more quickly applied and reapplied than a bandage and can be worn with the training unit if fluctuating stump girth is a major problem.

Disadvantages. Only the correct size can be worn. These socks have to be suspended by garters and a pelvic belt. Pelvic belts in some patients will not stay in place and often feel uncomfortable. Patients with protruding abdomens are unable to keep the belt properly in place.

If the stump shrinker sock is too long and unsuspended, the top rim often rolls into an elastic band. This elastic band will not only restrict circulation but also prevents the reduction of edema.

A shrinker sock which is too short will encourage the formation of an adductor roll in AK amputees. Stump shrinker socks are not suitable for bulbous stumps as the sock tends to form ridges in the tissue folds causing restriction of circulation.

Pressure Pump Applications

Intermittent compression therapy is often used for nonamputee patients in order to reduce lymphatic or venous edema. The swollen extremity is slightly elevated to permit gravitational edema backflow during pumping.

The pulsation of air compression and release is graded. The elevated position plus the intermittent compression assists in edema reduction.

Intermittent compression pump treatments for edematous lower extremity stumps, if the wound has completely healed and the skin shows no sign of infection, can be effectively carried out under controlled conditions (37). Such compression is not used routinely to achieve stump shrinkage and shaping because the amputee would be inactive for several hours during the day, however the pressure pump sleeve can be worn over the stump in a disconnected fashion over a long period of time. The applied pressure is then constant.

Advantages. This form of stump shrinkage method is advisable for some amputees, especially those with excessively bulbous stumps, where bandaging seems to be achieving a very slow rate of shrinkage. The stump sleeve will be pumped up to a maximum comfortable compression. A disconnection from the apparatus gives the patient freedom to move about and constant compression can be maintained over a long period of time.

Disadvantages. For a number of reasons this form of treatment is a selective one. The compression double-walled stump sleeve, which is marketed in one size only, will in the majority of cases merely apply lateral and not a distal pressure. The distal pressure is the one which aids primarily in stump shrinkage. Also, an AK amputee will have to hold the stump in an abducted and flexed position as the compression sleeve is bulky in its expanded state.

Should this patient spend time in the wheelchair, the sitting position would have to be altered with a pillow under the *sound* side, otherwise a pelvic tilt position, while sitting, is the result of the air-filled compression sleeve.

Young traumatic amputees with good standing balance often can effectively participate in ball games hopping on one leg with the sleeve attached to the stump. However, this form of treatment cannot be suggested for patients who have had circulatory disorders. Merely standing for a prolonged period of time on one leg is not possible for these amputees due to standing balance difficulties and ischemic reactions such as intermittent claudication. The remaining leg will not allow such activities. Furthermore, the posture of the AK patient's hopping, standing or walking on one leg during compression sleeve attachment is scoliotic in nature and not advantageous for future gait training posture.

Air Splints

In some centers, air splints are used for stump shrinkage and for early ambulation (41). An air splint is a double-walled, transparent, plastic, leg-shaped sleeve which surrounds the patient's stump. The double wall can be pumped up in order to give compression to the stump and to inflate the foot section. The air splint is capable of taking body weight up to approximately

25–30 lb (11–14 kg) if a compression of 30 mm Hg can be maintained. Some air splints are equipped with pressure gauge controls.

Advantages. An air splint protects the wound and permits compression and some end bearing. Moderate weight bearing is possible. The feedback from the ground contact through the air splint helps the amputee balance to some extent, thus avoiding holding the stump constantly in flexion to maintain balance. The suspension is controlled by the compression of the wall against the stump, therefore the longer the stump the better the suspension is maintained.

Disadvantages. One of the disadvantages of an air splint is air leakage. When this occurs the splint will collapse. The valve also may fail, causing decompression. Because the air splint is fabricated from plastic, the patient's perspiration cannot be absorbed adequately by the stockinette and, with excessive perspiration, skin friction may be experienced. Patients may find bed mobility activities awkward because of the bulk of the splint. As mentioned earlier, the suspension is poor and the leg position is stiff, necessitating hip hiking during swing phase. The unit has to be put onto the patient when he is in a lying position and body compression on the expanded splint will alter the leg length to some extent. The bulk of the air splint plus the positioning of the knee tend to encourage deviations in early ambulation activities (abducted gait, hip hiking, lack of knee flexion).

Gait Training Units

A gait training unit can be supplied to the BK as well as the AK amputee patient. The alternating weight bearing and nonweight bearing which occurs during the gait cycle provides an excellent method of stump shrinkage.

Training units usually consist of:

1. A temporary socket shell which can be supplied with or without a soft liner.
2. An adjustable pipe attachment connecting socket and foot.
3. A disc section between socket and pipe, permitting alignment alterations at the knee or ankle.
4. An adequate suspension system.

Sockets for gait training units can be fabricated from different materials:

1. Plaster of Paris. The device is then called a plaster pylon (*see* "Fabrication of Plaster Cast Sockets"). These plaster sockets are quickly and economically replaced if stump changes require a new socket. However, these sockets are not as durable as the ones fabricated from plastic materials.
2. Vitrathene. This lightweight malleable plastic is moulded over a positive cast mould to form the socket. Vitrathene's lightweight qualities are favored by the elderly and can be utilized for final fitting

but, as with any lightweight materials, they do not permit rugged use.

3. A preshaped modular plastic socket. This type of socket is quickly available but will not always provide the desired intimate socket fit.

Advantages. Shrinkage and shaping take place during early gait training. The patient is in an upright position (which has physical as well as psychological values) and can use voluntary graduated weight bearing. The gait training unit assists the patient in learning balance skills. He also can learn to judge the placement of the artificial foot. He may experience some piston action and thereby get a "feel" for locomotion. A further benefit for amputees with vascular problems is that the remaining leg has rest periods when the patient is standing on the gait training unit.

Disadvantages. Alignment adjustments are limited and with progression of stump shrinkage the socket diameter has to be altered frequently. If the therapist is not absolutely sure of gait training unit adjustments, the services of a prosthetist are frequently required. Changes in the socket diameter in BK gait training units are easier to control because shrinkage can be accommodated by extra socks. But when an AK stump shrinks, the socket walls of the quadrilateral, temporary, socket have to be adjusted by tightening or loosening the metal bands around the socket which has been split to accommodate shrinkage. This is not always easily performed. In order for the AK amputee to control the unit, the quadrilateral socket has to provide a medial-lateral stability. This requires that there be equal comfortable pressure over the whole lateral aspect of the stump (36). Should this socket firmness be applied only over a small area within the socket wall, the patient would then have pressure pain and would tend to abduct the stump against the socket wall and compensate with lateral trunk bending during stance phase. All temporary sockets need frequent alignment adjustments.

The suspension system of the training unit has to be functional to avoid excessive piston action and rotation of the socket on the stump. This is equally important for both the BK and AK amputation training unit.

Socket alignment errors or inadequate suspension will encourage gait deviations which are not desirable in any phase of gait training but especially not in this early phase of training.

Summary

Various stump shrinkage and shaping methods have been discussed. All methods can be used individually or in select combinations. One method may prove to be more successful with one amputee than another.

An often practiced combination is bandaging and the use of a gait training unit. The method used for shrinkage and shaping is up to the discretion of the physical therapist who will be able to observe during treatment how the individual patient responds to treatment.

OBSERVATIONS OF RESIDUAL LIMB DURING TREATMENT

Various signs and symptoms can be observed during the treatment and the physical therapist should be aware of the possible causes of these conditions before commencing treatment.

Skin

The stump of a diabetic patient probably will not have any hair growth, as the superficial circulation is impaired. The skin of the stump looks pasty and glassy and is prone to breakdown with very little pressure. More frequent bandage slippage occurs with this type of stump skin.

The stump of an arteriosclerotic patient can have hair growth, as the deep circulation is impaired while the superficial one might still be intact. This stump perspires, necessitating more frequent stump sock changes.

Dermatitis

If a patient has stump dermatitis, one usually can assume that this inflammation of the skin is either a contact dermatitis caused by friction or by piston action which is intensified by perspiration or an allergy to bandage, sock or socket materials. If the dermatitis were of a different nature, it would not be confined to the stump. This condition should not be confused with the reddish-bluish skin coloring which occurs after early weight bearing which may indicate "choking" of the stump in the socket. This choking of the stump in the socket recovers more or less rapidly when the socket is removed.

Venous Restriction

Venous restriction is recognized by discoloration. The stump is blue distally and red proximally with a small layer of white between. Should this be apparent in an AK stump, the quadrilateral socket design has to be checked. In rare cases, circulation restriction can occur when a patient sits on the ischial shelf.

A continental European AK socket shape, which is more oblong and oval and has a more triangular-shaped socket, may be indicated as the contours of this type of socket lessen the amount of compression under the ischial seat (16).

Dog Ears

A dog ear formation may occur at the distal lateral end of a stump with progressive stump shrinkage. This type of lapping will increase with further stump shrinkage and might develop into a skin fold which can create problems for the patient by folding when the stump enters the socket (Fig. 7.9). Another possible problem the dog ear formation can present is skin infection, as a result of perspiration settling into skin folds. This moist, dark

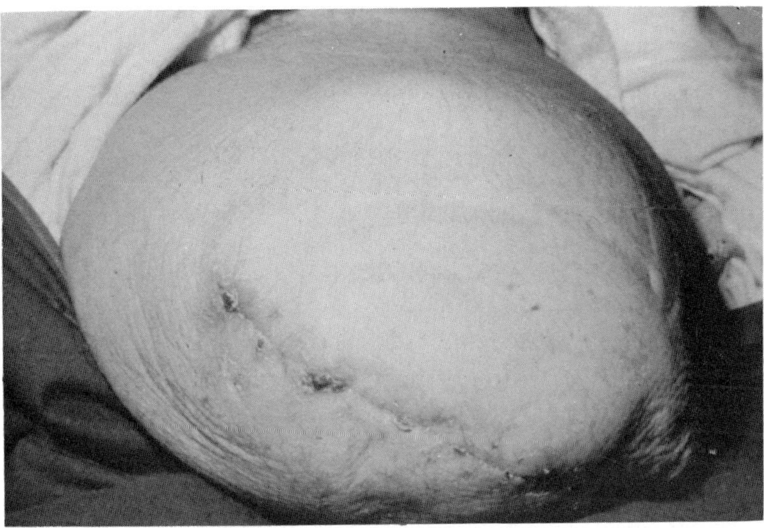

Fig. 7.9. A dog ear formation (*lower right*) may appear with progressive stump shrinkage.

area is an excellent environment for bacterial growth. Good stump hygiene is an essential prophylactic measure. The physical therapist can instruct the patient on how to control the dog ears by careful bandaging over the distal lateral portions of the stump. Proper bandaging can possibly reduce this situation to some extent.

Effect of Radiation Therapy

A patient who has undergone radiation treatment to the stump to arrest malignancy probably will have a very tender stump. Bandaging during the course of radiation is not advisable because, in addition to stump edema, the patient may have developed skin edema. These patients may present with a stump which looks red and is hot and tender to the touch.

Bandaging should start after the skin irritation has subsided. The physical therapist must use caution about the degree of bandage tension applied once the stump shrinkage treatment starts. Not all patients will respond to stump radiation treatment in this fashion. Patients receiving chemotherapy are not affected by this skin edema and can, therefore, continue their bandaging routines.

Early Ambulatory Pain

During early ambulation, intense generalized pain over the whole stump, even when protected by a nonremovable cast, might indicate a stump breakdown. This complaint has to be carefully followed-up, particularly if the amputation was performed at a marginal level. If severe pain persists, the cast should be removed and the wound evaluated. Following debridement, or stump revision if necessary, the nonremovable cast is reapplied and gait training is deferred.

Adductor Rolls

A common stump problem in elderly females with AK amputations is an adductor roll. An adductor roll is fatty tissue in the adductor area which creates biting, pinching and burning discomfort when the stump enters the socket. It also might prevent the patient from penetrating fully into the socket, giving the prosthesis the appearance of being too long. Gait deviations will result from this. This problem can be avoided almost completely if physical therapists, and nurses, stress correct bandaging techniques (*see* "AK Bandaging Procedure" under "Shrinkage and Shaping Techniques"). In the case of an unusually large adductor roll, the physical therapist either can incorporate an easily constructed Plastazote splinting shell which provides equal pressure over the area into the bandage (Figure 7.10) or fabricate an open-ended AK quadrilateral plaster of Paris socket with suspension straps. The patient can wear the plaster shell instead of the stump bandage. In most cases, this plaster shell will prevent edema but does not encourage further stump shrinkage due to its rigidity. This can be overcome by serial casting as the circumference of the stump decreases. In rare situations, uncontrollable and fatty tissue rolls can be surgically excised so that the stump will fit into the socket.

Summary

The physical therapist should observe the patient's stump carefully during exercise and gait training sessions. If any of the aforementioned conditions arise, the causes must be determined and, if indicated, the treatment adjusted accordingly.

Care of the Remaining Leg

The remaining leg in patients who experience vascular insufficiencies is not always a "good leg." Care of this leg is as important to the amputee as the care of the stump (3).

Physical therapists have to inspect this leg daily with an intensity equal to that given to the stump. The remaining leg is now the dominant leg which will be required to work harder. It must be stressed repetitively to the patient that proper care can help prevent future problems. It is the joint responsibility of the physical therapy and nursing staff to educate the patient concerning care of the remaining leg. When the patient is discharged, he should be competent in all phases of self-care.

Any abrasions, bruises or cuts should be reported to the physician, for

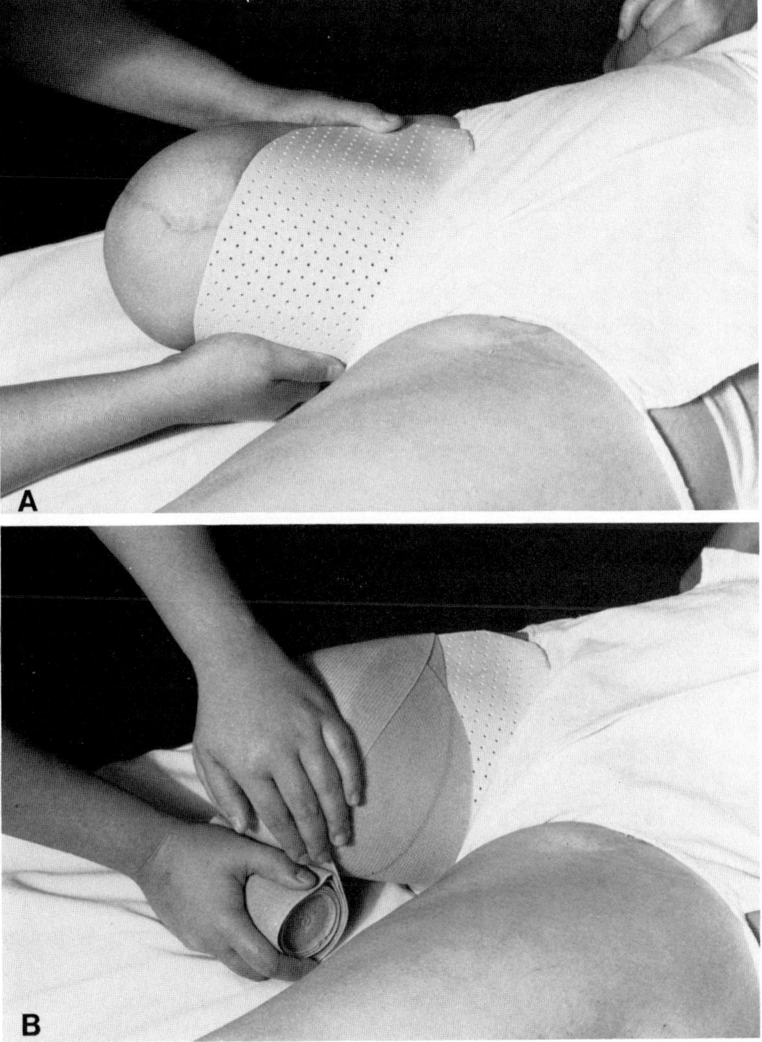

Fig. 7.10. *A*, A Plastazote splinting shell to avoid adductor roll; used under *B*, an elastic bandage.

these could cause complications at a later date.

Toenail cutting, if the patient is elderly, should be left to a skilled person. If toenails are thick, they should be soaked before cutting. Always cut straight across and not into the corners. Geriatric patients and diabetics often have impaired eyesight, poor eye-hand coordination and reduced sensation in the foot. Any injury caused by cutting toenails could have negative results.

Hygiene has to be meticulous:

1. Use soap, warm water and a towel to dry the skin thoroughly, including between the toes. Powder may be used on a daily basis, if indicated.
2. The remaining leg must always be protected by a well-supporting, comfortable shoe with a wide toe box.
3. Woolen socks are preferable as they help to absorb perspiration. Elastic rims should be avoided because these can restrict circulation.
4. If corns and callouses have to be removed, the patient must see his physician.
5. Walking barefoot or sitting in the wheelchair with merely a sock on, are definitely contraindicated. Any scrapes or abrasions could lead to infection and cause further problems.

The condition of the remaining leg, in vascular disorders, often will determine the level of independent ambulation and choice of ambulatory aids.

Daily monitoring of the remaining leg will permit prompt treatment of any problems which may arise. The therapist can assess such things as the need for appropriate external support to control swelling, the presence of any joint deformities which could hinder function, and the amount of activity which the patient can tolerate. The presence of ischemic pain on rest or after a short period of ambulation could affect the level of independent functioning.

Exercise is essential to maintain and increase the strength and joint range of motion of the remaining leg. Ambulation also achieves these goals but it is not a substitute for a specific exercise program.

The increased energy expenditure necessary to participate in the rehabilitation program also demands careful consideration for adequate rest periods. The condition of the remaining leg is one factor which will dictate the frequency and length of these rests.

The increased load which the remaining leg has to accommodate makes patient education and prophylaxis a major treatment concern.

Basic Rehabilitation Principles

BED

A firm bed permits correct body alignment and positioning. A soft mattress encourages a hip flexion contracture when the patient is supine because the hips, the heaviest part of the human body, will compress the soft mattress so that the hips remain slightly flexed during rest periods. A hip flexion contracture will give the patient a stooped position when he is upright.

OVERHEAD T-BAR

An overhead T-bar for the patient's convenience is generally not favored because pulling on the bar strengthens the biceps rather than the triceps which are necessary for use of any aids required for ambulation. If the patient is not provided with an overhead T-bar, then any movement which he attempts to make in bed will mean pushing down with his hands into the mattress in order to maneuver his body, thus utilizing his triceps.

There are, of course, exceptions to the rule. Should the patient be a bilateral amputee having difficulty attaining the sitting position or should bed sores be a problem, then an overhead bar can be of great assistance. If the patient is taught to hold on to the bar with one arm and use the other arm as the pushing arm, this will protect the skin over the sacral area and reduces skin irritation.

WHEELCHAIR

The most ideal chair for an amputee is an amputee wheelchair with the axis of the rear wheels set back to compensate for body weight loss in the front. In an ordinary wheelchair, the patient's feet act as counterbalance on the foot pedals and will prevent the chair from tipping. Antitipping devices for wheelchairs are available. An amputee chair should have a firm sitting surface for adequate pelvic support. Proper sitting support must be provided at all times in order to prevent a pelvic drop and spinal scoliotic compensation as both of these conditions can lead to fixed contractures. This condition will be more evident once the patient stands and begins ambulation. He will demonstrate uneven leg length and possibly secondary low back pain as a result of the fixed pelvic condition.

SITTING BOARDS

Wheelchairs have to be equipped with sitting boards; the ordinary wheelchair seat provides a hammock type surface which is undesirable for amputee patients. The AK amputee merely needs a square sitting board which gives good sitting support and prevents a pelvic drop. BK amputees need a board with an extension, either right or left, and a spring mechanism under the extension which will allow the board to be placed in a flexed or extended position (Figure 7.11). The stump should rest supported in extension during rest periods while the patient is in the wheelchair. However, when the patient tries to stand up or transfer from the wheelchair to bed or parallel bars, the extension should be released to avoid obstructing the patient's mobility. A thin foam cushion may be used for comfort.

PRONE LYING

Prone lying, a period of rest, is mainly intended for the AK amputee. This position has to be supervised and practiced several times daily. The length

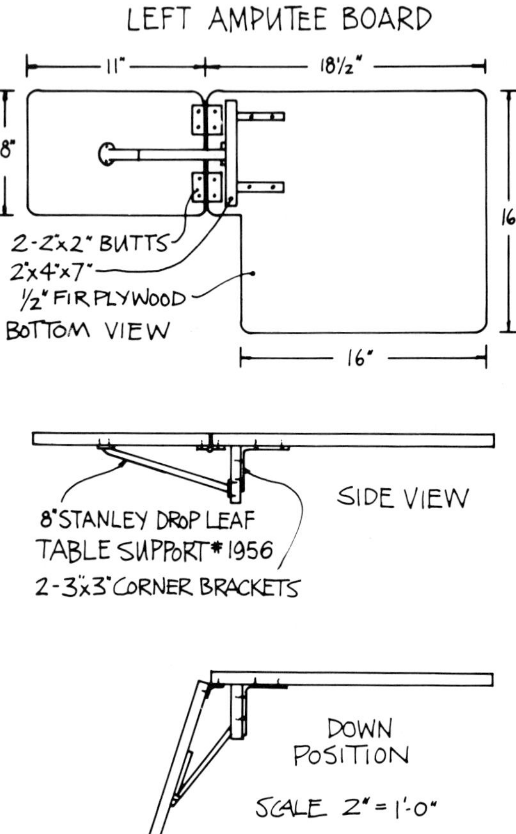

Fig. 7.11. The underside (*top*) of a wheelchair sitting board for a left below-knee (BK) amputee. The side views show the board in an extended position (*middle*), and in a down position (*bottom*). (Designed by Occupational Therapy Department, Chedoke-McMaster Hospitals, Chedoke Division, Hamilton, Ontario.)

of time in this position can be increased up to 1 hour, according to the patient's tolerance. The patient, when in the prone position, turns the head toward the sound side to avoid drawing up the affected hip. The purpose of prone lying is to keep the hip and the stump in a relaxed and stretched position. This procedure is done to give rest periods to the amputee and to counteract a possible hip flexion contracture. The bed has to be completely flat.

Should the patient have any respiratory disease such as emphysema or asthma and experience difficulty in breathing when they are in the prone position, then the bed is positioned in a reversed shock position and raised so that the head is higher than the hips. In this way, the patient will still remain in the correct prone position. An AK amputee may have difficulty in the prone position because of heavy breasts or a protruding abdomen. This problem can be overcome by utilizing pediatric pillows under the shoulders so that the prone position is comfortable and relaxing at all times. Support under the ankle of the remaining leg is indicated so that the toes are not causing irritation by pressing into the mattress. This support should be only underneath the ankle. The knee should lie flat on the mattress.

A close liaison between the physical therapist and the nursing staff will ensure that these principles are implemented both in the physical therapy department and on the ward.

Physical Therapy Modalities

Physical agents such as heat, light, water and electricity can be used in conjunction with an exercise program for amputees of all levels.

The physical therapist can apply these modalities to promote wound healing, to reduce stump pain, to provide the amputee with a feeling for body coordination, to increase circulation, and to encourage proprioception.

These modalities include the following.

TRANSCUTANEOUS ELECTRICAL NERVE STIMULATION

Transcutaneous electrical nerve stimulation (TENS) can be of some assistance in reducing or controlling chronic stump pain, provided the origin of pain is not caused by a febrile or infectious condition. It also has been helpful in the treatment of phantom pain. TENS is a symptomatic treatment and can help to some extent to substitute analgesic therapy (34).

Electrode placements can be segmental or local. The possible release of endorphins during stimulation is believed to provide temporary pain relief.

Not all amputee patients treated with transcutaneous nerve stimulation for stump pain experience permanent pain relief.

VIBRATORS

The use of a vibrator can be compared to an electrical massage. The device exerts short pulsating or gentle shaking motions over the tissues treated causing a soothing effect.

A vibrator, rarely used, is mainly indicated as a pleasant and gentle counter irritant when stump desensitization is desired.

HYDROTHERAPY

Young patients, traumatic amputees, and patients whose stump skin is intact will enjoy pool therapy. Thorough assessment including medical conditions which may contraindicate treatment must be done prior to commencing hydrotherapy. Water buoyancy allows freedom of movement of all body parts which is of tremendous benefit to these patients. Water activities can be programmed to assist or resist movement. The total body coordination achieved in the water will result in a feeling of well-being and contribute greatly to body coordination and balance on land.

WHIRLPOOL

A whirlpool bath at body temperature provides relaxation, an increase in circulation, a mechanical debridement of the wound and some desensitization of the stump. Savlon solution, which has disinfectant qualities, may be added to the water. This helps to cleanse the wound. One thousand milliliters of water shall contain 10 ml of Savlon, a proportion of 1:100 in order to achieve the required effect.

ULTRAVIOLET IRRADIATION

Ultraviolet light helps promote healing, increases circulation and helps destroy bacteria. Dosages to abscesses and their surrounding areas usually are administered with either a mercury vapor lamp or a Kromeyer lamp which has several attachments to facilitate entry into sinus wounds. The wound should be inspected carefully before calculating the appropriate dosages.

ULTRASOUND

The effects of therapeutic ultrasound applications are the production of heat in the body tissues and a micromassage effect due to the sound waves reflecting and refracting off tissue interfaces. The amount of heat produced depends on the frequency and the intensity applied and on the density of the tissues being treated. Ultrasound treatments have been used in an attempt to reduce pain due to neuromas but with questionable results. This seems to be due to the need to use low intensity. Ultrasound also can be used to reduce tissue adhesions. Applications of excessive intensity can produce necrosis in healthy tissues.

ELECTROMYOGRAPHIC BIOFEEDBACK

The electromyographic (EMG) biofeedback unit monitors muscle activity and can be used in several ways in the treatment of amputees. It can be used in conjunction with manual techniques to help release muscle tightness (4, 14). Placement of the electrodes on the bulk of the quadriceps will produce a visual or audio feedback to the patient when he contracts the muscle to straighten his knee (Fig. 7.12). The device can be adjusted so that maximal contractions are required to produce the feedback. This technique can be used when the BK amputee is participating in individual exercise sessions or when he is gait training.

Electrodes also may be specially implanted in the posterior wall of the AK quadrilateral training unit socket to teach the patient good stump extension which enhances knee stability from heel strike to foot flat. Care must be taken to remove the buttons on the electrodes because these can

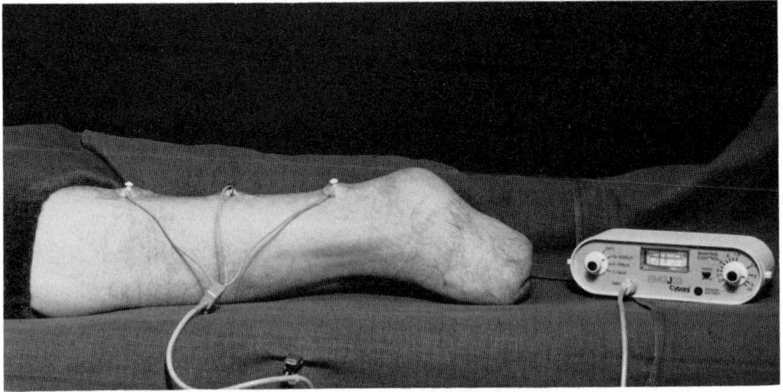

Fig. 7.12. An electromyographic (EMG) biofeedback unit in place on a below-knee (BK) amputee to monitor quadriceps muscle activity.

cause undue pressure on the stump and leave reddened areas on the stump skin. Again, the biofeedback unit can be used in individual exercise sessions with the AK amputee to encourage good stump extension to stretch hip flexion tightness.

Problems may be encountered getting an accurate feedback over the gluteus maximus if there is too much tissue coverage over the muscle. Research is still being done on more appropriate ways of placing the electrodes in the socket so that this method of treatment can be used more accurately and extensively in the gait training of amputees.

LIMB LOAD MONITOR

The limb load monitor is an electronic device which can be beneficial during gait training. It assists the amputee in learning to control the amount of weight bearing (4) (Fig. 7.13).

The patient experiences instant audio feedback indicating the weight he/she is exerting through the limb. In this way the patient can judge, respond, and self-control the amount of weight bearing. This feedback system reinforces to the patient and therapist that the patient can command the correct weight bearing on his prosthesis. It must be remembered that the limb load monitor is an adjunct to existing treatments and does not replace or eliminate other treatment procedures.

FRICTIONS

If, during healing of the surgical wound, scar tissue becomes adherent to the underlying tissues, one can attempt mobilization of these tissues by frictions. A mobile scar does not restrict stump mobility, whereas adherent tissues can produce undue stress on the stump due to their lack of mobility.

In order to attempt mobilization, the therapist should exert rotational

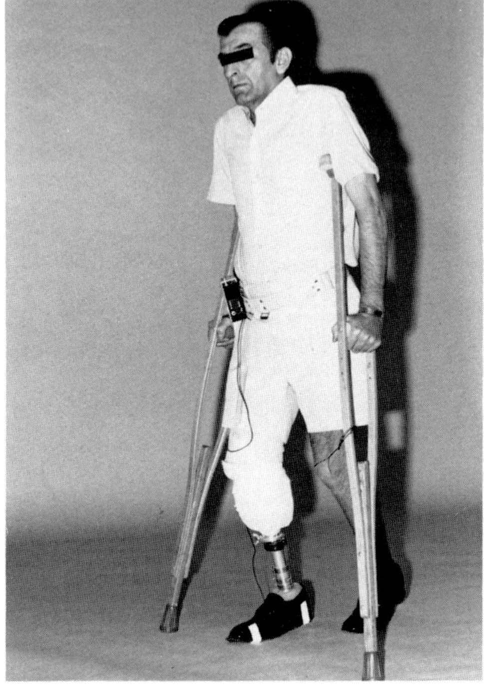

Fig. 7.13. A limb load monitor in place during gait training.

localized pressure with both middle fingers in a position parallel to the scar. Sliding motions over the skin are incorrect.

This increases the circulation of the underlying tissues and may help in breaking down adhesions. Frictions are not carried out over edematous skin areas or where inflammation is present.

SUMMARY

Although any of the physical therapy modalities and techniques discussed above may be used and are beneficial for amputees, the main emphasis in treatment should be on stump conditioning, exercising and gait training.

Exercises

Physical therapy activities start immediately following amputation surgery and exercise intensity gradually increases in order to prepare the patient for gait training and independence in activities of daily living.

Exercise tolerance and energy consumption are interlinked with the patient's cardiovascular system and the body's metabolism (6, 43, 45).

A traumatic amputee without other complications can cope with a vigorous routine; physical fitness improves emotional and physical well being. However, patients with peripheral vascular disease have to be monitored carefully to avoid undue fatigue following exercise activities. This can be indicated by breathlessness after exercise. Pulse and respiration rates should be checked frequently. Exercising and rest must be carefully balanced.

Another factor which has to be considered during exercise is increased perspiration. This is caused by the loss of skin surface (skin partially controls body temperature) by adaptation of circulation (establishing a collateral circulation in the stump), and by a higher energy output required to perform physical tasks (28). The body will adjust over a period of time and this increased perspiration will subside.

The amputee's basic needs include sitting, standing and walking balance. These objectives can be achieved by selective exercise programs which include general exercises for trunk and upper extremity strengthening, specific stump exercises and exercises for the remaining leg. All exercises must be meaningful. A brief explanation of the reasoning behind exercises often will gain the patient's cooperation, especially as some of the patients have not done exercises, as such, for years. Explanation for exercises also may improve the possibility of the patient's carrying on a maintenance exercise program after discharge from hospital.

GROUP EXERCISE

Bringing amputees together to exercise in a group is beneficial in several ways (15): it changes the environment for the patient because he has to come from the ward to the gymnasium for treatment; it encourages socialization, it makes him aware that he is not alone; it shows him that all amputees have to work hard in order to achieve goals; and it furthers togetherness and teaches him to adapt. Group exercises are a teaching tool for the therapist, for each exercise is done under controlled conditions for a specific reason.

Group activities can be done on exercise mats, sitting up in wheelchairs, or standing in the parallel bars. Ball games are excellent, whether in sitting or standing. They encourage group interaction, they demand a quick response to changes in motion. They encourage sitting balance and trunk rotation. They require functional movements which will help make the patient more independent and increase his confidence as his strength and balance improve. Ideally, patients should attend exercise class daily and then follow through with specific individual exercise programs and gait training.

INDIVIDUAL EXERCISE

Hands On

The therapist should guide the stump manually through the expected range of motion. In this way the patient can learn to master controlled stump motion. Manual feedback enhances proprioception and gives a sensory awareness of the position of the stump in relation to the rest of the body, and the intensity or speed in which the motion is performed.

If the patient can control the precise direction of the joint range, manual resistance can be given to increase muscle strength. The manual resistance technique has the advantage of allowing the therapist to actually feel the muscles contracting and judge both the smoothness of the initiating directive movement and the degree of fatigue which appears to follow repetitive resistive action.

STUMP MOBILITY

Each stump movement has a function in ambulation. When range of motion, stump strength or stump proprioception are decreased, gait deviations are demonstrated. The deviations caused by these problems can be observed by the physical therapist during treatment.

Motion: Stump Hip Flexion

Prime Mover. Iliopsoas.

Purposes. 1) To assist in accelerating the prosthesis; 2) to initiate control of the artificial knee joint; 3) trunk control from lying to sitting; 4) to assist in stair walking and inclines; and 5) to allow smooth movement in position change from sitting to standing.

Gait Observations. When walking, the patient leans forward and places his weight on the handles of the gait aid. This places the weight of the trunk on the handles and reduces weight bearing through the prosthesis. During gait, these patients tend to walk with excessive hip flexion and increased lumbar lordosis.

Comments. Active and resisted hip flexion does not need to be practiced with the same intensity as other stump motions. The amputee automatically uses his stump for balance when transferring or ambulating without his prosthesis. Stump flexion is a protective motion which brings the center of gravity in front of the hip joint, particularly in combination with trunk flexion. This helps to enhance the amputee's feeling of stability.

Motion: Stump Hip Extension

Prime Movers. Gluteus maximus. Some fibers also assist in abduction and adduction: semitendinosus; semimembranosus; and long head of biceps femoris.

Purposes. 1) To allow the AK amputee to hold the prosthetic knee in a position of stability during stance; and 2) to promote stability in ascending and descending stairs and inclines.

Gait Observations. AK and BK amputees with gluteus maximus weakness demonstrate an increased lumbar lordosis after heel strike of the prosthesis.

Short steps are taken in order to control the prosthesis during gait. In AK amputees, knee control is poor.

Comments. Weakness of the hip extensors encourages hip flexion. An overstretched, weak gluteus maximus cannot hold the AK stump and the artificial knee joint in stable extension. The amputee compensates by lurching, allowing a posterior displacement of the line of gravity on the amputated side at hip level. Weak hip extensors also cause hip instability when the amputee attempts to kneel.

If a knee flexion contracture or tightness is present in a BK stump it is more difficult to achieve full range of hip extension.

When exercising in the prone position a pillow under the pelvis provides a slight stretch on the gluteus maximus giving the muscle a better starting position from which to initiate muscle contraction.

Motion: Stump Hip Adduction

Prime Movers. Adductors longus, magnus, and brevis; gracilis; and pectineus.

Purpose. To assist in hip stability during stance by counteracting external rotation and abduction of the stump.

Gait Observations. The AK amputee tends to externally rotate the prosthesis giving his gait a "toeing out" characteristic. He is unable to maintain a correct foot position and may demonstrate a medial whip.

Comments. Prolonged sitting encourages hip abduction and external rotation as this position provides a good base for sitting balance. The AK stump externally rotates in sitting because it tends to follow gravity when relaxed and unsupported. Weak adductors can lead to a combination of hip abduction and external rotation contracture. This is more commonly observed in short AK stumps. Weak adductors are not as common as weak abductors.

When exercising in either supine or prone positions, the pelvis must be positioned at a right angle to the spine to avoid a pelvic drop or hiking during hip adduction.

Motion: Stump Hip Abduction

Prime Mover. Gluteus medius.

Purpose. To provide stability for the AK amputee in the stance on the prosthesis.

Gait Observations. The AK amputee will demonstrate a wide-based gait or lateral bending of the trunk. The patient leans the trunk toward the amputated side, the pelvis shifts downward and the patient's shoulder drops. A similar gait pattern may be observed in BK amputees who have short stumps with limited leverage.

Comments. The lateral aspect of the stump contracts against the socket wall in order to stabilize the hip during stance. During stance, the center of gravity shifts laterally over the stance leg. A positive Trendelenburg sign indicates a weak gluteus medius. Movements of stump abduction and external rotation are frequently combined because amputees have difficulty isolating these two motions.

Motion: Stump Hip Internal and External Rotation

Prime Movers. 1) External rotation—obturator internus; obturator externus; quadratus femoris; piriformis; gemellus superior; and gemellus inferior. 2) Internal rotation—gluteus minimus; and tensor fascia lata.

Purpose. To rotate the leg medially and laterally.

Gait Observations. These muscle groups alone do not present a major problem to amputees, however they make the gait appear stiff. The amount of internal and external rotation present at the hip determines the position of the prosthetic foot. A pelvic belt suspension will further restrict rotation. If an inverted or everted gait is demonstrated, foot alignment adjustments are necessary to accommodate for the patient's lack of ability to control the training unit, and to ensure comfort and a stable foot contact. A weakness in external rotation will be demonstrated by the patient using the stump as a stick, placed forward and in, during heel contact. During swing phase, the foot may demonstrate a lateral whip.

Comments. Weakness of the internal and external rotators is very rarely seen alone. It usually is combined with weakness of the flexors and extensors of the hip.

Motion: Knee Flexion

Prime Movers. Biceps femoris; semitendinosus; and semimembranosus.

Purposes. 1) To act primarily as a counterbalance to the quadriceps; 2) to decelerate the leg's foreward motion before heel contact; and 3) to assist in knee stabilization on weight bearing.

Gait Observations. Patients with weak hamstrings may use more power than necessary to produce knee flexion. This causes an uneven heel rise. Uneven step length is observed during gait, or hip hiking occurs to compensate for the loss of knee flexion.

Comments. A knee flexion contracture is particularly bothersome for the amputee with a short BK stump. Leverage is poor due to the length of the stump and lack of knee extension. These patients should never sit in wheelchairs without a BK sitting board.

Motion: Knee Extension

Prime Movers. Rectus femoris; vastus intermedius; vastus lateralis; and vastus medialis.

Purposes. 1) To promote good heel contact at heel strike; and 2) to enhance stability in stance.

Gait Observations. The patient with weak knee extensors will walk with a foot flat, bent knee, gait. They will take short steps and will have poor heel contact. When they reach stance they will have poor stability as the knee will tend to flex, unable to counteract the strength of the knee flexors and knee flexion movement.

Comments. This weakness is often combined with hip flexion because the lack of knee stability during stance makes the weight of the body accelerate in a forward and downward motion. Lateral shifting also may be observed during stance.

Summary

The foregoing has reviewed the problems which a BK and AK amputee may encounter with decrease of muscle strength or range of motion. However, at this point, one also must consider the transmetatarsal amputee. The therapist must encourage strong dorsiflexion and eversion of the ankle because the attachment of the tibialis anterior tends to pull the foot into inversion. Gait deviations are not marked because of equal leg length but the therapist may notice the amputee rocking on the lateral side of the foot with an abrupt toe off and exaggerated knee flexion. If this problem persists, ulceration or skin breakdown may occur on the lateral side of the foot.

For the purpose of clarity, ranges and weaknesses were discussed separately but it must be realized that locomotion involves total, synchronized body movement. For this reason, the problems are more commonly seen in combination rather than individually. The therapist must, therefore, consider the importance of exercise programs geared to the patient's individual needs.

CONTRACTURES

Contractures have a tendency to develop in the joint next to the level of amputation, immediately or soon after surgery. The position of most comfort to both the AK and BK amputees seems to be stump flexion. On rare occasions, recent peripheral vascular amputees can be observed in the sitting position, applying counter pressure to the distal end of the stump with their hands and compensating for the stump's rigid position with a trunk rocking motion. This position seems to reduce their pain. Rehabilitation of these patients is marginal, as their stump tenderness often will make them dependent on walking aids. Prolonged maintenance of this flexed position, to relieve pain, encourages the development of contractures.

Some joint restrictions, manifested by muscle tightness, can be released by exercising, stretching, splinting, normal mobility and walking (29, 39). Others are fixed and, to a certain extent, can be accommodated for in the alignment of the prosthesis.

Knee Flexion Contractures

Some knee flexion contractures present marked, visible, hamstring tightening. In testing, assisted knee extension comes to a rigid stop. This is usually an indication that contracture release cannot be completely achieved. The patient's socket will have to be set in flexion to accommodate this joint fixation. This will result in a tiring gait as the quadriceps have to be in synergistic control at all times during stance in a flexed position.

Test Position and Technique for Measurement.

1. The patient is placed in the prone position to eliminate hip motion.
2. The patient is asked to bend and straighten the knee as far as he can (22).

Goniometer readings at the end of each range will indicate the range of movement in degrees. A tape measure also can be used, in which case total distance is measured from the bone end perpendicular to the bench. A decrease in distance measurement indicates an increase in range of motion.

Hip Flexion Contractures

A hip flexion contracture is often associated with a lumbar lordosis. Unfortunately this combination rarely can be corrected. Supervised prone lying will help counteract a hip flexion contracture.

Test Position and Technique for Measurement.

1. The patient is placed in the supine position.
2. Using the Thomas test position, the patient is asked to flex the hip and knee of the remaining leg as much as possible. He then fixes the position by hugging the flexed extremity. This decreases the amount of lumbar lordosis.
3. The patient is then asked to extend the stump as far as possible (17).

Measurement of hip extension can again be done in degrees by goniometer readings or by measuring the distance from the bone end perpendicular to the bench.

Pelvic Tilt Contractures

A pelvic tilt also can result in a fixed contracture, but initially this is not as readily observed as other contractures. Measurement of this contracture is very difficult since a lateral pelvic drop is usually seen in combination with pelvic rotation. Prevention is the best remedy for this type of contracture. When walking, the amputee will demonstrate dropping, usually of the amputated side. The patient also may demonstrate a compensatory scoliosis which can produce low back discomfort.

Abduction Contractures

Abduction contractures also can be observed, more commonly in AK amputees. The condition tends to be accentuated in bilateral AK amputees because of the nature of their sitting position, with stumps in abduction and external rotation.

Test Position and Technique for Measurement.

1. The patient is placed in the supine position.
2. Using the anteriosuperior iliac spines as a guide, the therapist ensures that the pelvis is level.
3. One arm of the goniometer is placed in line with the axis and the other is placed in line with the femur, using the bone end as a guide.
4. The patient is then asked to adduct the stump as far as possible.

Stretching of Contractures

Young amputees do not have to cope, to the same extent, with fixed contractures caused by muscle and ligamentous shortening. However, the older amputee, whose posture is already more "set," tends to allow the stump, following amputation surgery, to draw into the more comfortable, flexed position. Preventive measures such as positioning and exercise must be practiced.

Should a contracture occur, then stretching is indicated. It is important to remember that stretching should be done only within the pain-free range. Overstretching can cause joint inflammation or establish a protective reaction which causes the stump to flex more to compensate for the pain which the patient feels.

Two stretching methods can be practiced, one with the patient actively participating or another with the patient completely relaxed during a passive muscle stretch (29).

In both methods, the therapist feels the amount of stretch indicated. Stretching is more effective if the stump is warm and comfortable. For this reason a preliminary application of heat, after skin sensation testing, may be indicated. Combined, repetitive stretching and relaxing are more effective than prolonged constant stretching. The constant stretch causes tissue fatigue and sets up the protective counter reaction.

Contractures will respond best to ambulation activities, with the necessary prosthetic alignment adjustments. A hip flexion contracture is stretched each time the patient goes from midstance to toe off, provided the patient is doing adequate weight bearing. A knee flexion contracture is stretched at heel strike, encouraging the patient to increase the step length on his prosthetic side. As one can see, this type of stretching occurs within the pain-free range and has the qualities of stretch followed by relaxation.

Position and Technique for Stretching Knee Contractures.

Patellar mobilizations:

1. Patient supine with sandbag under knee for support.
2. The therapist faces the distal end of the stump with the heel of the hand at the proximal patellar border. The fingers grip the distal patellar border.

3. The patella then can be moved in a proximal-distal or medial-lateral direction (21).

Restriction of patellar mobility can cause restrictions in knee range:

1. With the patient supine, the therapist faces the patient's knee and stabilizes the tibia with one hand.
2. After stabilizing the femur and pushing the patella distally with the other hand, a slow controlled dorsal pressure is applied within the patient's tolerance (21).

Position and Technique for Stretching Hip Flexion Contractures.

1. The patient is positioned in side-lying position, on his sound side, with the hip and knee flexed. The bent leg stabilizes the patient and flexes the lumbar spine.
2. The therapist works from behind, fixing the position by kneeling against the patient's buttock.
3. With one hand holding the patient's knee in flexion, the AK stump is stretched into extension without compensation occurring in the lumbar spine.

These stretches are gently repeated. Prone lying can follow as soon as the stump can relax in the extended position.

Contract-relax and hold-relax techniques also can be used for both BK and AK contractures. This technique works on the principle of reciprocal inhibition. Manual resistance is advised to allow the therapist to accurately gauge the amount of resistance given. Range measurements before and after treatment are suggested.

Another method which may be used to maintain achieved range, is the bivalved plaster cast. This form of treatment can be utilized only if the knee flexion contracture is not combined with a hip flexion contracture. If the hip is contracted as well, the patient will further flex his hip during sleep in order to overcome the stretching effect of the cast on the knee joint. Serial casting must be done in order to accommodate the increase in achieved extension range. This is a very good method of maintaining range while permitting regular rehabilitation activities during the day.

Contractures are very debilitating because they necessitate walking with a very tiring gait. For this reason, prevention and control through any appropriate means are very important parts of treatment.

Gait Training

Gait training is an indispensable phase in amputation rehabilitation and consists of more than training alternating leg motions. It involves total body movement (23). Gait training is preceded by an intensive and individual conditioning program.

A well controlled prosthetic gait is the safest; requires the least amount of energy output; and is, therefore, the most efficient. Although one always analyzes and strives to improve gait, one has to realize that moderate gait deviations have to be accepted provided the gait is safe and requires a minimum of energy consumption. These deviations may have been part of the amputee's former gait habits.

Each person's gait, although demonstrating an underlying basic pattern of locomotion, has a "personality" which cannot be built into a prosthesis. Furthermore, the gait cycle is basically symmetrical. The human body, however, is not symmetrical. It displays an accepted and normal asymmetry (44) which is more pronounced in some people than others (*e.g.* facial sides differ from right or left). This holds true for extremities, dexterity, mobility and shape. A locomotor asymmetry is apparent during gait training.

Gait, therefore, will differ greatly in individuals. It is important to remember that one is dealing, following amputation, with a mechanically abnormal gait, and the goals should be to achieve the best results that the patient's individual capabilities allow.

WALKING AIDS

Parallel bars, lightweight walkers (also called walking frames), various types of crutches, and canes can be used as ambulation aids.

Parallel Bars

The patient holding onto the bars can stand, walk, and shift body weight and correct his posture while seeing himself in the mirror in front of him. Verbal and manual guidance by the physical therapist can correct early gait deviations. Any type of gait pattern can be taught in the parallel bars as the patient can rely on the stability of the parallel bars for balance. Ambulation faults can be corrected with the therapist standing on the side of the patient giving manual assistance or resistance where needed.

Walkers

Most lightweight aluminum frames can be adjusted in height so that the patient can achieve a comfortable stance with something stable around him. This form of walking aid is frequently used following surgery. A walker provides stance stability particularly when the patient stands for the first time. Most of the patient's body weight is pushed through his arms and hands onto the walker while the patient adjusts to the feeling of standing on one leg. Although the emphasis in treatment is placed on the patient looking up and forward in order to assist experiencing the upright posture, initially he is permitted to look down occasionally. The visual feedback helps him improve his feeling for balance. As soon as balance with visual cues has been achieved the patient is then encouraged to look up and forward.

Initially during gait training sessions, walking without supervision is not advised. Each time the patient takes a step with his remaining leg and his training unit, the walker must be moved. This encourages unequal step length and an irregular gait pattern.

Crutches

Wooden crutches have an axillary section, often erroneously called the arm rest, a handle and a safety crutch tip. They must be fitted to correct height. During crutch length measurements, the elbow is held in slight flexion. This permits full elbow extension when the patient pushes his body weight through the crutch handles thereby allowing swing through with the body. Body weight must not be carried by axillary tissue. If these tissues are compressed, crutch palsy can result.

Wooden crutches tend to restrict rotational trunk mobility. Metal elbow crutches, on the other hand, permit a wider range of body mobility.

Canes

Many amputees manage to walk after completion of their rehabilitation program unaided. Elderly patients, however, should be encouraged to use a cane for safety. In all probability, these patients would have relied on a cane had they not had an amputation.

A cane provides that extra stability when needed (*e.g.* coping with bus steps, getting on and off escalators, walking in winter conditions).

GAIT ACTIVITIES

Gait training activities include, in addition to locomotion, such skills as: donning and removing the prosthesis; gait practice; analysis of common gait deviations; transfers from bed to chair, to the washroom, into a car; coping with stairs, inclines, uneven ground and obstacles; and falling and getting up off the floor (5, 26).

The amputee's gait speed is an individual matter. The higher the level of leg amputation, the slower the patient's walking speed. During gait practice sessions, one should concentrate and correct sequential motions and permit the amputee to find his own speed (43).

If a metronome is used initially, it may confuse the amputee as he is trying to concentrate on the actions needed to control his training unit. However, when his gait pattern becomes more automatic, then rhythmic assistance, using music or a beat is beneficial.

Donning and Removing the Prosthesis

A prosthetic socket may be compared to a shoe, in that it must fit well and be comfortable. Stump socks, as with ordinary socks, must be wrinkle free to promote comfort while walking.

Below-Knee Applications. When the amputee dons his/her prosthesis, the stump and the anatomical landmarks within the socket have to be aligned to assure a precise contact fit. The stump sock is pulled on and held firmly, anteriorly, in order to compress the tissues thus avoiding stress on the suture line. The stump is initially flexed and after entry into the socket it is extended. This motion is followed by an initial stance period so that the amputee can feel if stump and socket are in correct contact. A malaligned socket causes stump pain, and with pain the amputee cannot walk efficiently.

Should the BK prosthesis be fabricated with a socket insert, then the amputee puts the stump sock on first, then the insert, and then places the stump into the socket.

Above-Knee Application. An AK amputee places his/her stump, with the sock on, into the socket observing the adductor longus tendon groove and the artificial foot position so that he/she sits comfortably on the ischial shelf. If the patient has problems with bunching of the sock, especially in the groin area, the sock can be placed in the socket first, overlapping the outside of the socket wall. The amputee then inserts the stump into the sock-lined socket.

Whichever method is utilized, the patient must make sure that the adductor longus tendon enters next to the medial socket wall to avoid pinching during gait. The ischial tuberosity also must be on the ischial shelf, otherwise the prosthesis will appear too long.

The patient must exert weight onto the prosthesis when fastening the suspension belt otherwise the leg will internally rotate, thus causing a gait deviation when the patient ambulates.

If stump piston action is observed, the socket fit is loose and extra stump socks must be added to accommodate for the lack of fit between the stump and socket wall.

In cases of bulbous stumps, a stockinette may be used to pull the stump into the socket.

The gait training unit or the prosthesis must fit comfortably before gait training can commence.

Gait Practice

Gait training sessions begin between parallel bars, in front of a mirror. In this way the patient can see what he is doing using the stability of the bars to compensate for any lack of confidence due to poor balance.

Stance with feet 10–15 cm apart, weight equally distributed on both feet with an upright posture, and hands placed on the bars, is the correct starting position.

Balance and body coordination are essential for weight bearing and stepping. Control during weight shifting is a prerequisite for locomotion.

Step Positions. Step positions (26) are practiced before commencing locomotion. This helps the amputee to feel his body position over the training unit.

Balance exercises with changing foot positions help increase the patient's confidence. The prosthesis should be placed alternately in abduction and adduction, internal and external rotation. Knee flexion and extension, and pivoting on the heel also must be practiced. The sound leg practices the same motions individually or in unison with the training unit. All exercises have to be carried out in a slow and precise fashion so that the patient learns to completely control these motions. Control of knee motion by placing body weight anterior and posterior to the knee joint enhances stump proprioception.

Raising both arms well above the head stretches the trunk and places the center of gravity over the legs with the hips in extension (32). This is a necessary exercise as it counteracts the stooped position which one observes when amputees walk with a walker or crutches. It is most important for the AK amputee as this permits active hip extension control which aids in locking the artificial knee joint during stance.

Gait. Actual walking between the bars is initiated when the patient is able to control balance and weight shifting. Increased weight bearing through the training unit is encouraged.

The anteroposterior weight-shifting exercise is then progressed to gait with the amputee concentrating on maintaining the upright position and bringing his pelvis forward over the training unit before stepping through with the sound leg.

Common postural errors demonstrated during early gait practice are: remaining on the prosthesis too long; not overstepping with the sound leg which causes unequal step length; excessive hip flexion, bringing trunk weight forward only; holding the prosthesis off the ground before attempting heel contact; leaning trunk backwards to initiate swing phase; avoiding weight-bearing; and inability to unlock artificial knee in AK amputees.

If these gait faults are detected, they must be corrected early; otherwise they may become fixed habits. Progressing to crutches will be attempted only if the physical therapist is satisfied with the patient's previous gait performance between the parallel bars. If the amputee demonstrates poor locomotor control, he should return to the parallel bars for further practice of balance, weight shifting and stepping.

Following each practice session the stump shall be inspected.

Increased reddened areas accompanied by discomfort may indicate improper weight bearing. This, however, should be differentiated from the generally increased pink color of a recently amputated limb which is caused by the contact of the socket wall on the stump skin. This occurs in early stages of rehabilitation before the stump has toughened. This accepted pinkness will subside when the training unit is taken off.

One also should feel if the distal end of the stump is cooler to touch after walking. This temperature change accompanied with a feeling of tightness around the distal end of the stump may indicate "choking." This condition can be relieved to some extent by adjusting stump socks or increasing the socket diameter. This condition should not be confused with the generalized coolness of the stump which is often present in amputees with peripheral vascular disease.

Locomotor faults are sometimes difficult to isolate and to correct. They are associated with the amputee's medical-surgical condition, with existing prosthetic conditions (alignment, weight of prosthetic components) or can be caused by poor postural control.

Descriptive, accepted terminology and standard recording procedures are used to record these gait deviations (26), *e.g.* abducted gait, circumducted gait, medial or lateral whip, etc. (*see* "Prosthetic Gait Deviations," in Chapter 8). Most of these observations are based on leg motions.

Therapists will analyze, on an ongoing basis, the amputee's gait performance and discuss the reasons for any gait fault with the physician and the prosthetist.

Analysis of Common Gait Deviations

Table 7.1 lists typical *postural* faults, only, which are related to body motion and locomotion and which can, to some extent, be controlled and corrected by training. Deviations specific to certain levels of amputation are indicated.

Again it must be stressed that certain gait deviations have to be accepted (23). The patient's gait prior to amputation may have demonstrated gait deficiencies which cannot be corrected after amputation surgery, *e.g.* arthritic joints, limitations in joint ranges, unequal leg length, etc. It also is important to remember that gait training sessions include teaching of some unnatural or motion restricted gait patterns.

Examples.

1. The gait of an AK amputee is always an unnatural gait because he/she can only weight bear on an extended artificial knee. In normal gait, the knee is slightly flexed during stance. The artificial knee, however, has to be kept extended during stance and therefore provides a stiff-legged gait. This unnatural phase within the gait cycle proves, for some patients, to be difficult to learn, because hip extension has to be held longer on the prosthetic side than in normal gait.

2. In normal locomotion the trunk accommodates the opposing acceleration and deceleration swing pattern of legs and arms thus counter-rotating from side-to-side with each step.

When a patient depends on crutches he/she cannot utilize this natural counterbalancing trunk rotation as the crutches fix him/her into one plane, restricting him/her to a mere back and forth motion which is unnatural to normal gait (32).

TABLE 7.1. *Analysis of Common Gait Deviations*

Commonly demonstrated gait deviations by AK[a] and BK amputees	Reasons for these postural and locomotor gait deviations
Abducted gait	Wide stance base to control poor balance
	Adductor roll pinching (AK)
	Stump not completely inserted into socket (AK)
	Fear of knee instability
	Inability to extend hip adequately
Trunk forward flexion	Hip flexion contracture
	Inability to lock artificial knee with hip extension (AK)
	Low back pain
	Quadriceps weakness
	Gluteus maximus weakness
	Fear of knee instability (AK)
Feather weight bearing	General stump discomfort
	Deliberately avoiding knee flexion and extension
	Loss of proprioception
Keeping knee in flexion	Knee flexion contractures (BK)
	Heel contact missing
	Weak gluteus muscles allows knee to collapse (AK)
Heel contact missing	Knee flexion contracture (BK)
	Weak quadriceps muscle
	Poor control of prosthesis during swing phase allows artificial knee to flex by gravity before heel contact takes place (AK)
Hip hiking	Inability to cope with weight of prosthesis
	Clearing ground with stiff knee
	Osteoarthritis of hip
	Unequal step length
	Poor control of prosthesis resulting in carrying prosthesis through gait cycle instead of activating it properly (AK)
	Incorrect initiation of swing phase
Lateral trunk bend on stance	Weak abductors
	Unsure of control of knee
	Short AK stump
Lateral and medial heel whips	Mobile stump tissues which roll around bone
Foot pivoting	Active external or internal rotation of the hip
	Prosthesis incorrectly worn, rotated when fastening belt suspension without exerting weight through prosthesis (AK)
Lack of toe off	Short steps with sound leg
	Inability to activate artificial knee (AK)
	Hip flexion contracture
Inability to initiate prosthetic knee flexion	Very long stumps with the knee axis set lower than anatomically desired; hav-

TABLE 7.1. *Continued*

Commonly demonstrated gait deviations by AK[a] and BK amputees	Reasons for these postural and locomotor gait deviations
	ing an over-stable knee and, with full weight bearing, patient cannot activate knee flexion (practice toe off)
Stiff legged gait	Very short stumps tend to keep knee in extension caused by poor leverage Fear of knee instability (AK)
Uneven step length	Long step with prosthesis indicates poor proprioception Hesitant gait, patient will not step forward with sound leg to shorten stance period on prosthesis Overstepping of prosthesis is avoided due to stump pain
Shoulder elevation unilateral	Preexisting scoliotic spine or spinal postural compensation Walking with cane, holding trunk rigid and not using natural pendular motion of the arms Shifting balance over prosthesis
Lack of trunk mobility	Decreased mobility enhanced by previous crutch walking Fear of falling Motion restricted to avoid shift of center of gravity
Analysis	
See figure 7.14, Mrs. X	*See* figure 7.15, Mrs. X
Patient progressing in an angle to the line of progression Small steps, hesitant gait Prosthesis held in internal rotation Cane carried too far out Postural forward flexion which places center of gravity too far forward to assist the feeling of knee stability Right arm held rigidly at side during gait Lateral bend which shifts center of gravity over prosthesis Shoulder elevated to compensate for lateral bend	Postural correction by manual feedback Note, the therapist places her foot against prosthesis to counteract abduction of prosthesis when trunk is guided
See figure 7.16, Mr. X	*See* figure 7.17, Mr. X
Excessive trunk flexion with head looking down Trunk weight on walker Learning to extend stump and bring pelvis forward simultaneously by correcting the position passively Center of gravity in front of knee joint for stability	Learning to maintain the trunk in upright position before attempting to initiate hip and knee flexion

[a] The abbreviations used are: AK, above-knee; and BK, below-knee.

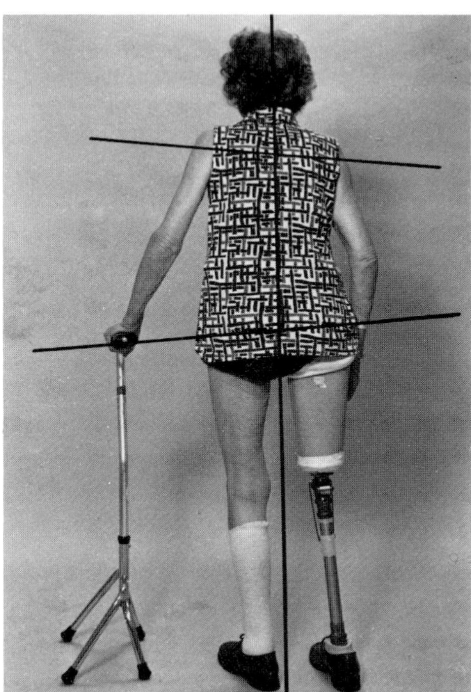

Fig. 7.14. A commonly demonstrated gait deviation on Mrs. X, an above-knee (AK) amputee (*see* "Analysis" in Table 7.1).

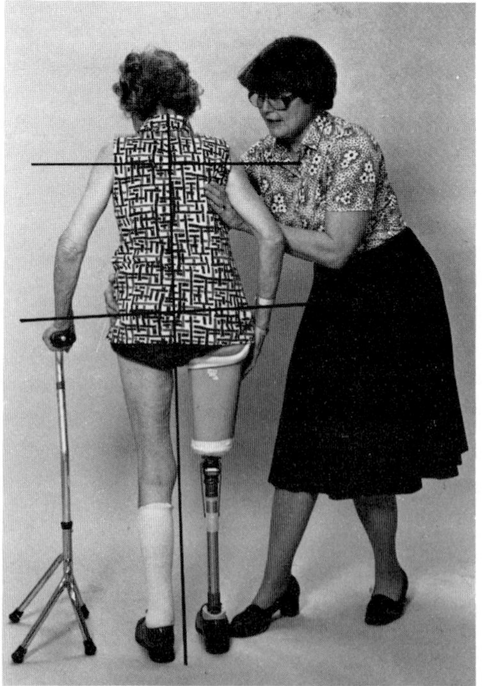

Fig. 7.15. Postural correction with manual feedback by the therapist on the same patient shown in Figure 7.15 (*see* "Analysis" in Table 7.1).

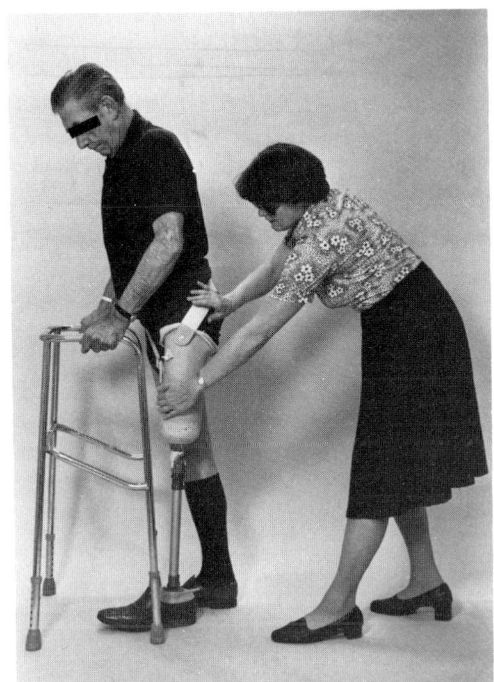

Fig. 7.16. An excessive trunk flexion with head looking down as seen on Mr. X, an above-knee (AK) amputee (*see* "Analysis" in Table 7.1).

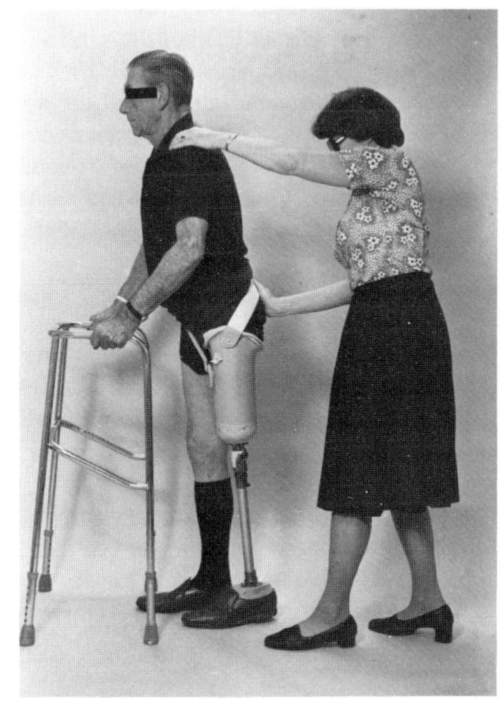

Fig. 7.17. Trunk correction with manual feedback by the therapist on the same patient shown in Figure 7.17 (*see* "Analysis" in Table 7.1).

3. A stiff-legged gait demonstrated by a patient with a very short BK stump is caused mechanically by too short a lever. This gait compensation may be demonstrated by the patient raising the pelvis and abducting at hip level, allowing the thigh on the involved side to rotate inward in order to lift the prosthesis off the ground.

The initiation of swing phase is tiring to this patient as he uses his hip flexors only. He loses out on the double pendular action which controls acceleration and deceleration of the swinging leg. He is inclined to keep his knee stiff during stance phase, as well, so that he can place his stump directly over the socket on weight bearing. This gives him a feeling of security but he then walks like a person wearing a long leg cast. A stiff knee gait increases energy consumption while normal knee flexion minimizes the energy output required during a gait cycle (38).

Transfers

Getting from the bed to a wheelchair, to the bath or into a car requires arm strength, abdominal muscle control, balance and forward placement of the center of gravity.

Basic transfer from bed to wheelchair for unilateral amputees:

1. Secure brakes;
2. Place chair at an angle to the bed, the sound leg should be closest to the bed;
3. Bed and chair height should be level;
4. Patient sits at side of bed;
5. Places sound leg on the floor:
6. The hand closest to the chair holds onto the arm rest farthest from the patient while the other hand pushes on the bed;
7. Standing is accomplished by leaning trunk over the transfer leg;
8. Stump is held in flexion for balance (only if prosthesis is not worn);
9. Pivoting on sound leg toward the chair will bring the patient to the position to sit.

The bilateral amputee, transferring without his prostheses, may encounter more difficulties. For these amputees, good arm strength will aid in transfers.

1. The wheelchair is positioned facing the side of the bed;
2. The patient sits on the bed with his/her back facing the chair;
3. He reaches back for the arms of the chair and lifts himself/herself into the chair;
4. If assistance is required, attendants stand on either side of the patient, holding him/her under the arms and lifting him into the chair.

Another method which can be utilized for the geriatric amputee is the side-sliding transfer.

1. Place wheelchair beside the bed and remove the arm of the chair closest to the bed;
2. Position a sliding board between the bed and the chair;
3. The patient holds on to the arm of the chair and, and using push-pull technique, slides himself into the chair.

Variations of individual transfer techniques depend on the patient's needs. These are taught together with activities of daily living by occupational therapists who decide what type of aids (transfer boards, seat adjustments, etc.) may be beneficial to the amputee (*see* Chapt. 9).

Stairs, Inclines, Uneven Ground, Obstacles

When climbing stairs, both AK and BK amputees will use the same procedure (1, 2, 26).

Up. Standing close to the bottom step, the sound leg steps up first. It performs the harder muscle work of bringing the body up. The prosthesis follows and is placed on the same step.

Climbing is done one step at a time (not overstepping) with the sound leg always leading.

Crutches accompany the prosthesis, their function is to support the prosthesis. If a railing is used, the prosthesis is centered between railing and crutches, which are both held on the opposite side of the rail.

Down. The pattern is reversed. Prosthesis and crutches step down first. The sound leg again performs the harder work of supporting the body until the prosthetic leg is stable, then it is placed on the same step. Descending is done one step at a time.

Inclines. Any sloping surface requires the amputee to adapt his gait pattern. In an upward approach, stepping sideways, the sound leg precedes the prosthesis, similar to stair walking, only the amputee turns 45° to the line of progression. In the downward direction the pattern is reversed.

Turning the body sideways to cope with inclines is necessary, particularly when going down hill, otherwise the prosthesis would buckle in a forward direction following foot contact as the slope contributes in accelerating the prosthetic foot into foot flat and thus causing unexpected early knee flexion.

Uneven Ground. When the amputee demonstrates adequate prosthetic control, balance and has stump proprioception, he can start with more difficult tasks such as gait on uneven ground. Gravel surfaces and lawns provide an excellent change from walking on a smooth floor. The patient will experience a different feedback sensation in the stump. When he adjusts his stance accordingly, the leg is then becoming part of him. He should be advised to carry a cane during nature hikes or when surface conditions indicate that assistance may be necessary (snow).

Obstacles. If the obstacle is big in nature the most practical way to overcome it is by stepping on top of it using the stair-walking technique. A smaller obstacle, if there is no other way of avoiding it, is approached by overstepping. Both feet are placed parallel a few centimeters away from the obstacle. The weight is transferred onto the sound leg, the prosthesis is swung forward by stump flexion and placed on heel contact past the obstacle (26). When prosthetic control is present, the sound leg follows.

AK amputees need more practice time as the artificial knee will flex before heel contact is accomplished if the overstep motion is not performed smoothly.

Falling and Getting Up

Falling. In theory, amputees should know how to protect themselves when falling. The actual fall is seldom practiced by geriatric amputees for fear of further injury. As soon as the amputee realizes his balance is lost and he is about to fall, he should remember two basic rules:

1. Drop walking aids;
2. Flex body if hands cannot be used to cushion impact.

Any advice, as to what to do in a forward/sideways or backward fall, is not realistic as the amputee hardly has enough time to decide which technique he should select while falling.

Getting Up.

1. Sitting position: on floor;
2. Sound leg: knee flexed all the way with arm support close to trunk;
3. Motion: turning toward sound side with momentum-pivoting on sound foot, into low stance using double hand support and hoisting trunk up. Prosthesis follows through (26).

These techniques will act as a guide to the therapist, however, modifications may be necessary as individual situations arise.

Sensitive and Painful Stumps

During prosthetic fitting and gait training, one can encounter problems with sensitive and painful stumps. Examinations will indicate if the socket alignment is correct, or if the stump is merely sensitive on weight bearing and has to toughen with time. Methods used to investigate socket alignments are:

Pressure Sensitive Dye-Filled Microcapsules. A pressure-sensitive stump sock made of polyurethane foam impregnated with pressure-sensitive dye-filled microcapsules can be of use (7). On weight bearing, these capsules break, marking the sock and, therefore, indicating where weight is taken. This form of testing proves particularly useful for patients who undergo stump expansion during the day and reduction of stump circumference at night.

X-Rays. Radiological examinations, including lateral and anteroposterior views of the patient weight bearing and nonweight bearing in his prosthesis, also can be of value. Determining the distribution of weight on the stump, and amount of piston action, and the possible presence of a "bell clapper" effect of the stump can be seen and recorded. The bell clapper effect occurs when the distal socket walls lose their contact with the stump producing hypermobility of the distal stump within the socket. The patient often will experience pain on the anterior distal aspect of the socket if this condition is present.

If X-rays are taken with the prosthesis on, the technologist has to use a higher level of exposure in order to penetrate through the fiberglass sockets of the prosthetic device. Exposure readings cannot be suggested as the thickness of the prosthetic wall is not standard (40).

Videotaping

To provide visual feedback to patients during gait training, videotaping can be used. During "instant replay" the amputee can see himself from front, side and back. The therapist then can point out postural habits and locomotor performance. Such observations as stance, position of feet, upright posture, step length, initiation of swing phase, posture at double support, line of progression, etc., then can be explained.

Videotaping can be repeated several weeks later and, by comparison, actual performance improvement can be documented.

DEFINITIVE PROSTHESIS—PROSTHETIC CHECK-OUT

When the stump has matured and girth measurements have stabilized, then consideration is given to ordering the definitive prosthesis.

The team members observe the amount of control which the amputee has over his training unit and his stability during ambulation. Final alignment and socket adjustments are considered at this time as well as the patient's vocational and avocational requirements.

The prescription is written considering all of the patient's needs and fabrication of the prosthesis commences. The patient will visit the prosthetic department several times for casting, fitting and adjustments.

When the patient receives his prosthesis, whether he has been discharged from the center or he is still an inpatient, it is the physical therapist's responsibility to perform a prosthetic checkout. As for the initial physical therapy assessment, availability of a standardized form will facilitate collection of data.

The therapist will evaluate such things as:

Below-Knee Prosthesis

1. Is the socket comfortable?
2. Is the anteroposterior alignment correct?
3. Is the mediolateral alignment correct?
4. Is the prosthesis the correct length?

5. The amount of piston action present.
6. Are the socket walls of adequate height?
7. Is the patellar tendon bar correctly placed?

If Patient Has Thigh Corset.

8. Do the uprights conform to the flares above the condyles?
9. Are the knee joints too close to the condyles?
10. Does the thigh corset fit properly?
11. Are the functions of the thigh corset met?

In Sitting.

12. Can the patient sit comfortably with knees flexed to 90°?

While Walking.

13. Are the socket and suspension systems comfortable?
14. Does the knee cuff maintain its position?

Cosmesis.

15. Does the prosthesis function quietly?
16. Are the size, contours and colors of the prosthesis approximately the same as those of the sound limb?
17. Does the patient consider the prosthesis satisfactory?

Above-Knee Prosthesis

1. Is the socket comfortable?
2. Is the adductor longus tendon properly located in its channel?
3. Does the ischial tuberosity rest on the ischial seat?
4. Is the prosthesis the correct length?
5. Is the knee stable on weight bearing?
6. Are the suspension attachments correctly located?
7. Does the pelvic belt accurately fit the contours of the body?
8. Is the center of the pelvic joint correctly located?
9. Is the patient comfortable in sitting and does the socket maintain position while the patient is sitting?
10. Does the prosthesis operate quietly?
11. Does the patient consider the prosthesis satisfactory as to comfort, function and appearance?

These are some of the basic observations which are made during a BK and an AK prosthetic check-out (26). However, special consideration must be given for supracondylar suprapatellar sockets, total contact sockets and different suspension systems.

The level of activities of daily living (ADL) function is also included in this check-out. Any apparent gait deviations are noted at this time.

After completing the assessment, the therapist meets with the physician and the prosthetist to discuss possible means of correction of any problems which have become evident as a result of the physical therapy evaluation. Close correlation of the individual assessments of the team disciplines will result in the fabrication of a prosthesis which is cosmetically acceptable and will allow the amputee optimum function.

Bilateral Amputees

Treatment goals and treatment procedures for bilateral amputees differ according to circumstances. The amount of independence to be achieved depends on the levels of amputation and the individual.

Functional ambulation can be achieved if several conditions are met. Patients must have endurance, arm strength, balance and contracture-free, healed stumps. These amputees have to work very hard mastering sitting balance, transfer techniques and wheelchair activities prior to commencing gait training. Locomotion on two prostheses is energy consuming and exhausting to many patients (28). To promote stability for ambulation, the height of the prostheses may be lowered to bring the center of gravity closer to the ground.

An elderly bilateral amputee with medical problems may manage to get about under supervision while in hospital, but may regress to wheelchair mobility once they have returned home and regular treatment supervision is no longer available.

When rehabilitating bilateral amputees, one must remember that previous unilateral amputees who have undergone amputation surgery for the second leg must await healing of the recent stump before walking commences. It is also biomechanically inadvisable to stand and ambulate on one prosthesis because the amputee would hold the prosthesis centrally under him, which produces a postural misplacement. Body weight would exert tremendous forces on the stump. Balance cannot be achieved because the prosthesis is not aligned to allow correct balance in this position.

BELOW-KNEE—BELOW-KNEE

One can assume that a bilateral BK amputee will walk because he still has his knee joints. Bilateral BK amputees adapt to a wider standing base, demonstrate slow velocity and usually need walking aids, but are able to cope with stairs, get in and out of cars, and can handle ADL.

From Sitting to Standing.

1. Secure brakes on wheelchair;
2. Sit as far forward on seat as possible;
3. Place prosthetic feet firmly on ground with knees bent more than 90°;
4. Place trunk weight over prosthesis;

5. Push on arms of wheelchair with hands and come to standing position;
6. Stabilize stance before commencing to walk.

BELOW-KNEE—ABOVE-KNEE

The amputee with a combination of an BK and AK amputation also can ambulate. His BK stump serves as the dominant leg. His remaining knee has to perform all major tasks such as stability to reach standing, being the lead leg when climbing stairs, etc. The range of knee flexion during sitting periods should not exceed 90°; this position avoids restricting stump circulation. The higher the level of amputation, the slower the walking speed.

Gait is taught with a wide base and balance work is intensive. These amputees spend a long time training in the parallel bars before proceeding to walkers or crutches.

From Sitting to Standing.

1. Secure brakes on wheelchair;
2. Sit diagonally as far forward on seat as possible, with the BK stump turned toward the sitting edge;
3. Place BK prosthetic foot firmly on ground with knee bent more than 90°;
4. Place AK prosthesis forward in extension;
5. Lean trunk weight over BK prosthesis;
6. Push on arm rests and come to standing, pulling the AK prosthesis under the trunk;
7. Lock artificial knee on foot contact;
8. Make sure stance base is stable before commencing walking.

While rising, marked trunk flexion over the BK stump is necessary to place the body's center of gravity forward so that the quadriceps muscles can extend the knee.

ABOVE-KNEE—ABOVE-KNEE

Some young, healthy bilateral AK amputees will be able to master gait. Geriatric amputees with underlying medical pathology will not be able to accomplish this task on an ongoing basis. No matter how long and how intensive the rehabilitation program may be, walking on a regular basis is not a realistic goal.

Bilateral AK amputees have multiple problems which need to be overcome. The higher the level of amputations, the harder it is to learn to walk; the greater the energy output will be (28, 43, 45), and the heavier the prostheses will be.

Special prosthetic prescriptions are indicated such as one safety knee (probably on the side of the shorter stump) and one free swinging knee. Two safety knees are not safe as it deprives the amputee of the necessary knee motion should he fall. Knee stability also can be achieved by setting the knee axis posteriorly, however, this makes it physically harder for the amputee to activate his artificial knee.

The physical efforts of donning two AK prostheses, having both suspension systems in place and being able to stand up, and then walk, activating two artificial knees, is difficult and cumbersome. For these reasons, consideration for wheelchair independence becomes more realistic for the geriatric amputee. The distance which the patient is able to walk with two prostheses is limited, and the energy consumption is high. Wheelchair mobility is achieved at a lesser energy expense and the amputee reaches the desired location faster. The amputee's hands are free for ADL activities. Useful and pleasant activities such as reading, stamp collecting, needlework, telephoning etc., can be carried out from a wheelchair.

The treatment goals for most bilateral AK amputees differ from those of a unilateral AK amputee, but are still functional and realistic.

From Sitting to Standing.

1. Wheelchair placed facing parallel bars;
2. Secure brakes;
3. Sit forward on seat;
4. Place both feet firmly on ground and lean forward;
5. Reach out with one arm placing hand on bar;
6. The other hand rests on the chair arm;
7. Use pull-push technique to elevate trunk;
8. Lock artificial knees at the same time.

Bilateral Above-Knee Gait Characteristics.

1. Wide stance to aid balance;
2. Marked lateral trunk bending during locomotion to place center of gravity over stance leg;
3. Trunk flexion position if walker is used;
4. Trunk held in lumbar lordosis with pronounced arm swing without the use of walking aids.

During the initial assessment, nearly all bilateral amputees will express the wish to walk with two prostheses. In their minds, it is easy to imagine being up and about, as locomotion at one time was an effortless part of their existence. The clinic team has to evaluate the bilateral amputee's potential with utmost care to be able to serve him in his best interests. Rehabilitation trial periods will often be initiated to permit better judgement as to what the treatment outcome will be. Sometimes it may be necessary to fit a bilateral amputee with a prosthesis even though the clinic team may believe that prosthetic ambulation is unrealistic. Through this process the patient, himself/herself, will decide to abandon prosthetic ambulation as a realistic goal.

Conclusions

Amputation rehabilitation can be challenging to both the amputee and the physical therapist.

The treatment aim is to achieve the highest level of independence possible—physically, socially and emotionally.

The physical therapist's responsibilities include more than exercising, positioning, bandaging, teaching transfers, crutch walking, and gait training. The nature of the underlying disease process, such as circulatory disorders, metabolic deficiencies, malignancy, infections and the implications of each to treatment, must be taken into consideration. Surgical procedures, socket designs, weight-bearing distribution, prosthetic alignment and the physical endurance of the individual also must be fully understood.

Each patient must be thoroughly assessed and the treatment program formulated to meet the individual needs and problems. As the patient progresses, treatment must be evaluated and changed constantly. Although the treatment approach is practical, one must not overlook the amputee's psychological needs, anxieties, fears, frustrations. Listening to problems and reacting with kindness and understanding is an important part of treatment.

The amputee, an active participant in his treatment program, must know that the best aligned prosthesis will not overcome poor gait habits. The amputee's physical ability, his motivation as well as his determination, will control his level of independence in gait and activities of daily living. He is the key to success in his own rehabilitation.

REFERENCES

1. ALEXANDER, A. *Amputee's Guide, Below the Knee.* Medic Publishing Co., Bellvue, Wash., 1975.
2. ALEXANDER, A. *Amputee's Guide, Above the Knee.* Medic Publishing Co., Issaquah, Wash., 1978.
3. BANERJEE, S. N. Assessment and Management of the Ischemic Foot. *Can. Fam. Physician 25:* 842–846, 1979.
4. BASMAJIAN, J. V. *Biofeedback: Principles and Practice for Clinicians.* Williams & Wilkins, Baltimore, 1979.
5. BATZDORFF, J., AND FRANKEL, B. Initial Gait Training of the Patient with Above-Knee Amputation. *Phys. Ther. 58:* 575–578, 1978.
6. BLESSEY, R. Energy Cost of Normal Walking. *Orthop. Clin. North Am. 9:* 356–358, 1978.
7. BRAND, P. W., AND EBNER, J. D. A Pain Substitute Pressure Assessment in the Insensitive Limb. *Am. J. Occup. Ther. 23:* 479–486, 1969.
8. BRAND, P. W. Management of the Insensitive Limb. *Phys. Ther. 59:* 8–12, 1979.
9. BURGESS, A. M. *The Management of Lower-Extremity Amputations: Surgery, Immediate Postsurgical Prosthetic Fitting, Patient Care.* Veterans' Administration, Washington, D.C. 1969.
10. BURGESS, E. M., AND ALEXANDER, A. G. The Expanding Role of the Physical Therapist on the Amputee Rehabilitation Team. *Phys. Ther. 53:* 141–143, 1973.
11. CHUSID, J. G. *Correlative Neuroanatomy and Functional Neurology.* 16th ed. Lange Medical Publications, Los Altos, Calif. 1976.
12. COLTHURST, A. J. B., AND FALCONER, K. A. *Manual Muscle Testing.* University of Toronto Press, Toronto, 1973.

13. FISHMAN, S. Amputee Needs, Frustrations, and Behavior. *Rehabil. Lit. 20:* 322–329, 1959.
14. GAARDER, K., AND MONTGOMERY, P. *Clinical Biofeedback: A Procedural Manual.* Williams & Wilkins, Baltimore, 1977.
15. GILLIS, L. *Artificial Limbs.* Pitman Medical Publishing, London, 1957.
16. HABERMANN, H., JR. *Continental Above-Knee Socket.* Paper presented at Advanced Course on Above-Knee Prosthetics. Copenhagen, November 1978.
17. HOPPENFELD, S. *Physical Examination of the Spine and Extremities.* Appleton-Century-Crofts, New York, 1976.
18. HUANG, C., JACKSON, J. R., MOORE, N. B., FINE, P. R., *et al.* Amputation: Energy Cost of Ambulation. *Arch. Phys. Med. Rehabil. 60:* 18–24, 1979.
19. HUSNI, E. A., ZIEMENES, J. O. C., AND BOYETTE, E. M. Elastic Support of the Lower Limbs in Hospital Patients. A Critical Study. *JAMA 214:* 1456–1462, 1970.
20. JEANS, M., STRATFORD, J. G., MELZACK, R., AND MONKS, R. C. Assessment of Pain. *Can. Fam. Physician 25:* 159–162, 1979.
21. KALTENBORN, F. M. *Manual Therapy for the Extremity Joints. Specialized Techniques: Tests and Joint Mobilisation.* 2nd ed. Olaf Norlis Bokhandel, Oslo, 1976.
22. KENDALL, H. O., AND KENDALL, F. P. *Muscles—Testing and Function,* 1st ed, Williams & Wilkins, Baltimore, 1949.
23. KOERNER, I. The Gait of the Amputee. *J. Can. Physiother. Assoc. 19:* 321–329, 1967.
24. KOERNER, I. Clinic Experiences and Interpretation of the Phantom Limb Phenomenon in Amputee Training. *J. Can. Physiother. Assoc. 21:* 90–100, 1969.
25. KUBLER-ROSS, E. *On Death and Dying.* Collier-Macmillan, London, 1969.
26. *Lower Extremity Prosthetics.* New York University Postgraduate Medical School, Prosthetics and Orthotics, New York, 1971.
27. MACMILLAN, A. H. Personal communication.
28. MCCOLLOUGH, N. G., 3rd. The Dysvascular Amputee: Surgery and Rehabilitation. *Curr. Probl. Surg.* 1–67, 1971.
29. MEDEIROS, J. M., SMIDT, G. L., BURMEISTER, L. F., AND SODERBERG, G. L. The Influence of Isometric Exercise and Passive Stretch on Hip Joint Motion. *Phys. Ther. 57:* 518–523, 1977.
30. MELZACK, R. Phantom Limb Pain: Implications for Treatment of Pathologic Pain. *Anesthesiology 35:* 409–419, 1971.
31. MENSCH, G. Cast Applications Below-Knee and Above-Knee Amputees Prior to Prosthetic Fitting. In *Proceedings of the Sixth World Confederation for Physical Therapy,* pp. 404–412. Amsterdam, 1970.
32. MENSCH, G. Prosthetic Gait Observation: Comparison of Bipedal and Quadrupedal Locomotion. *Physiother. Can. 31:* 269–672, 1979.
33. MENZIES, H., AND NEWNHAM, J. Semi-Rigid Dressings: The Best for Lower Extremity Amputees. *Physiother. Can. 30:* 225–228, 1978.
34. MILES, J., AND LIPTON, S. Phantom Limb Pain Treated by Electrical Stimulation. *Pain 5:* 373–382, 1978.
35. MITAL, M. A., AND PIERCE, D. S. *Amputees and Their Prostheses.* Little, Brown, Boston, 1971.
36. RADCLIFFE, C. W. Biomechanics of Above-Knee Prostheses. In *Prosthetic and Orthotic Practice,* edited by G. Murdoch, pp. 191–211. Edward Arnold, London, 1970.
37. REDFORD, J. B. Experiences in the Use of a Pneumatic Stump Shrinker. *Inter-Clinic Information Bull. Prosthet. Orthotics 12:* 1–7, 1973.
38. SANDERS, J. B., *et al.* The Major Determinants in Normal and Pathological Gait. *J. Bone Joint. Surg. 35A:* 543–548, 1953.
39. SARMIENTO, A. Postoperative Management. *Orthop. Clin. North Am. 3:* 435–446, 1972.
40. SEEBER, J. J., MAGILNER, A., AND REYES, T. Radiologic Technique to Evaluate Patellar-Tendon-Bearing Prosthesis. *Arch. Phys. Med. Rehabil. 53:* 65–69, 1972.
41. SHER, M. H. The Air Splint: an Alternative to the Immediate Postoperative Prosthesis. *Arch. Surg. 108:* 746–747, 1974.

42. SHIPLEY, D. E. Clinical Evaluation and Care of the Insensitive Foot. *Phys. Ther. 59:* 13–18, 1979.
43. SULZLE, H., PAGLIARULO, M., RODGERS, M., AND JORDAN, C. Energetics of the Amputee Gait. *Orthop. Clin. North Am. 9:* 358–362, 1978.
44. WALL, J., AND ROSENROT, P. Department of Human Kinetics, University of Guelph. Personal communication.
45. WATERS, R. L., HISLOP, H. J., PERRY, J., AND ANTONELLI, D. Energetics: Application to the Study and Management of Locomotor Disabilities. Energy Cost of Normal and Pathologic Gait. *Orthop. Clin. North Am. 9:* 351–356, 1978.
46. WINTER, D. A. Energy Assessments in Pathological Gait. *Physiother. Can. 30:* 183–191, 1978.

8

Normal Locomotion and Prosthetic Gait Deviation

V. NANDA KUMAR, M.D.

Human locomotion is a phenomenon of the most extraordinary complexity. Although the primary objective of locomotion may be simply stated as the translation of the body from one point to another by means of a bipedal gait, its analysis requires the collection of large amounts of data in order to follow the entire cycle of events. Full description of locomotion involves consideration of both kinematics and kinetics of the extremities in all their manifold details. Even this complete description would be of little value to the physician unless it were integrated to evolve a concept of locomotion from which deductions can be drawn and applied to the analyses of the clinical problems (17).

Fundamental determinants of gait can be obtained with the aid of a variety of techniques. Since a study of locomotion involves the recording and the measurement of the magnitudes, directions, and rates of changes of the translations, rotations, and forces occurring in the body with respect to the three coordinate axes in space, a number of methods have to be employed. No single technique can provide all the required information. Selection of a particular technique depends on such factors as the simplicity of recording, the ease of deduction of the data, and the accuracy of the findings. Eberhart *et al.*, (7) in their detailed study, described various techniques, which include interrupted light techniques (to study displacement in sagital plane), insertion of pins into the bones (to study the transverse rotations of the limb segments), electromyography, and use of force-plate (to study the gravitational and muscle forces) (Fig. 8.1).

Center of Gravity

The force of gravity acts on the body and its component parts at all times. The limbs may be ragarded, therefore, as weightless levers of the body under static conditions. The center of gravity of the body has been determined by a number of methods. It was found in cadavers by the familiar

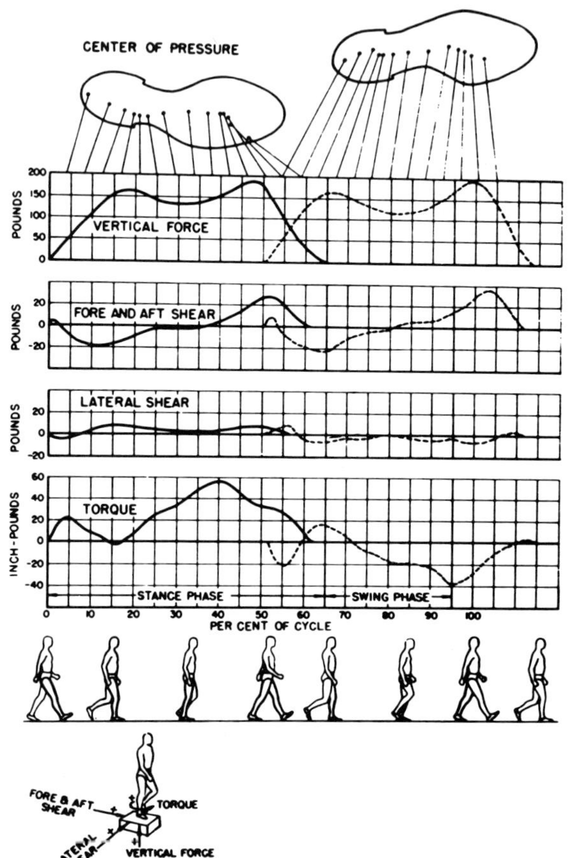

Fig. 8.1. Study of various forces during various phases of gait cycle. (Courtesy of Bennett Wilson, Jr.)

experimental technique of double suspension and in living subjects by the use of a balanced beam. In grown-up men and women, it is found that the center of gravity of the body lies in the midline at a distance from the ground corresponding to about 55% of the total height (SD 1.25%), and it is slightly anterior to the second sacral vertebra.

Gait Cycle

The gait cycle is defined as the sequence of events in the lower extremities from the heel strike of one foot during ambulation to the next heel strike of the same foot. It is subdivided into the stance phase and the swing phase. The stance phase, comprising 60% of the gait cycle, is the time when the foot is touching the ground. The swing phase, comprising the remaining 40% of the gait cycle, is the time when the foot is off the ground, swinging through toward the next heel strike. During this period, the opposite foot is in the stance phase. Between the stance and swing phases, there is a moment when both feet are on the ground supporting the body weight (double support). This moment becomes progressively shorter as the speed of walking is increased. Running is defined as locomotion without this moment of double support.

The normal gait cycle starts at heel strike at 0%, the foot is flat on the ground; at 10%, the heel lifts off; at 45%, the knee bends in preparation for forward acceleration of the leg; and at 60%, the toe lifts off. During the swing phase, both the hip and knee are flexed and the foot is dorsiflexed in order for the toes to clear the ground. At 100% the gait cycle is completed as the heel strikes again.

Displacement of Center of Gravity

The rhythmic up and downward displacement of the body is a feature of locomotion which is familiar to all. These movements reflect the displacement of the center of gravity in the vertical plane. The line described by the center of gravity in the plane of progression is a smooth undulating or sinusoidal curve. This curve can be seen where a small boy holding a piece of chalk against his body at the level of his center of gravity scratches a wavy line on a wall as he walks parallel to it.

In normal locomotion, the amount of vertical displacement in grown-ups is about 2″. Individual variations are negligible. The summits of these sinusoidal waves occur at 25 and 75% of the gait cycle, each corresponding to the middle of the stance phase of the supporting limb; the opposite limb is at this time in the middle of the swing phase. At 50%, or the middle of the cycle, the center of gravity falls to its lowest level (double support).

The center of gravity of the body also is displaced laterally in the horizontal plane. Relative to the plane of progression, the center of gravity describes a sinusoidal curve, the summits of which alternately pass to the right and to the left in association with the support of the weight-bearing limb. The curve is smoothly undulating without irregularities and it is similar in form to that of the vertical displacement. The size of horizontal displacement in normal level walking is about 2″.

When the vertical and horizontal displacements of the centers of gravity of the body are combined and are projected on the coronal plane, they are found to describe an almost perfect figure-8, occupying a 2″ square since the vertical horizontal deviations are almost equal (Figs. 8.2 and 8.3).

Determinants of Gait

PELVIC ROTATION

In normal locomotion on level ground, the pelvis rotates alternately to the right and to the left, relative to the line of progression. At the usual cadence and stride of average persons, the magnitude of this rotation is about 4° on either side of the central axis, or a total of some 8°. Since the

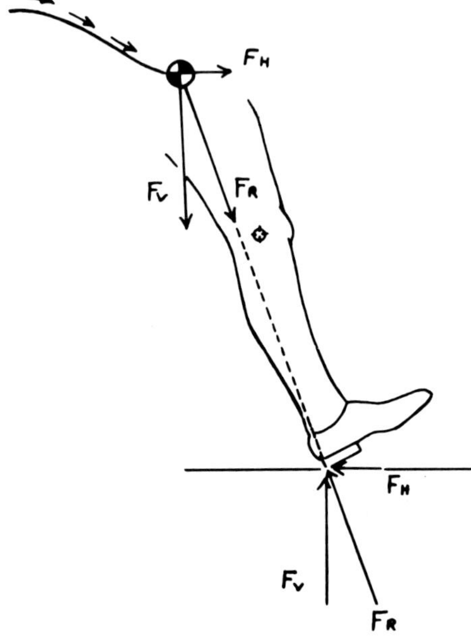

Fig. 8.2. Effect of the forward and downward forces of the center of gravity at heel strike.

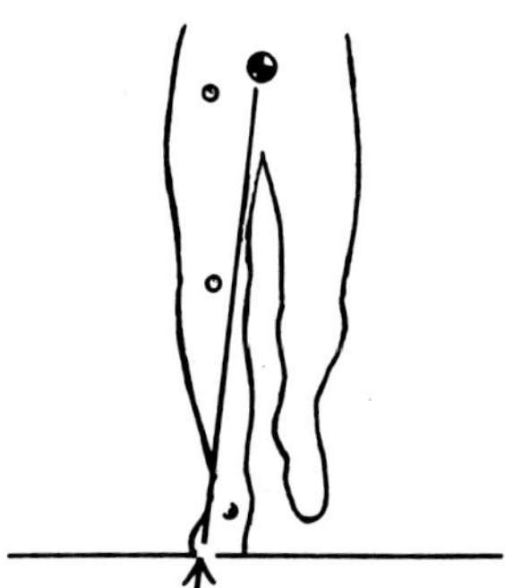

Fig. 8.3. Analysis of mechanical forces in frontal projection.

pelvis is a rigid structure, the rotation occurs alternately at each hip joint which passes from relative internal to external rotation during the stance phase.

PELVIC TILT

In normal level walking, the pelvis is tilted relative to horizontal plane on the same side of the swinging leg (positive Trendelenburg). The alternate angular displacement is about 5°. As a result, the position of the center of gravity is about 0.5 cm lower than it would be otherwise.

KNEE FLEXION IN THE STANCE

In normal locomotion, passage of the body weight over the supporting limb occurs while its knee joint is undergoing flexion. The supporting extremity enters the stance phase at heel strike with the knee joint in full extension. Thereafter, the knee joint begins to flex and continues to do so until the foot is flat on the ground. The average size of this flexion is 15°. This flexion effectively shortens the length of the supporting limb during the stance phase and lowers the normal center of gravity from its highest position (midstance) by about ½″.

The above three determinants of gait all act in the same direction by flattening the arc through which the center of gravity of the body is translated. The relative lengthening of the extremities reduces materially the range of flexion and extension at the hip joint required to maintain the same length of stride. The relative elongation of the limbs plays an important role in permitting increased velocities of gait at slight increases in energy cost, since greater velocities of locomotion are achieved by the lengthening of the stride rather than by increasing in cadance.

FOOT AND ANKLE MOTION

On heel strike, the ankle arcs down to its lowest position as the entire foot is on the ground. As the heel lifts off, the ankle arcs up to its highest position at toe off. During the swing phase, the ankle does not normally influence the center of gravity. Ankle motion is synchronized with the movement of the center of gravity so that it smooths out the abrupt change in its direction at the lowest portion of the curve, thereby reducing declaration and acceleration.

ANKLE AND KNEE MOTION

Synchronization of ankle and knee motion is considered the fifth determinant.

LATERAL DISPLACEMENT OF PELVIS

Lateral displacement of the pelvis produces horizontal movement of the center of gravity. Since weight is shifted from one foot to the other when walking, balance is maintained by moving the center of gravity alternately over the base of support, which is each foot during stance phase. If femur and tibia formed a straight line from the hip joint to the foot, the lateral shift of the center of gravity would be considerable. The femoral neck-shaft angle and femoral-tibial angle reduce the amplitude of this diplacement. In women, the femoral-tibial angle is greater because of a wider pelvis. In locomotion, the alternate horizontal movement of the center of gravity traces a sinusoidal path with an amplitude of less than 2″.

Any change in kinematics alters the determinants of gait and affects the path traced by the center of gravity, either by an increase in amplitude or, more likely, by more rapid acceleration or deceleration, which will increase energy consumption, or by both.

AXIAL ROTATION

During the gait cycle there is also axial rotation of the lower extremity the extent of which is dependent on the speed of walking. At the normal rate of ambulation, the total rotation is about 22–23°, but at a faster rate, it may exceed 35°. The total rotation is divided as follows: 5° of pelvic rotation, 9° of rotation of the femur and 9° of rotation of the tibia. During the swing phase, progressive axial internal rotation occurs, continuing into the stance phase to full weight bearing. At this point, a rather sudden reversal into axial external rotation occurs just about as the foot is to leave the ground. In addition, the subtalar angle moves toward eversion during the first third of the stance phase and reverses toward inversion of the foot during the later part of the stance phase; the total angular change in eversion and inversion is approximately 6° (13).

Muscle Activity During Gait Cycle

Muscle activity powers the gait cycle (10). None of the muscle groups are working full time. During gait cycle, each muscle contracts for a short time. These intermittent contractions facilitate blood flow, as it increases while the muscles are relaxing. The muscles then recover sources of energy for further contraction. The various muscle activity described below is in a subject with normal cadence of 100 steps/min.

At heel strike, the dorsiflexors of the foot are maximally contracted. The ankle joint is in neutral position (90°), the knee is fully extended (180°), and the hip is at 25° of flexion. The extensors of knee and hip also are active (Fig. 8.4).

As the cycle progresses into foot flat, the dorsiflexors of the foot let the foot down gradually by a lengthening contraction, which functions like a shock absorber. During this process, the ankle is 15° plantar flexed, the knee develops 20° flexion, and the hip flexion decreases to 20–22°. The extensors of knee and hip continue to be active (Fig. 8.5).

During midstance, the dorsiflexors are minimally active as the activity shifts to the plantar flexors. The ankle tends to develop a small amount of dorsiflexion (2–3°), the knee is in 10° flexion, and the hip is in 10° flexion. The quadriceps continue to be active, and the hip flexors start contracting, (Fig. 8.6).

As the gait progresses to heel off, the calf muscles, primarily gastrocnemius and soleus, are active maximally, providing strong plantar flexion of the foot which lifts the body and propels it forward. The ankle tends to stay in about 15° of dorsiflexion, the knee stays in minimal flexion of 2° and the hip stays in 10° extension. At this point, the hamstrings contract to maintain the hip extension and to prevent the knee from buckling under (Fig. 8.7).

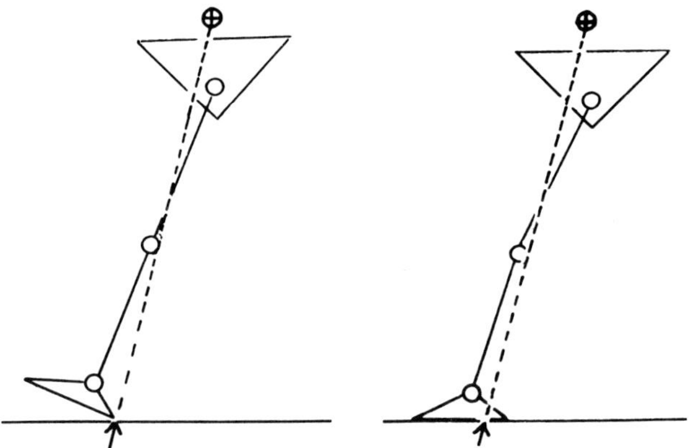

Fig. 8.4. (*Left*) Analysis of mechanical forces at heel strike. Fig. 8.5. (*Right*) Mechanical forces at foot flat.

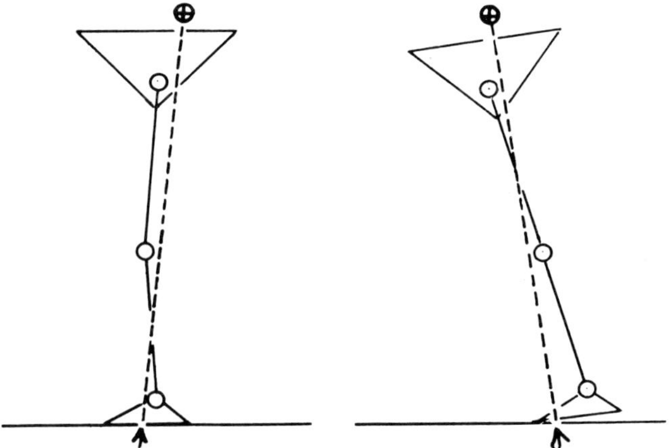

Fig. 8.6. (*Left*) Mechanical forces in midstance. Fig. 8.7. (*Right*) Mechanical forces at heel off.

During toe off, the plantar flexors are maximally contracted (concentric), with peroneal muscles as stabilizers of the ankle joint. The ankle goes into 20° of plantar flexion, the knee develops 40° of flexion and there is 10° of hip flexion. The eccentric contraction of quadriceps helps maintain the flexion at knee, and the hip flexors are active in preparation for the acceleration phase (Fig. 8.8).

Accleration phase occurs at the end of the stance phase when the rectus femoris contracts, producing hip flexion and forward acceleration of leg. Hamstrings participate with a lengthening contraction to prevent excessive heel rise. The dorsiflexors of the foot tend to be active in an attempt to

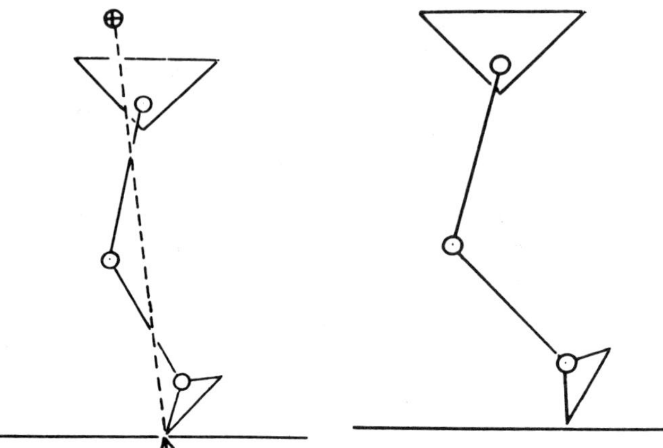

Fig. 8.8. (*Left*) Mechanical forces at toe off. Fig. 8.9. (*Right*) Position of joints in acceleration phase.

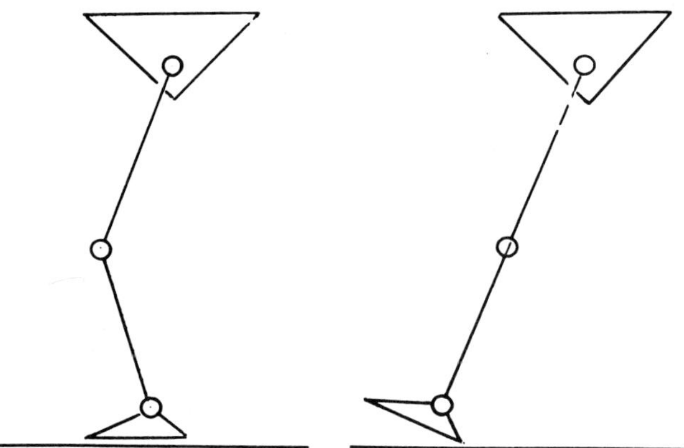

Fig. 8.10. (*Left*) Position of joints in mid-swing. Fig. 8.11. (*Right*) Deceleration phase.

clear the toes off the ground. Initially, the ankle is in 20° of plantar flexion, the knee is in 65° of flexion, and the hip is in 5° of flexion (Fig. 8.9).

In midswing, the ankle reaches a neutral position (90°) with dorsiflexors still active. The knee continues in flexion (65°) with early initiation of extension movement. The hip flexion increases to 25° with increased activity of hip flexors (Fig. 8.10).

Finally, the deceleration sets in with the ankle at 90° (dorsiflexors still active), and the knee reaches full extension (180°) with strengthening contraction of hamstrings. At this point the hip extensors are active as the hip remains flexed at 25° (Fig. 8.11).

Analyzing the gait in a frontal plane, varus and valgus forces can be studied at different joint levels. At the subtalar joint, varus stress occurs between heel strike and foot flat and between heel off and toe off. The main muscles which are active are peroneus longus and peroneus brevis. Valgus stress appears between foot flat and heel off and the main muscles which are active are posterior tibial, flexor digitorum longus and flexor hallucis longus. In the knee, varus stress occurs at heel off and this stress is controlled by lateral collateral ligament. No valgus stress is noted at the knee during normal gait. At the hip, considerable varus stress occurs and muscles responsible to counteract this force are gluteus minimus, gluteus medius, and tensor fasciar latae. No valgus stress is noticeable at the hip as the line of resultant force is medially placed.

Prosthetic Gait Deviations

It is very important that deviations in gait be analyzed in a systematic fashion. Snap judgements should not be made from seemingly similar patterns. For any deviation from normal, it is most important to determine not only what the deviation is and what parts of the body it involves, but also at what point it occurs during the gait cycle.

The examiner should do a general appraisal of the gait observing the following: 1) symmetry of movements of any part of the body and of any phase of the gait cycle, such as length of stride, arm swing, movement of the trunk, and rise of the body; 2) smoothness of movements; 3) normal-based, narrow- or wide based gait; and 4) presence of pain, noting when and where it occurs.

The examiner also should observe the patient from side, front and back to get a three-dimensional view of the gait pattern.

Gait Analysis of Above Knee Amputee

1. *Abducted gait:* This is a very wide-based gait with the prosthesis held away from the midline at all times.
   a. Prosthetic causes:
      1) Prosthesis could be too long.
      2) Too much abduction may have been built into prosthesis.
      3) High medial wall may press on pubic ramus causing amputee to hold prosthesis in an abducted position.
      4) Poorly contoured lateral wall can fail to provide adequate support for femur.
   b. Amputee causes:
      1) Abduction contracture.
      2) Habit pattern.
2. *Lateral bending:* Lateral bending of trunk is characterized by excessive bending laterally from the midline, usually to the prosthetic side.
   a. Prosthetic causes:
      1) Prosthesis could be too short.

2) High medial wall, producing pressure and discomfort to crotch area.
3) Poorly contoured lateral wall which provides inadequate support for femur.
4) Prosthesis aligned in abduction may cause wide-based gait, leading to lateral bending in gait.

b. Amputee causes:
1) Poor balance.
2) Abduction contracture.
3) Stump may be painful.
4) Very short stump may fail to provide a sufficient lever arm for pelvis.
5) Habit pattern.

3. *Vaulting:* This is characterized by a rising on the toe of the normal foot permitting the amputee to swing the prothesis through with little knee flexion.
   a. Prosthetic causes:
   1) Prosthesis could be too long.
   2) Socket suspension may be inadequate.
   3) Excessive stability in alignment of prothesis.
   4) Limitation of knee flexion such as a knee lock or a strong extension aide.

   b. Amputee causes:
   1) Fear of stubbing toe.
   2) Stump discomfort.
   3) Habit pattern.
4. *Circumducted gait:* In this gait, the amputee swings the prosthesis laterally in a wide arc during swing phase.
   a. Prosthetic causes:
   1) Prothesis could be too long.
   2) Prosthesis may be having too much friction in knee, making it difficult to bend knee in swing through.

   b. Amputee causes:
   1) Abduction contracture of hip on the amputated side.
   2) Muscle weakness, leading to patient's hesitance to flex prosthetic knee.
5. *Medial or lateral whip:* These are observed best when the patient walks away from the observer. A medial whip is said to be present when the heel moves medially on initial flexion at the beginning of swing phase. A lateral whip is present when the heel moves laterally.
   a. Prosthetic causes:
   1) Medial whip may result from excessive external rotation of knee.
   2) Lateral whip is result of excessive internal rotation of mechanical knee.

3) Socket may fit too tightly, thus reflecting stump rotation.
4) Excessive valgus in mechanical knee.
5) Malaligned toe break in a conventional foot may cause twisting on toe off.

b. Amputee causes:
1) Faulty habit pattern.

6. *Foot Slap:* This is a too rapid descent of the anterior portion of the prosthetic foot.
a. Prosthetic causes:
1) Plantar flexion resistance is too soft.
b. Amputee causes:
1) Driving prosthesis down rather forcibly to assure extension of knee.

7. *Rotation of prosthetic foot on heel strike:*
a. Prosthetic causes:
1) Too much resistance to plantar flexing by plantar flexion bumper or heel wedge.
2) Too much toe out may have been built into prothesis.
3) Loosely fitting socket.
4) Gluteus maximus too tight in socket.
b. Amputee causes:
1) Too vigorous extension of stump at heel strike.
2) Poor muscle control of stump.

8. *Uneven heel rise:* This is characterized by the prosthetic heel rising markedly and quickly when the knee is flexed at the beginning of swing phase.
a. Prosthetic causes:
1) Knee joint has insufficient friction.
2) Knee joint has inadequate extension aide.
b. Amputee causes:
1) Using more force than necessary to force knee into flexion.

9. *Uneven timing:* This is characterized by steps of unequal duration, usually a short stance phase on the prosthetic side.
a. Prosthetic causes:
1) Improperly fitting socket causing pain may result in desire to shorten the stance phase on prosthetic side.
2) Weak extension aide of insufficient friction in prosthetic knee can cause excessive heel rise and result in uneven timing because of a prolonged swing through.
3) Knee may be buckling due to faulty alignment.
b. Amputee causes:
1) Weak musculature of stump.
2) Poor balance.
3) Fear and insecurity.

10. *Uneven arm swing:* This is characterized by the arm on the prosthetic side held close to the body during locomotion.
    a. Prosthetic causes: None.
    b. Amputee causes:
        1) Poor balance.
        2) Fear and insecurity.
        3) Habit pattern.
11. *Instability of the mechanical knee:* This could cause patient to fall.
    a. Prosthetic causes:
        1) Knee joint is too anterior to the trochanter-knee-ankle reference line (TKA alignment).
        2) Initial flexion built into socket may be insufficient.
        3) Plantar flexion resistance may be too great, causing knee to buckle at heel strike.
        4) Failure to limit dorsiflexion can lead to incomplete knee control.
    b. Amputee causes:
        1) Hip extensor weakness.
        2) Severe hip flexion contracture.
12. *Terminal swing impact:* This is characterized by rapid forward movement of the shin piece allowing the knee to reach maximum extension with too much force before heel strike.
    a. Prosthetic causes:
        1) Knee extension aide may be too strong.
        2) Inadequate knee friction.
    b. Amputee causes:
        1) Deliberate and forced extension of stump to get knee in full extension.
13. *Long prosthetic step:* This is noted when the patient takes a longer step with the prosthesis than with normal leg.
    a. Prosthetic causes:
        1) Inadequate initial flexion in socket.
    b. Amputee causes:
        1) Flexion contracture which cannot be accommodated prosthetically.
14. *Drop off at the end of stance phase:* This is characterized by a downward movement of the trunk as the body shifts forward over the prosthesis.
    a. Prosthetic causes:
        1) Limitation of dorsiflexion of prosthetic foot may be inadequate.
        2) Heel of a SACH type foot may be too short.
        3) Socket may have been placed too far anterior in relation to foot.
    b. Amputee causes: None.
15. *Excessive trunk extension:* This occurs during stance phase in which the amputee creates an active lumbar lordosis.

a. Prosthetic causes:
   1) Inadequately moulded posterior wall may cause forward rotation of pelvis to avoid full weight bearing on ischium.
   2) Initial flexion built into socket may be inadequate.
b. Amputee causes:
   1) Hip flexor tighteness.
   2) Weak hip extensors and amputee may be substituting lumbar erector spinae.
   3) Weak abdominal musculature.
   4) Moving the shoulders backward in an effort to obtain better balance.

Energy Costs of Gait

The professionals involved in prosthetic rehabilitation of lower limb amputation require a good working knowledge in 1) how to increase the amount of work the patient can do with the residual functional parts of his/her body, and 2) how to decrease the amount of work required by the use of adaptive devices and environmental manipulation (3). This knowledge helps the rehabilitation worker to set realistic goals for his/her amputees in their daily activities.

The terminology used in this area should be clearly defined and units of measurements well understood. The commonly used terms are: work is equal to force, times distance. In walking, the force is mainly the gravity and friction plus the inertia of acceleration and deceleration. The distance is the up-and-down motion of the body and its separate parts. Power is the rate of doing work:

$$\text{Power} = \frac{\text{Force} \times \text{Distance}}{\text{Time}}$$

The power available, *i.e.* the rate at which a patient can expend energy for the work of walking, usually limits walking speed.

The only source of energy that the human body can utilize is the chemical energy contained in complex food molecules (2). The oxidation of these to simpler substances such as water and carbon dioxide is an exothermic reaction:

$$\text{Glucose} + O_2 = \text{Water} + \text{Energy}$$

A variety of body functions, such as maintenance of a pressure gradient in the arterial system, breathing, maintenance of body temperature, etc., need energy expenditure, even at rest. The efficiency of muscle action rarely exceeds 25% and average closer to 10%, so most of the energy expended during physical exertion is lost as heat.

The units of measurement of work are expressed in kilocalorie or "large calorie." The units of power are expressed in kilocalories ("large calorie")/ min. One kcal/min is approximately the basal metabolic rate for an average sized adult (3).

TECHNIQUES OF MEASURING ENERGY COSTS

The common technique used is called indirect calorimetry. This involves measurement of oxygen consumed and was introduced by Atwater during the late 19th century. An average of 4.83 kcal of energy is released when 1 liter of oxygen is consumed to oxidise an ordinary diet. In most systems used to measure human oxygen consumption, the expired air is collected, its volume measured, the expired oxygen concentration determined, and the expired volume of O_2 subtracted from the oxygen in the inspired ambient air.

The method of collecting expired air is in a rubber-impregnated canvas Douglas bag or a neoprene bag, especially when studying moving patients (amputee gait).

In 1970, Corcoran and Brengelmann (4) described another system for evaluating energy cost of ambulation which was safe, permitted precise measurement of speed and oxygen consumption and allowed use of the subjects' usual walking environment. This system is called SCRAM (speed-controlled respirometer for ambulation measurement).

During the test the subject breathed room air through a rubber mouthpiece with his nose held closed by a spring clip. Low resistance one-way flutter valves were placed close to the mouthpiece to keep respiratory dead space to a minimum. A lever was connected to a three-way valve so that turning it upward at the desired time initiated a collection of expired air which passed directly to a 120-liter neoprene balloon. The same valve simultaneously diverted inspired air through one of two previously calibrated standard gas meters, mounted on the SCRAM to measure ventilatory volume. The subject walked beside the SCRAM which was pushed by the investigator at a preset speed. Expiratory tubes of lightweight plastic connected the subject to the SCRAM.

The investigator controlled the speed on the basis of two sources of auditory signals fed to a set of earphones. One earphone received a click each time a switch was triggered by a lug on one wheel of the SCRAM. This switch discharged a capacitor causing one click to occur for every complete revolution of the wheel. To the other earphone was fed a steady clicking rate from an electronic signal generator set at a predetermined frequency, corresponding to the desired speed. The operator pushed the SCRAM at a speed so that the two clicks from the two signals were synchronous. This method of speed control has less than 2% variation, exceeding the accuracy of many motor driven treadmills (4).

ENERGY COST DURING AMBULATION

Large numbers of subjects were studied and the data on the energy cost of ambulation was analyzed by McDonald (11). In his study he found heavy persons using more energy at a specific walking speed, but when corrected for the weight of the subjects, the metabolic cost of walking is similar to lighter, normal subjects. Age and height have no effect, but female subjects usually show about 10% lower energy expenditure at a given speed.

The energy costs of ambulation increase as walking speed increases. This relationship is curvilinear; at faster walking speeds a further increment in speed will necessitate a greater increase in oxygen consumption than at lower speed (15). The amount of work done in walking a given distance is greater at very slow speeds than at ordinary walking speeds. It is known that the calorie cost of walking a given distance is lowest at a walking speed of around 3 mph and does not exceed the 5 kcal/min limit for sustained work without accumulating an oxygen debt. Bard and Ralston (1), found that patients with abnormal ambulation also tend to select the walking speeds at which the work of walking the desired distance is minimal. This optimal speed may not be possible if the energy costs exceeds 5 kcal/min, or if the cardiovascular or respiratory capacity is diminished (5).

The energy cost of ambulation on a 10% gradient is about double the energy cost of ambulation on level ground; on a 20–25% upgrade, the rate of energy cost is tripled. On down grades the energy cost is lowest at a 10% grade and rises again on steeper down grades.

Extra weight added to the subject in the form of extra weight or clothing and equipment causes a linear increase in the energy cost of ambulation. Added loads are carried most efficiently on the head, somewhat less efficiently on the back, and still less efficiently in the hands, and least efficiently on the feet. The addition of 2½ lb. to shoe weight can increase the energy cost of ambulation by 5 to 10%. This is due to the greater gravitational force exerted during the up and down excursions of the feet during the gait cycle, as well as to the greater mass that must be accelerated and decelerated at the end of the limb. The implications for prosthetic design are obvious (3). Soft or uneven ground can increase the energy demands by 40% or more. Climbing stairs requires from 6–12 kcal/min depending on body weight and speed. Descending stairs required only one-third as much energy.

ENERGY COSTS OF AMBULATION IN LOWER EXTREMITY AMPUTATIONS

Several studies have shown that people spontaneously select a comfortable walking speed (CWS) that coincides with the lowest caloric cost (4, 5, 15). The comfortable walking speed of below-knee amputees was found to be 3.5 ft/sec, which is approximately 22% slower than normal (4–5 ft/sec). The energy costs at these two speeds were approximately equal, meaning that a below-knee amputee spent as much energy walking at 3.5 ft/sec as a normal subject walking at 4.5 ft/sec Gonzalez and associates (9) studying a group of unilateral below-knee amputees with various stump lengths found stump length had no influence upon comfortable walking speeds. Both the short stump and long stump groups had CWS of 3.5 ft/sec (2.4 mph or 3.86 km/hr) which was 22% slower than normal. However, a statistically significant negative correlation between length of stump and increase in energy expenditure was obtained. Patients with long stumps average a 10% increase, whereas those with short stumps averaged a 40% increase in energy expenditure above normal. In this study, however, other major determinants affecting speed, such as age, sex, duration of amputation, general physical condition, associated other medical conditions, and the prosthetic type and fit were not considered in the analysis.

Studying (19) various subgroups in lower limb amputations, it was found that the CWS (expressed as a percentage of the average value for the normal group of controls) for vascular amputees was 66% at Symes amputation level, 59% at the below-knee level, and 44% at the above-knee level. In traumatic amputees it was 87% in the below-knee level and 63% at the above-knee level. The traumatic amputees walked faster than patients with vascular amputation above- or below-knee, primarily because of the differences in age. Cummings and associates (6) studied energy costs of below-knee prosthesis using two types of suspension. They are cuff suspension and side-joint-thigh corset suspension which add some extra weight but provides extra stability. They found no clear cut difference between the energy costs of supracondylar cuff *versus* side-joint-thigh corset.

The data on energy costs of ambulation in above-knee amputees is rather scant and the samples studied are small. Ralston (16) in a study of 17 above-knee amputees more than 50 years of age, using a prosthesis, found 55% above normal oxygen consumption. Miller and Hettinger (12), reported 24%–50% above normal oxygen consumption in three traumatic amputees from 30–38 years of age. Erdman *et al.* (8), studied 9 above-knee amputees from 18–65 years of age, comparing axillary crutch walking without a prosthesis, and prosthetic ambulation. They concluded that poor ambulators consumed less O_2 using axillary crutches without a prosthesis than with prosthetic walking. They added that there is an increase in the pulse rate of 39% with crutch walking, which would cause a heavier work load on the heart.

In a more controlled study (18) of the above-knee amputees, it was found that crutch walking (62% above normal) and prosthetic ambulation (65% above normal) require the same energy expenditure. There was no significant difference between the energy requirements of ambulating with knee locked (59% above normal) or unlocked (67% above normal). More energy (65%) was required at approximately one-half the normal speed of ambulation for the above-knee amputee as compared to a normal person. Wheelchair propulsion with no prosthesis required 47% less oxygen consumption than ambulating with the prosthesis.

A hydraulic knee unit requires the same energy expenditure as a constant friction knee joint at comfortable walking speeds (2.1 mph), but about 10% less energy at 2.7 mph, and permits a higher maximum walking speed (3.3 mph) (14). The speed of an above-knee amputee is limited by the resonance frequency of the prosthesis. Patients automatically select the step length at which the energy cost is minimal (12).

REFERENCES

1. BARD, G., AND RALSTON, H. J. Measurement of Energy Expenditure during Ambulation, with Special Reference to Evaluation of Assistive Devices. *Arch. Phys. Med. Rehabil., 40:* 415–20, 1959.
2. BROWN, A. C., AND BRENGELMANN, G. Energy Metabolism. In *Physiology and Biophysics*, 19th ed., pp. 1030–1049. W. B. Saunders, Philadelphia, 1965.
3. CORCORAN, P. J. Energy Expenditure During Ambulation. In *Psysiological Basis of Rehabilitation Medicine*; edited by J. A. Downey and R. C. Darling, Chap. 10, pp. 185–197. W. B. Saunders, Philadelphia, 1971.
4. CORCORAN, P. J., AND BRENGELMANN, G. L. Oxygen Uptake in Normal and Handicapped Subjects in Relation to Speed of Walking Beside Velocity-Controlled Cart. *Arch. Phys. Med. Rehabil., 51:* 78–87, 1970.
5. CORCORAN, P. J., JEBSEN, R. H., BRENGELMANN, G. L., AND SIMONS, B. C. Effects of Plastic Metal Leg Braces on Speed and Energy Cost of Hemiparetic Condition. *Arch. Phys. Med. Rehabil., 51:* 69–77, 1970.
6. CUMMINGS, V., MARCH, H., STEVE, L., AND ROBINSON, K. G. Energy Costs of Below-Knee Prosthesis Using Two Types of Suspension. *Arch. Phys. Med. Rehabil., 60:* 293–297, 1979.
7. EBERHART, H. D., INMAN, V. T., SAUNDERS, J. B., LEVENS, A. S., BLRESLER, B., AND MCGOWEN, T. D. *Fundamental Studies on Human Locomotion and other Information Relating to Design of Artificial Limbs. A Report to the National Research Council, Committee on Artificial Limbs.* University of California, Berkeley, 1947.
8. ERDMAN, W. J., HETTINGER, T., AND SEZ, F. Comparative Work Stress for Above-Knee Amputees Using Artificial Legs or Crutches. *Am. J. Phys. Med., 39:* 225–232, 1960.
9. GONZALEZ, E. G., CORCORAN, P. F., AND RODOLFO, L. R. Energy Expenditure in Below-Knee Amputee: Correlation with Stump Length; *Arch. Phys. Med. Rehabil., 55:* 111–119, 1974.
10. KLOPSTEG, P. E., AND WILSON, C. D. Presenting Results of Engineering and Medical Studies of Human Extremities and Application of Data to Design and Fitting of Artificial Limbs and to Care and Training of Amputees. In *Human Limbs and Their Substitutes*, edited by P. E. Klopsteg and P. D. Wilson. Hafner, New York, 1969 Repr. of 1954 edition.
11. MCDONALD, I. Statistical Studies of Recorded Energy Expenditure of Man and Expenditure of Walking Related to Weight, Sex, Age, Height, Speed and Gradient. *Natl. Abst. Rev., 31:* 739–762, 1961.
12. MILLER, E. A., AND HETTINGER, T. Arbeits Physiologiche Unterswchwngen Verschiedener Oberschenkel—Kunstbeine. *Z. Orthop, 81:* 525–545, 1952.
13. PIEZER, E., WRIGHT, D. W., AND MASON, C. Human Locomotion. *Bull. Prosthet. Res.*, pp 10–12; 48–105, 1969.
14. RADCLIFFE, C. W., AND RALSTON, H. J. *Performance Characteristics of Fluid Controlled Prosthetic Knee Mechanisms, Report No. 49.* University of California Biomechanics Laboratory, San Francisco, 1963.

15. RALSTON, H. J. Energy-Speed Relation and Optimal Speed During Level Walking. *Int. Z. Angew. Physiol, 17:* 277–283, 1958.
16. RALSTON, H. J. *Conference on Geriatric Amputee, Publication 19,* pp 151–153. National Academy of Sciences—National Research Council, Washington, D.C., 1961.
17. SAUNDERS, J. B., INMAN, V. T., AND EBERHART, H. D. The Major Determinants in Normal and Pathological Gait. *J. Bone Jt. Surg., 35A:* 543–358, 1953.
18. TRAUGH, G. H., CORCORAN, P. J., AND REYES, R. L. Energy Expenditure of Ambulation in Patients with the Above-Knee Amputations. *Arch. Phys. Med. Rehabil., 56:* 67–71, 1975.
19. WATERS, R. L., PERRY, J. P., ANTONELLI, D., AND HISLOP, H. Energy Cost of Walking of Amputees: The Influence of Level of Amputation. *J. Bone Jt. Surg., 58A:* 41–46, Jan. 1976.

9

Adaptive Devices for Amputees and Training of Upper Extremity Amputees

A. Training of Upper Extremity Amputees

HANNA HEGER, O.T.(C)

To achieve successful vocational and social rehabilitation of the amputee the coordinated effort of all members of the rehabilitation team is necessary. The training is designed to meet the specific needs of the individual amputee. This includes assistance in his/her psychological adjustment to the amputation and the prosthesis. Careful assessment of personal and social needs, interests, abilities and pertinent physical factors is necessary to ensure provision of a prosthesis that will meet the specific demands and provide optimum service. The training facilitates acceptance of the artificial limb by encouraging the amputee to learn to use it to its full potential and providing him/her with guidance for developing the necessary skills.

It is essential that the amputee is seen as a whole person with all the needs he/she presents. The amputee also needs to be seen as a member of the treatment team, provided with pertinent information and encouraged to actively participate in his/her rehabilitation.

In order to promote acceptance and good use of the prosthesis it also is important that the amputee be fitted with a prosthesis as early as possible to let him/her reestablish a bilateral work habit before he/she becomes adapted to a single-handed mode of life. Even in a well motivated amputee a long delay between amputation and prosthetic fitting may result in considerable reluctance to accept the prosthesis as a useful appliance since the functional gain that it provides may not be immediately apparent to the amputee. He/she has to change those acquired motor habits and overcome the initial awkwardness encountered in learning to use the prosthesis, as well as adapt to the discomfort caused by weight and harness.

Psychological Adjustment

Of all of the intricate functions of hand and arm, the prosthesis can only replace basic functions of grasp, push, pull, lift and carry, while sensation remains lacking. For the unilateral amputee the prosthesis is a practical aid for the remaining hand and can provide relative cosmetic compensation. For the bilateral amputee the prostheses are indispensable to achieve independence in daily living activities. To establish a satisfactory relationship between the amputee and his/her prosthesis the limb must be integrated into the amputee's sphere of activity and become part of his/her body image.

The loss of a limb and prosthetic replacement result in a change of body image, self-concept and social interaction and may necessitate considerable changes in the life style of the amputee. The response to this loss and to the required adjustment can vary greatly. The therapist needs to understand the normal adjustment process which follows traumatic injury and physical disability and recognize the reactions of the amputee and his/her individual schedule of the adjustment process. Encouraging a positive attitude towards self in present and future situations will aid the amputee in adjusting to the new circumstances and enhance a successful return to vocational and social roles. The therapist needs to be interested in the whole person and needs to listen with empathy, facilitating acceptance and verbal and nonverbal expression of feelings. Support may be necessary to help the amputee develop appropriate ways of dealing with feelings of anger and resentment. Without this, repressed feelings can have a detrimental effect on training and successful rehabilitation.

The amputee needs to feel accepted by others and to accept and respect him/herself as the whole person he/she still is, in spite of the amputation and the imposed limitations. Support in mourning the loss and accepting the limitations may be necessary. The amputee also may need to be made aware of accomplishments and the satisfaction they provide. He/she needs to develop remaining or latent abilities and to learn to choose realistic goals. Focusing on strengths and assets, assisting the amputee in gaining independence and providing him/her with opportunities to accomplish successfully familiar and new tasks will help him/her to increase self-confidence and reduce anxiety.

Working successfully alongside other patients in the occupational therapy department can help the amputee to regain self-assurance in social contacts. There also may be the opportunity to observe other amputees and gain from their experience. Care should be taken to structure the program to individual needs and evaluate performance independently. Although competition occasionally can be a useful aid, an amputee should not be compelled to compete with other amputees if this could be detrimental to his/her progress.

Pre-Prosthetic Training

The preprosthetic training covers the period from amputation to fitting with a prosthesis. During this time the patient receives information about the prosthesis and the rehabilitation program. The stump is prepared for prosthetic fitting and the patient's general physical condition is maintained or improved. Independence in self-care activities is stressed. The training period is used to gather information for prosthetic prescription. Any accompanying injuries are treated as necessary.

ORIENTATION

The amputee will appreciate information about specific aspects of his/her rehabilitation program such as the stages of prosthetic fitting and training, the length of the training, the nature of vocational and financial assistance. He/she needs to know what will be expected of him/her and what he/she may expect from the therapist and the other members of the treatment team. Often the amputee has only a vague idea about a prosthesis. In order to form realistic expectations about its appearance and function he/she needs to be informed about the basic components of the prosthesis and the mode of control, as well as the functional use and inherent limitations. If possible, the amputee should be shown a sample of the type of prosthesis he/she will receive. He/she also should be made aware of the available options and be informed about new developments in the prosthetic field.

To develop in the patient a positive attitude towards the artificial limb, the therapist needs to be aware of the concerns of the amputee in terms of function and cosmesis. The prosthesis should be presented in a meaningful way such as a helping limb—a tool to accomplish tasks otherwise impossible or more difficult to do—and as an extension of the body that the amputee may learn to integrate into his/her body image.

PHANTOM SENSATION

Most amputees seek information about the phantom sensation, however, some may be afraid for fear of being regarded as crazy or as having hallucinations. They are usually relieved to hear that it is a common natural phenomenon in amputees, which is usually caused by impulses from the cut nerve endings to the brain. These sensations should not be referred to as phantom pain, as many amputees tend to do, unless the sensations are painful. Supportive counselling, use of the stump and early fitting with a prosthesis have a positive effect. The amputee also is encouraged to consciously relax the phantom hand, without trying too hard, and to "exercise" it by opening and closing the hand and by moving the fingers and wrist for a few minutes at a time. Many amputees find this helpful in diminishing unpleasant sensations of cramps, tightness etc.

CARE OF STUMP

The amputee is instructed in the daily care of his/her stump: to wash the stump, exercising particular care in the folds of the skin; to dry it thoroughly by blotting and not by rubbing the skin; and finally, to inspect the stump for any evidence of irritation.

If the amputee objects to the word "stump," other words such as "arm" or "remaining arm" can be used.

PREPARING STUMP FOR PROSTHETIC FITTING

Bandaging

An effective program of bandaging with tensor bandages aids in preventing and reducing edema, in reducing subcutaneous fat, in promoting circulation in conjunction with exercise and in forming the stump for prosthetic fitting. All stumps shrink through disuse tissue atrophy. However, the use of bandaging in conjunction with a temporary prosthesis maximizes the shrinkage in the first 3 months after the amputation, thereby permitting a better fit of the permanent prosthesis.

Gentle bandaging can be started over the dressing about 3–4 days after the operation. After the stitches have been removed the bandage can be applied directly with normal tension, barring any contraindications such as a skin graft. For best results, the bandage is worn continuously, except later when the amputee wears the prosthesis. It is reapplied three times a day or whenever the tension is lost. The amputee is taught to apply the bandage her/himself (Figs 9.A-1–9.A-4) and the therapist checks it periodically. The stump should be measured at regular intervals to assess the amount of stump shrinkage.

Instructions for Bandaging

Before applying the tensor bandage, make sure that the stump is clean. The skin will break down if hygiene is neglected.

Use a firm clean bandage of the correct size (3″–4″), single or double length depending on the size and length of the stump.

Change bandages regularly for maximum elasticity.

Bandage all areas of the stump firmly leaving no bulging areas; this ensures even shrinkage.

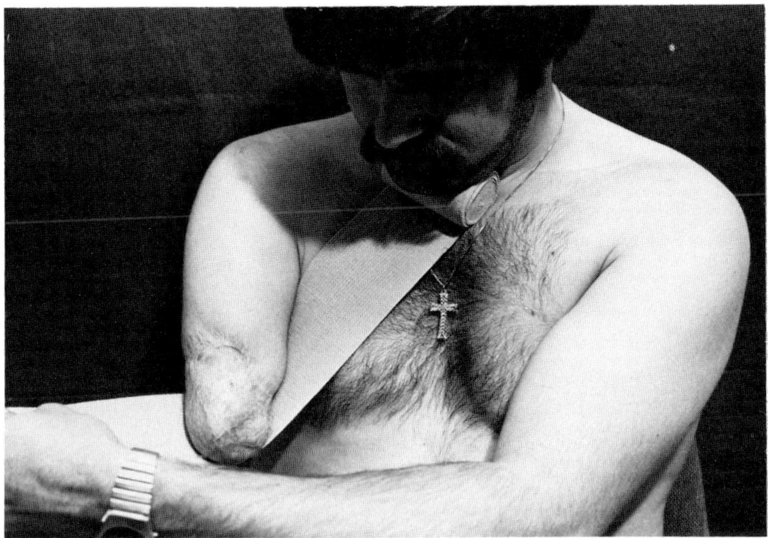

Fig. 9.A-1. The amputee bandages his stump by himself.

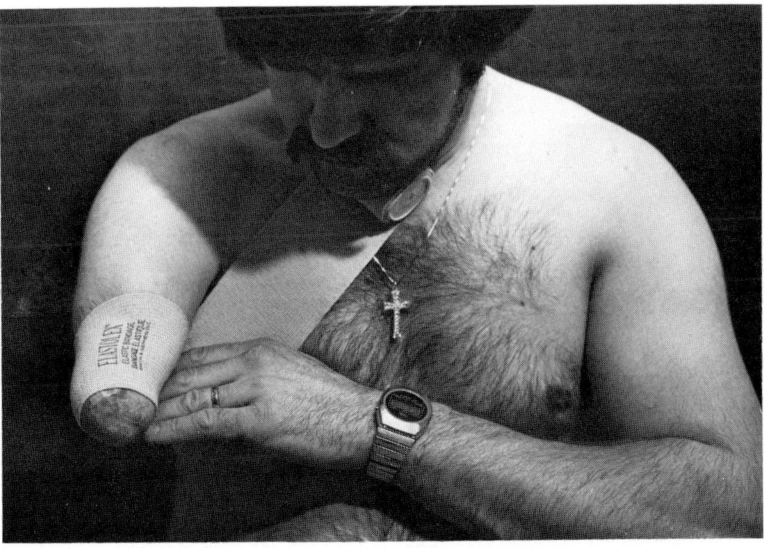

Fig. 9.A-2. He tucks the end of the bandage under the stretched part of the bandage, making sure that the bandage is applied in a diagonal direction.

Control tension carefully and graduate pressure evenly, applying the greatest pressure at the stump end.

Avoid wrinkles, pleats, tucks or infolding of the skin, as this will cause discomfort.

Make certain the bandage extends high enough on the arm and stays

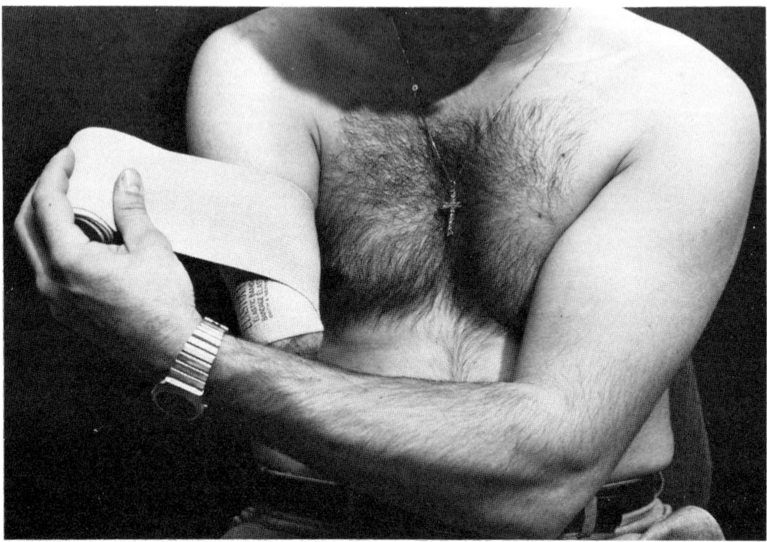

Fig. 9.A-3. He takes the roll of bandage in his hand and applies it in diagonal, figure-8 turns.

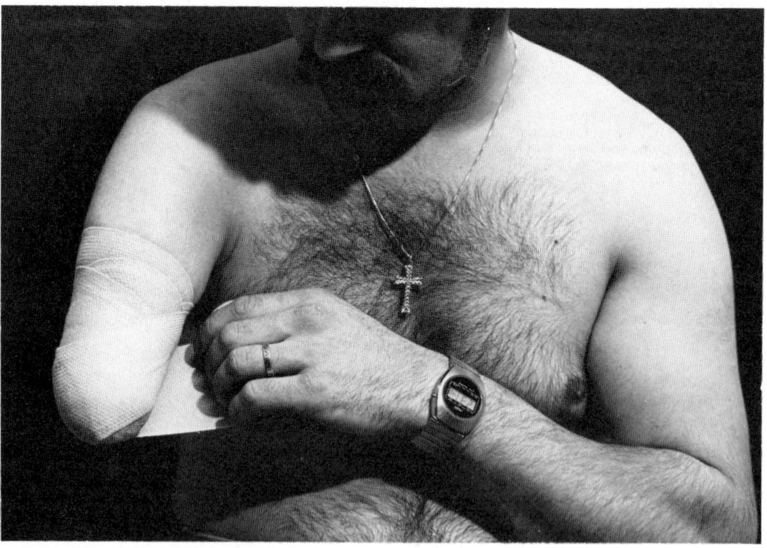

Fig. 9.A-4. Finishing off the bandaging.

in position. In case of a short stump, a few turns above the proximal joint help to hold the bandage in place.

Apply the bandage in spiral diagonal figure 8 turns; avoid circular turns since they cause constriction and can result in a bulbous stump end.

Apply the bandage with the amputee holding the stump in a good position to prevent deformities.

Fasten the bandage securely and ensure that the clips do not irritate the stump.

The amputee is cautioned to remove the bandage if the stump starts to feel uncomfortable, and to reapply it after approximately 20 min. If the amputee cannot tolerate the bandage at night, he/she can take it off, because sound sleep is more important than accelerated stump shrinkage. The stump should be checked daily for blisters, sores and other signs of skin irritation.

The amputee also is instructed in the care of the bandage. The bandage should be washed daily with mild soap in lukewarm water. The water is squeezed out gently, not wrung out, and the bandage is hung over the shower pole to dry. It should not be stretched or ironed.

Additional Modalities

In addition to the bandaging program, treatment with an intermittent compression pump may be used to control and reduce edema. The pump is applied for periods of 30 min twice a day. The pressure should never exceed the diastolic blood pressure. The pump is contraindicated if the amputee has circulatory or cardiac impairment.

From experience it was found that if the stump is covered with extensive skin grafts an individually fitted Jobst elastic pressure stocking can be used instead of the tensor bandage. The pressure of the bandage may cause repeated skin breakdown whereas the tension of the pressure stocking is usually tolerated better and results in accelerated maturation of the skin graft.

CONDITIONING PROGRAM

During the immediate postoperative period the patient is encouraged to perform gentle, active exercises with the stump, within the limits of his/her pain. This helps maintain range of motion and strength and prevents contractures that inhibit the operation of the prosthesis. It also prevents the formation of adhesions, improves stump circulation, controls edema and helps diminish stump sensitivity.

Following removal of the stitches, from about the 10th–14th postoperative day, the patient is progressed to a conditioning program in the physical therapy department. The primary objectives of this program are to reduce traumatic and postoperative edema in the stump, to maintain or to reestablish full range of motion in the remaining joints, to specifically condition the injured limb to maximum potential and generally condition the patient to preaccident levels. Secondary objectives are to help reeducate the patient, in cases where the dominant arm is lost, to transfer dominance in terms of coordination and skillful movement; to encourage endeavor and to rehabilitate psychologically; and finally, to foster independence and ambition in the new physical circumstances. In some cases, exercise helps to absorb anger and frustration and redirect the amputee's energy output to productive channels.

In the initial stage, free active exercises are used to stimulate and maintain the range of motion of joints. The amputee is encouraged to move the stump in all ranges and planes of motion, working within pain tolerance. In some cases, either passive assistance or autoassisted circuits in the form of slings, springs and pulleys may be utilized. In the progressive stage, when wounds and skin have attained sufficient maturity, the therapist can give resisted exercises using various "hands on" techniques, such as "hold-relax." This resisted stage also may involve springloaded resistances in the form of various sleeve or cuff pulleys. Velcro resistance belts also are used to produce static and isometric muscle work. Following prosthetic fitting, exercises are directed at activities involving the prosthesis. They are selected to increase dexterity and speed in using the artificial arm with the hook and include picking up varied objects and throwing and catching bean bags or rubber rings.

At all times before and after prosthetic fitting, the amputee is given activities to challenge his/her abilities which, in the spirit of the "complete person" concept, are directed at recreational activities as well as toward future work. Games, like badminton and paddle ball, and swimming are used, and if the amputee is keen to pursue a particular hobby such as golf, billiards, fishing, the exercises are focused on these hobbies as well.

Amputees may use swimming as part of their conditioning program providing the skin is soundly healed and there are no vulnerable sites for potential infection. Swimming encourages full range of motion and general mobility. It stimulates cardiovascular fitness which for the lower extremity amputees is particularly difficult to achieve since they cannot run. While lower extremity amputees swim as well if not better than before their amputation once their new balance in water is found, upper extremity amputees have to adapt more to their loss as swimming depends essentially on arm power. Below-elbow amputees often use floats to assist propulsion. For unilateral amputees this is usually a swim cuff; for bilateral amputees inflatable cuffs are more suitable as they allow the amputee to rest in a floating position. Above-elbow amputees swim best with a side stroke or back stroke. The stump is used for counter balance, the hand performs an additional whip stroke for directional guidance. Swimming provides additional benefits such as allowing plenty of hard exercises in a safe environment, where loss of balance is not a disaster and, most of all, it provides fun and recreation as well as a challenge that is possible to meet.

INDEPENDENCE IN ACTIVITIES OF DAILY LIVING

The amputee is questioned about his/her independence in activities of daily living (ADL) and if necessary, self-help devices are supplied or specific instructions on one-handed performance are given. Most activities in self-care can be accomplished with one hand. Occasionally a few self-help devices are used such as a rocker knife for cutting meat, a hand brush with suction cups, nail clippers mounted on a board, elastic shoe laces and Velcro fastenings instead of buttons. Some devices, such as a card holder, can be made by the amputee. Furthermore, these devices are usually only temporary for a unilateral amputee; once he/she has received the prosthesis he/she is encouraged to use it for self-care.

Bilateral below-elbow amputees are provided with special washing mitts and bath towel (Figs 9.A-5–9.A-6). Drying also can be accomplished with a snugly fitting bath robe or with a commercially available hot air body dryer. Bilateral above elbow amputees can be fitted with a special bathing device that consists of sockets to which adjustable metal rods with terry cloth-covered foam pads are attached (5). Bilateral below-elbow amputees can be supplied with eating utensils, if necessary with a swivel, which are fixed to forearm cuffs. However, it is advisable to fit bilateral amputees early with temporary prostheses, even before stump shrinkage has stabilized, to allow as much independence as possible, even if this requires repeated fittings as the stumps shrink.

USE OF STUMP

The amputee is encouraged to use the stump, if possible, for stabilizing in various activities such as working on simple carpentry projects, drafting and collating, to maintain a bilateral work habit. This also helps to desensitize the stump and to maintain strength and range of movement in the arm. It

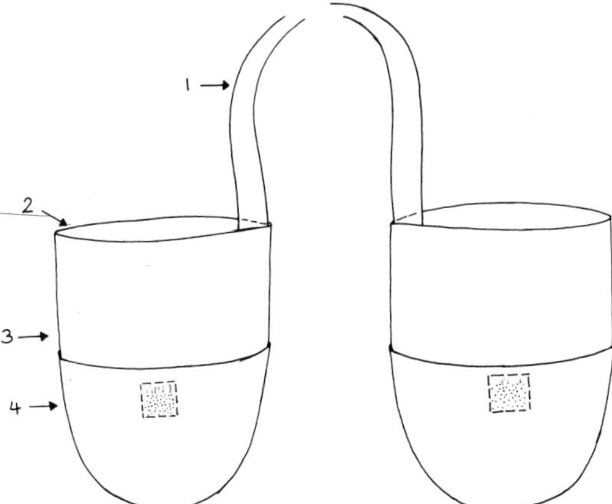

Fig. 9.A-5. Washing Mitts for bilateral below-elbow amputees. *1*, measure around neck. Strap must be long enough to allow movement but short enough to hold mitts on; *2*, circumference of stumps; *3*, length; and *4*, add pocket for soap, with Velcro closure.

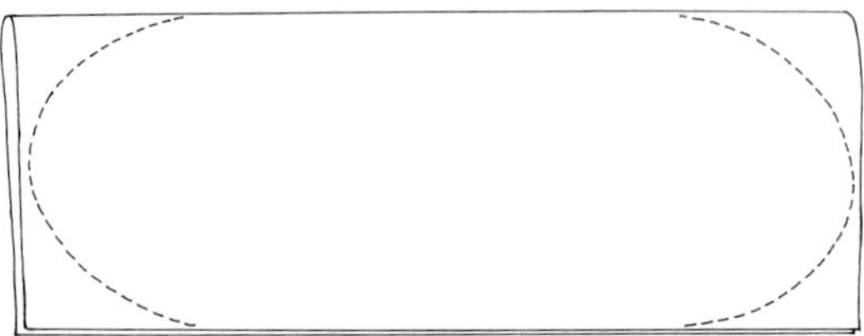

Fig. 9.A-6. Adapted bath towel for bilateral below-elbow amputee. Fold bath towel and stitch along *dashed-lines*.

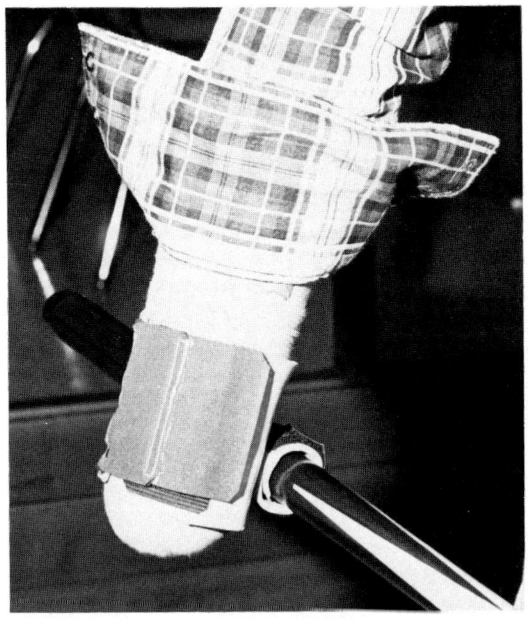

Fig. 9.A-7. A temporary device such as a pool cue holder can be made of Sansplint. The cue handle fits into a sleeve that is closed tightly with a Velcro strap and fastened on to the cuff with a rivet. This allows sufficient rotational movement for the motion of the arm in guiding the cue. The cuff is closed with a Velcro strap as well. The device is worn over the bandage.

encourages the amputee to hold and use the stump in a normal relaxed manner. If necessary, utensils can be inserted into the bandage or fastened to a cuff made of Sansplint which is held on with Velcro straps, to provide added function until the prosthesis is fitted (Fig 9.A-7).

CHANGE OF DOMINANCE

If the dominant hand is amputated, the patient is given a variety of activities from gross motor tasks to fine manipulative tasks to improve the dexterity in the remaining hand. The below-elbow amputee can be given a choice when considering the change of dominance in writing. Depending on his/her wishes and future requirements, *e.g.* study, clerical work where a great deal of writing may be encountered, he/she is taught to write with the subdominant hand, since writing with the prosthesis tends to be more tiring (1, 2, 4). Related activities such as drawing, doodling and typing are useful in increasing fine motor skills. However, the above-elbow amputee usually has little choice but to change his/her dominance to the remaining subdominant hand. For bilateral amputees, the longer stump is usually trained as the dominant one unless there is little difference in length or unless the longer stump is less suitable due to limited range of movement or strength or greater pain, in which case normal dominance is retained.

Some patients are easily discouraged or expect to be able to accomplish the change of dominance rather quickly. They need to be encouraged to practice regularly and to accept a reasonable period of time for acquiring the necessary skill.

INFORMATION FOR PROSTHETIC PRESCRIPTION

Based on discussions with the amputee about the physical requirements of vocational and recreational activities, his/her needs for cosmesis of the prosthesis and the condition of the stump, information is gathered for the prescription of the prosthesis with regard to components, terminal devices and modifications of socket and harness. Recommendations then are made to the treatment team.

Since the prosthesis is basically a tool, it must be functional and designed for the job it is intended to do. For example, if a below-elbow prosthesis is to be used for heavy work it can be equipped with metal hinges, heavy duty steel cable, steel wrist unit and shoulder pad harness. For lighter tasks such as clerical duties or housework, flexible hinges, a figure 8 harness and a lightweight or neoprene-lined hook may be sufficient. Lightweight hooks also usually are prescribed for amputees with short or weak stumps who find the steel hooks too heavy. Occasionally a job may require a specific component such as an insulation cable for an electrician. Amputees who use tools often for work or recreation may be supplied with a suitable hook such as the Dorrance hook No. 6 or 7 (farmer's hook) as well as a simpler hook so that they can interchange them depending on the requirements of the tasks. Tools also may be modified to fit directly into the wrist unit, or special devices may be designed to meet specific needs.

FITTING WITH A TEMPORARY PROSTHESIS

The amputee is best fitted with a temporary prosthesis as soon as the stump is fully healed and not grossly edematous. This has several advantages. The time between amputation and prosthetic fitting is shortened, enabling the amputee to reestablish his/her bilateral work habit sooner. The socket promotes additional shrinkage of the stump preparing it for a better fit with the permanent prosthesis. It accustoms the amputee to wearing a prosthesis and assists in desensitizing and strengthening the stump.

The temporary prosthesis can be fabricated out of Sansplint in a few days. It is inexpensive and can be modified easily. It has great utility as a trial for the prescription of the permanent prosthesis in terms of modifications, components and terminal devices since it contains the standard prosthetic components. It is more cost efficient since it is used during the period of rapid stump shrinkage, thus allowing postponement of fitting of the permanent limb until the stump has stabilized. The amputee uses the temporary prosthesis for several weeks. Following the initial training phase, more time is needed for continued stump shrinkage and for the manufacturing of the permanent prosthesis. At this time, the amputee is encouraged to use the temporary prosthesis in the home environment to try various activities and to acquaint his/her family with its appearance and function.

The temporary prosthesis is suitable for below-elbow and long-to-medium above-elbow stumps. It is not possible to fit amputees with higher levels of amputation successfully with a temporary prosthesis. They are, therefore, measured for their permanent limb as soon as the condition of the stump allows this.

Functional Training

The functional training with the temporary and/or permanent prosthesis has the following goals:

1. Initial evaluation of the prosthesis;
2. Familiarization of the amputee with all prosthetic components, as well as maintenance of the limb;
3. Teaching of the active and manual controls;
4. Instructions in the practical use of the limb in self care, recreational and work tasks;
5. Ongoing functional evaluation, and if necessary, modification of the prosthesis;
6. Final evaluation of the prosthesis prior to discharge.

Amputees vary considerably in their initial response to their new prosthesis. Some look forward to it impatiently while others may be hesitant. Some may even experience an emotional shock when they first receive their prosthesis, particularly if they have problems with acceptance of the amputation or have unrealistic expectations of the limb. This also can happen if they see the prosthesis in the early fitting stages, *e.g.* an electric shoulder disarticulation prosthesis without cosmetic cover. To promote acceptance of the prosthesis, amputees will benefit from expressing and discussing their feelings of ambivalence or disillusionment. The role of the prosthesis needs to be clarified.

The therapist aids the amputee in developing the necessary skill in using his/her new tool so that it will substitute the lost function as much as possible and assure self-sufficiency for the amputee. She/he guides the amputee by selection of suitable activities that can be successfully completed, with consideration of his/her individual style of learning, and by encouragement to use the device efficiently. The training provides the basis for a good functional use of the prosthesis. Thereafter, the skillful handling of a prosthesis is an ongoing learning process as new tasks are encountered. The purpose of the training should be explained to the amputee. Cooperation and motivation to learn to use the prosthesis is essential for a successful training. Motivation can be encouraged by creating incentives for the amputee, formulating desirable goals with the amputee and assisting him/her in progressing towards those goals. The goals most amputees strive for are independence in self-care, ability to return to the former job or a better one with subsequent social acceptance and financial security, ability to return to the enjoyment and satisfaction of preferred or new recreational activities, and improved appearance through efficient inconspicuous control of the prosthesis.

The amputee will accept the prosthesis more readily if it provides maximum function with a minimum of discomfort, effort or sacrifice of cosmesis. The functional training period is used for evaluating the prosthesis and, if necessary, modifying it to provide greater comfort and function. The initial evaluation is performed when the amputee receives the prosthesis. If the prosthesis is satisfactory, training is begun immediately. If however, some adjustments are required, they should be reported to the prosthetist and completed before commencing training.

FAMILIARIZATION WITH PROSTHESIS

The amputee is first made familiar with the components of the prosthesis, their use and correct terminology. This enables him/her to communicate effectively with the prosthetist if repairs or parts are required.

PUTTING ON AND REMOVING PROSTHESIS

The unilateral amputee puts the prosthesis on by holding it in front, slipping the stump under the Y-strap medial to the harness, then pushing the stump into the socket. The hand slides into the loop of the figure 8 harness as into a coat sleeve. Another method can be used where the harness is held in front of the body while the hand slides into the loop and pulls the harness over the head like a sweater.

Bilateral amputees can put on the prostheses in the following manner. They lay out the prostheses on a bed or table, put the dominant stump in the socket by approaching the cuff from the medial side with the harness lying across the stump shoulder, allow the opposite prosthesis to dangle down at the back, then slip the other stump into the other socket similar to getting into a coat, and shrug the harness into place. They take the prosthesis off by pushing off the axilla loops from the shoulders with the opposite hook and slip out of the harness, again, similar to getting off a coat. If necessary, the hook can be placed around a solid object in a way that the socket can be pulled off. It also is possible to put the prostheses on in sweater fashion by sliding into both sockets with the harness lying across the chest, then lifting the harness strap up with the opposite hook and sliding it over the head, shaking the harness into place. They can be removed in the reverse way as well. Both these methods require some practice before they can be easily accomplished. Amputees can pull the stump socks on with their teeth, or with the aid of hooks or furniture through loops sewn on the socks. For bilateral above-elbow amputees, a special board made to put on the stump socks and the prostheses can be of considerable assistance (3) (Figs. 9.A-8 and 9.A-9).

MAINTENANCE AND CARE

The harness is checked for proper adjustment during the training, since it may stretch through use and necessitate adjustments. The amputee is taught how to adjust the harness and how to exchange the control cable and the harness. The harness straps may be marked with indelible ink to make the reattachment and adjustment of straps easier after washing. The amputee also is shown how to add elastic rubber bands to the hook with the rubber band spreader. The amputee is instructed in the care of the prosthesis and the stump socks (Table 9.A-1) and is shown how to make a stump sock dryer (Fig. 9.A-10). The amputee should be supplied with a spare harness, a spare cable, a supply of stump socks, elastic rubber bands and a rubber band spreader before discharge.

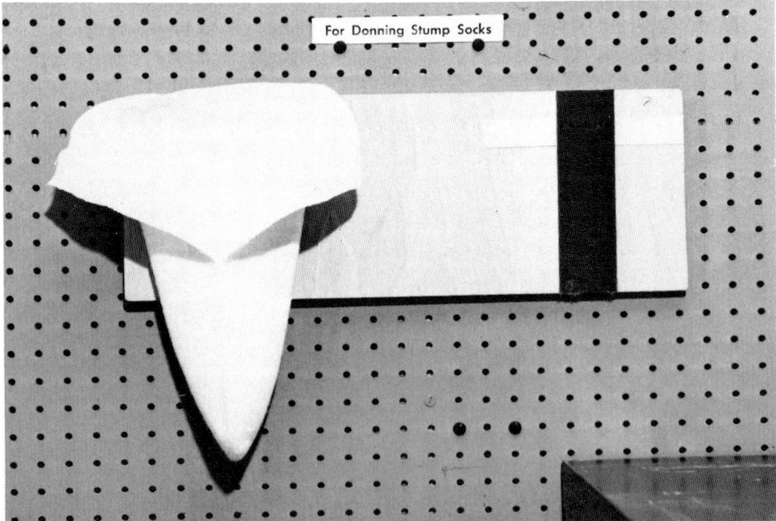

Fig. 9.A-8. Device for donning stump socks. Two strips of Velcro hook are glued to a board which is mounted on the wall below shoulder height. A strip of Velcro pile is sewn on the lateral side of the stump sock. The amputee places the stump socks using his/her stumps or mouth, on the board. The Velcro straps hold the socks in place while the amputee pushes his/her stumps into the socks.

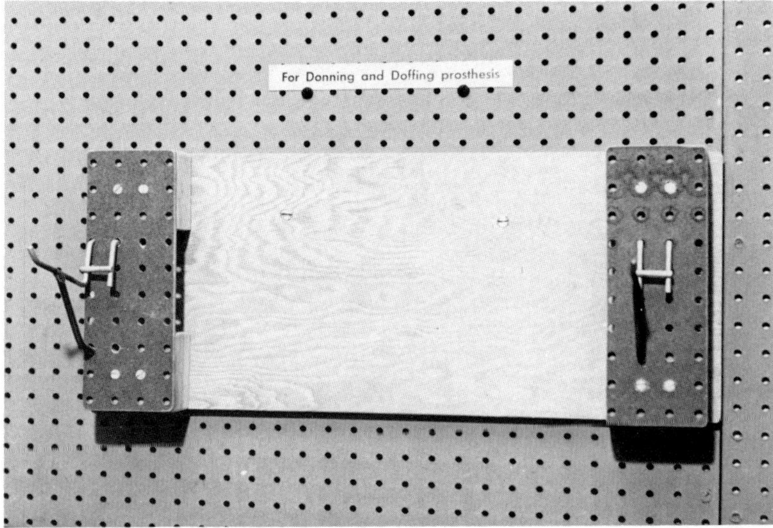

Fig. 9.A-9. Device for donning prostheses for bilateral above-elbow amputee. Two hooks are attached to a board which is mounted on the wall at shoulder height. Two leather loops are fastened to the top of the prosthetic sockets. The amputee stands with his/her back to the board, maneuvers the hooks into the loops and then slips the stumps out of the sockets. To put the prostheses on the procedure is reversed.

TRAINING IN CONTROL OF PROSTHESIS

The therapist must be familiar with the efficient control and use of the prosthesis. To gain a more direct understanding of the sensations and experiences that an amputee encounters in using a prosthesis, a special prosthesis can be made out of Sansplint that can be worn and operated by the therapist.

Active Controls

The amputee is taught the basic body movements necessary to control the prosthetic components and coordinate them effectively to operate the prosthesis efficiently and gracefully. Awkward and inefficient movements need to be eliminated before use training is begun. The control training period also is used to detect any deficiencies in the harness and control system and to rectify them before continuing the training.

The basic control motion to operate the terminal device is flexion of the shoulder on the amputated side, a "reaching out" movement. Scapular abduction can be added. When the figure 8 harness is used, the opposite shoulder acts only as a stabilizer to resist the force transmitted through the harness. The control motion opens the voluntary opening device and closes the voluntary closing device.

TABLE 9.A-1 . *Patient Instruction Form*

Care of Stump Socks

Use stump socks made of wool; in case of allergy use cotton.

Put a freshly washed sock on every day; change more often in warm weather.

Wash the stump socks in lukewarm water with a mild soap or detergent.

Do not rub during washing; it felts the wool.

Rinse in lukewarm water and squeeze out the excess water. Do not wring—this may break threads.

It is best to dry the stump socks on a flat surface or on especially built sock dryers in a cool shaded atmosphere. Drying on a radiator will harden the finish of the stump socks.

Following these precautions will prolong the useful life of the socks and their comfort to you.

Care of Prosthesis

Wipe out socket and inside cuff with a *damp* cloth daily, first with mild soap and then with plain water.

Clean the leather parts with saddle soap (purchased from any shoe store) and a damp cloth. Ordinary soap hardens and cracks the leather.

Any dacron parts of the harness can be washed with a mild detergent.

When the prosthesis is not being used hang it on a hook by its harness; do not hang it by its cable or cable strap.

Water will not harm the hook but will rust your wrist unit and elbow unit. If these parts come in contact with water, put a few drops of oil into them immediately.

Never pry or hammer objects with your hook. This causes it to go out of alignment, shortens its life and damages the wrist unit.

A T-shirt worn under the harness keeps the harness cleaner, absorbs perspiration and protects the skin.

Examine the cable and harness periodically. When the parts are worn or cut have them repaired by your prosthetist.

Below-Elbow Amputee. This control motion is demonstrated to the below-elbow amputee who then practices it with the arm in various positions until he/she is able to control the terminal device fully throughout the range of arm movement. The amputee is made aware of the feedback of tension that is felt through the harness as indication of terminal device operation.

Above-Elbow Amputee. The dual control system of the above elbow prosthesis requires the serial teaching of the control motions necessary to operate elbow lock, elbow flexion and terminal device opening. First the principle of the elbow lock is explained and demonstrated. Starting with the forearm held in flexion with the arm adducted and the elbow unit unlocked, the forearm is pushed back until a click indicates locking of the elbow unit. The forearm is then returned to the neutral position until a second, fainter, click indicates that the lock is in neutral and ready for the next cycle in the operation. The motion is repeated to unlock the elbow unit. The amputee

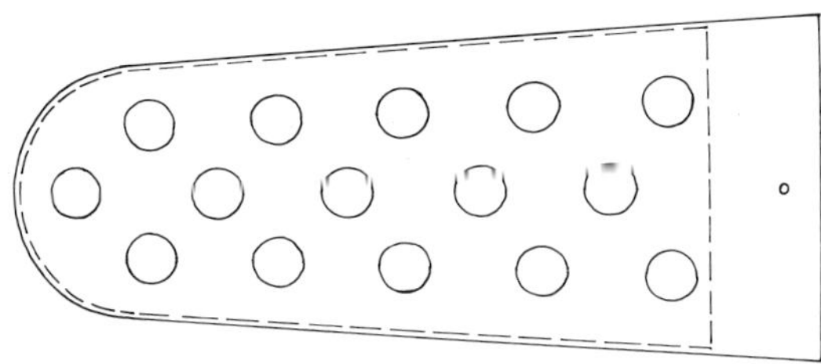

Fig. 9.A-10. Stump sock dryer. The stump sock dryer can be made out of masonite or 1/4″–3/8″ birch plywood, using the latter for larger sizes. The board is cut approximately 1/8″ larger and 2″ longer than the stump sock. Large holes for ventilation are drilled into the board; the holes should not be too close to each other or to the edge of the board to avoid weak areas in the board. The board is sanded well and several coats of sealer and varnish are applied for water proofing.

is asked to repeat the procedure using humeral extension while the elbow is fully extended. When the amputee can operate the elbow lock in this way he/she is instructed to add shoulder protraction to the motion to decrease the amount of humeral extension necessary to operate the elbow lock. Further reduction of arm extension is achieved by combining shoulder depression (pushing the stump into the socket) with the two previous movements.

When the amputee is able to perform this movement pattern satisfactorily, control of forearm flexion is practiced. With the elbow unit unlocked, humeral flexion results in flexion of the forearm. This movement has to be performed slowly and cautiously since strong flexion can elevate the prosthetic forearm too quickly and result in the terminal device hitting the amputee's face. To extend the elbow, the arm is brought back slowly to the neutral position. A quick release of tension on the cable will result in the elbow falling into extension. The next step is to lock the elbow unit in various positions of elbow flexion. Since the tension on the control cable releases when the arm is extended for the operation of the elbow lock, the forearm is returned to neutral by gravitational force. Humeral abduction is therefore added to the combination of humeral extension, shoulder protraction and depression to keep the elbow in the flexed position. The amputee practices these control motions until he/she can lock the elbow unit smoothly in various positions of flexion.

The control of the terminal device is added by applying further humeral flexion when the elbow unit is locked. This is practiced with the elbow locked in different positions. Full opening of the terminal device at full elbow flexion may not be possible initially due to the slack of the control cable in this position. Lack of strength in the stump or experience of pain may limit terminal device opening as well.

If the amputee can initially tolerate only one or two tension bands on the terminal device, the flexion of the elbow unit will be impeded through the unintentional opening of the hook as a result of the low resistance. This problem is, hopefully, quickly overcome with the strengthening of the stump.

Shoulder Disarticulation Amputee. For the shoulder disarticulation amputee, the control motion for elbow flexion and terminal device operation is shoulder protraction and chest expansion. The elbow lock cable is usually attached to the waist band and operated by shoulder elevation on the amputated side. The amputee is usually restricted in the ability to open the terminal device fully due to the limitations in the range of excursion, particularly when the cable is slack through elbow flexion. The training starts with control of elbow flexion and extension by protracting the shoulder and then relaxing it again, letting the elbow return smoothly to the extended position. Then elevation of the shoulder is practiced to lock and unlock the elbow in the extended position. Following this exercise, forearm flexion is combined with elbow lock operation by holding the shoulder protracted while elevating it. This is practiced with the elbow locked at various angles. Operation of the terminal device is added by protracting the shoulder further when the elbow unit is locked.

Bilateral Amputee. Bilateral amputees who are fitted with two prostheses perform the same control motions as unilateral amputees. However, since both control systems are usually attached to the same harness an additional effect, called cross-control, may be evident. The force produced to control one prosthesis may be transmitted through the harness to cause a partial control of the opposite prosthesis. This is particularly common in bilateral above-elbow prostheses with dual control where the position of the forearm changes the effective cable excursion considerably. When the elbow unit on one side is locked in full flexion with the arm held adducted, the resultant slack in the cable and harness necessitates a greater excursion on the other side to flex the elbow fully, or to open the terminal device. The reverse is happening when the elbow unit on one side is locked in full extension.

This control effect has to be taken into consideration when activities require maximum flexibility in one prosthesis and detrimental effects, such as loss of prehension on the other side, have to be avoided. To minimize the effects of cross-control, the prehension force in one terminal device can be increased. Adjusting the harness so that it is slightly looser, or using a Northwestern ring-type harness which provides more independent control, are useful measures as well. The amputee can revise the basic control motions by bringing one arm closer to the body as well as shift or stabilize the harness in various ways to suit each particular situation.

Manual Controls

Following the training in controlling the prosthesis actively, the amputee receives instructions in controlling the manual components of the prosthesis. The positioning of the terminal device for efficient grasping is explained. In a friction wrist unit, the terminal device is rotated to the desired position. If a quick-change wrist unit is used, the amputee positions the terminal device by pressing the release button lightly, rotates the device, and locks it by pushing it into the wrist unit. The terminal device is exchanged by applying heavier pressure on the release button in the direction of the stump, which allows the terminal device to be pulled out completely. The cable is disconnected and attached to an alternate device which is then pushed into the wrist unit while the release button is pressed simultaneously. This maneuver usually requires some practice and should be repeated periodically until it is performed smoothly.

The above-elbow and shoulder disarticulation amputee also is instructed in the purpose of the turntable to rotate the forearm to a suitable working position closer to the midline of the body and to return it to the neutral position to allow the arm to swing clear of the hip when walking. The amputee can rotate the turntable with the elbow flexed at 90° by moving the forearm with the sound hand or by pushing it against an object. The position of the shoulder joint in a shoulder disarticulation or forequarter prosthesis also is controlled by hand or by pushing the arm against an object.

Bilateral amputees are fitted with wrist flexion units as well. The positioning of the terminal devices and of the flexion units requires considerable training. Aside from using the opposite hook they can also use their body, *e.g.* by pushing the hook against the knee, or furniture, to assist them in this task.

Prehension Training

Since the terminal device provides no sensory feedback, all control is based on eye-hand coordination. The prosthetic hand often obscures the object being handled. It also is heavier than a hook and its prehension force cannot be adjusted easily to the tolerance of a new stump. It is therefore best to start the training with a hook. Although some amputees object to the hook for cosmetic reasons, they are encouraged to use it for the training, but can be supplied with a prosthetic hand for social events.

The prehension force on the hook is determined by the amount of force that the amputee can generate in accordance with the resistance he/she can tolerate in the stump and in other pressure areas such as the axilla in the figure-8 harness. It also is influenced by the prehension force that is required to perform necessary tasks. The prehension force should be lower initially. It is increased gradually as tolerance is built up, causing minimal discomfort and fatigue, until the optimum prehension force is reached. On voluntary opening hooks two or three tension bands are usually used in the beginning (Fig. 9.A-11). New bands are added as required by the training tasks and tolerated by the amputee (Fig. 9.A-12). If a more gradual increase is necessary due to a weak or painful stump, the tension bands can be cut into

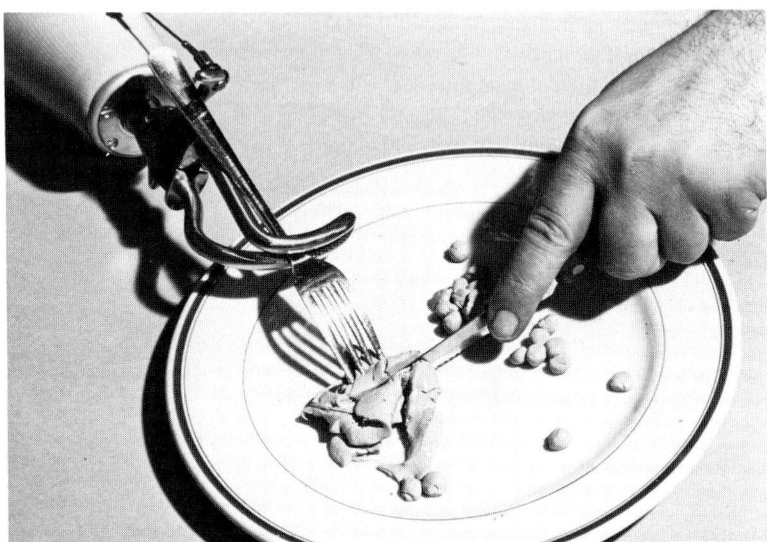

Fig. 9.A-11. The fork is held in the hook to stabilize the meat while cutting it. This grip is adequate even when the amputee can tolerate only a few tension bands.

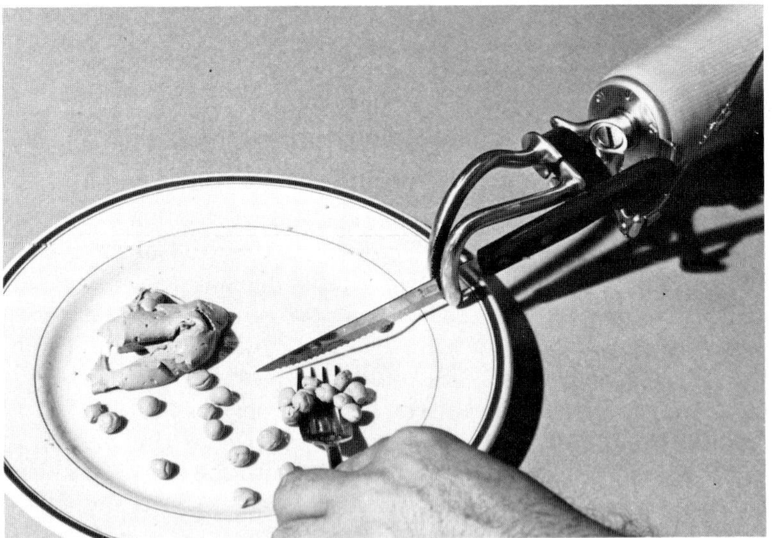

Fig. 9.A-12. The knife is held in a similar way but more tension bands are necessary to provide a solid grip.

smaller bands. The tension bands need to be replaced when they lose their strength through oxidization or if they become affected by oil, solvents, heat, etc.

The amputee now learns to grasp and hold objects effectively in the

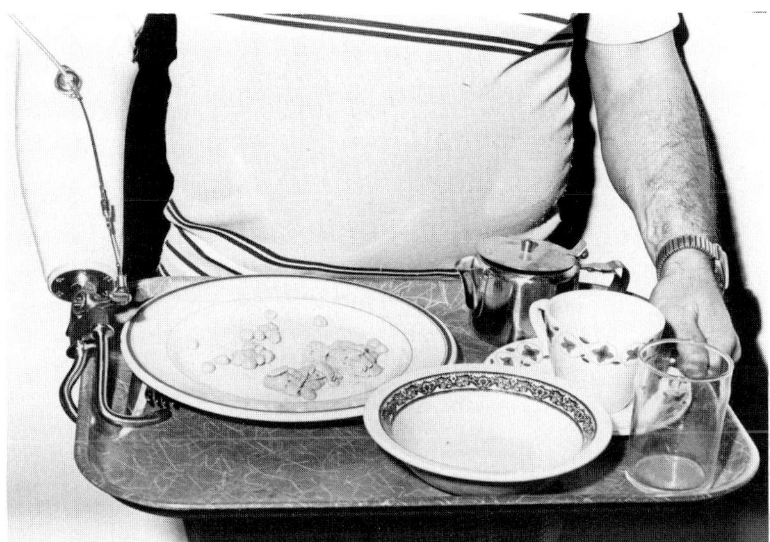

Fig. 9.A-13. When carrying a tray, a good grip and balance is obtained by sliding the hook in as far as possible and holding the tray closer to the distal edge. While picking the tray up or setting it down, it is pushed slightly over the edge of the table so that the hook can approach or release it freely.

terminal device. He/she practices this by grasping and releasing objects of various shapes and weights. This is done from different heights, including the floor, and from a standing and sitting position. The hook, as well as the elbow unit in a higher level prosthesis, is prepositioned as necessary to avoid awkward compensating body movements when gripping the objects. Energy conservation is practiced by opening the hook only as far as necessary. To practice maintaining control of tension on the cable, the amputee picks up crushable objects such as a paper cup and moves the arm through the range of movement, observing the change in tension and the required adjustment in the control. The various methods of holding objects in the hook with a stable grasp by utilizing all parts of the hook are demonstrated (Figs. 9.A-11 and 9.A-13–9.A-15).

Training Considerations

Training in the control of the prosthesis is comparatively easy for the below-elbow amputee and may take only a short time. An above-elbow amputee, however, may require a few days before he/she is able to perform well coordinated movements. Although it is imperative that the amputee learns to control the prosthesis effectively without undue exertion or attention, it is equally essential that he/she experiences the satisfaction of being able to perform practical tasks with the new limb early in the training. The controls training period should, therefore, not be too long; the training in

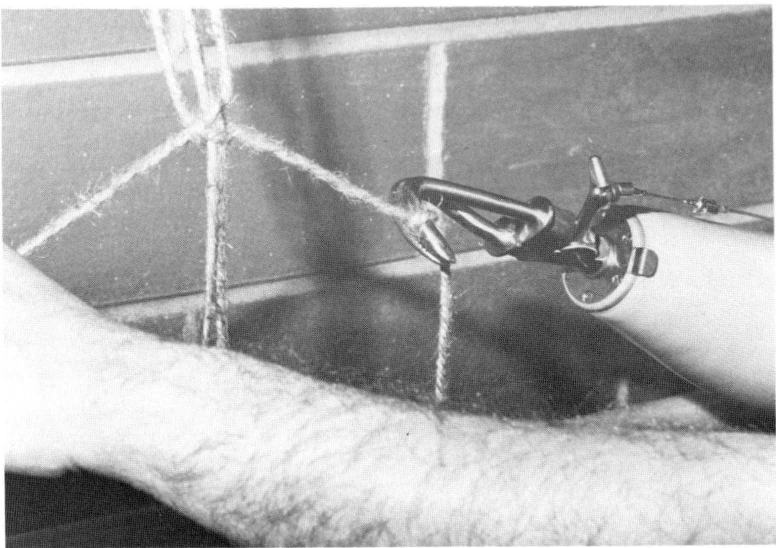

Fig. 9.A-14. To prevent the string from sliding through the hook when insufficient prehension force is available, the string is wound around the hook finger once.

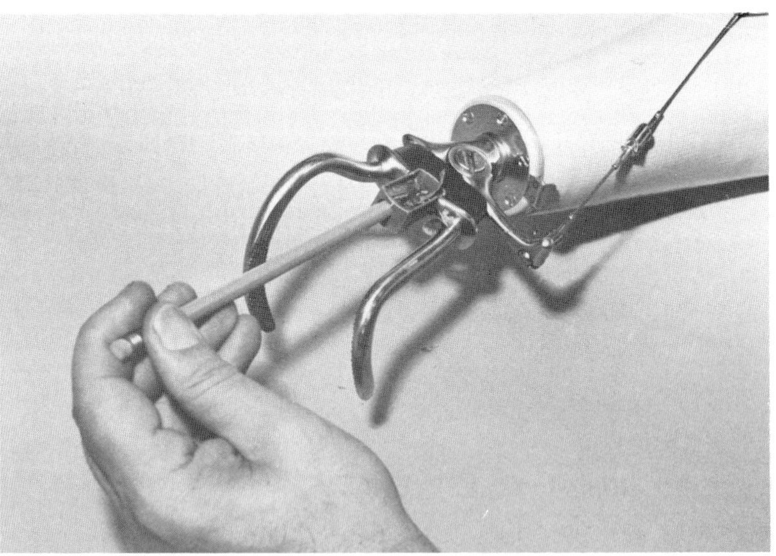

Fig. 9.A-15. The cutout at the base of the hook fingers can be used for holding some utensils.

the use of the prosthesis can sometimes be started even if the amputee has not mastered all controls as well as desired, provided that the operation of controls are reviewed and checked on a daily basis until they are performed satisfactorily.

The amputee should use the prosthesis outside the clinic or at home only after he/she has mastered the controls and has begun to use the limb for self-care activities and other functional tasks in order to avoid frustration, the development of bad habits and breakdown of the stump due to incorrect use of the prosthesis.

The training periods are limited by the amputee's tolerance for wearing and operating the prosthesis. They usually start with a period of up to 1 hr of intermittent activity and increase gradually as tolerance improves until the amputee can wear the limb for the full day. Overdoing activity in the beginning can cause discomfort and edema of the stump and discomfort in the pressure areas of the harness with subsequent setback.

TRAINING IN USE OF PROSTHESIS

In this phase of the training the amputee is familiarized with the potential value of the prosthesis and encouraged to use it in a practical way. The role of the prosthesis needs to be evaluated in each task to achieve full utilization. Based on the mechanical range of function, the prosthesis is mainly used as a stabilizing tool during bilateral activities, while the remaining hand performs the more complex aspects of activities. If the dominant hand is amputated, amputees usually will transfer their dominance to the remaining hand but may continue to perform certain activities of dominant function with the prosthesis such as writing or handling some tools. Limitations of the prosthesis need to be taken into consideration when choosing activities for training, particularly initially, when low tolerance to resistance may restrict the prehension force that can be applied. Finding alternate ways of gripping, or applying practical tricks, may occasionally compensate for limited prehension force (Fig. 9.A-14 and 9.A-15). Special devices and adaptations also can be used in the prosthesis for specific tasks.

The emphasis in the training is on practical, purposeful activities to demonstrate meaningful application of the prosthesis and terminal device. They include the amputee's individual needs in ADL, employment and recreational interests. This gives the amputee a sense of achievement and progress toward a goal, demonstrates the usefulness of the prosthesis and thereby ultimately assists in its acceptance. The sequence of activities is geared to a gradual progression in the complexity of the tasks, the frequency of gripping required and the resistance encountered in the performance to facilitate increase of tolerance and skill. When possible, the amputee is encouraged to practice specific activities during the time he/she spends at home to extend the use of the prosthesis to all areas of life. Motivation, functional gain and successful performance will determine an amputee's use of his/her prosthesis.

Presenting the amputee with as many bilateral tasks as possible encourages her/him to practice using the prosthesis to the best advantage and to develop coordination and skill in using the terminal device. He/she is allowed to experiment and test his/her own ideas when approaching new tasks. This leads to the development of a *problem solving attitude*, and the habits of analyzing prospective tasks and evaluation of the efficient use of the prosthesis. This skill will increase the amputee's confidence and assist him/her after completion of the training whenever new tasks have to be mastered. Where necessary, specific *instructions* are given and activities are repeated to ensure effective use of the prosthesis in order to avoid undue frustrations or time-consuming work habits. The amputee will benefit from *feedback*—reassurance when he/she performs well, as well as correction of incorrect or inefficient actions, to avoid uncertainty. There are proven techniques for many tasks, but some activities can be performed successfully in several ways. The amputee will choose the one which feels comfortable to him or her. In cases where specific instructions for a task are not available, either because of marginal function of the amputee, the uniqueness of the task or the lack of experience of the therapist, both amputee and therapist work together until a successful method is developed. This is followed by feedback and specific instructions from the therapist.

It is important to help generate a *sense of accomplishment.* Rewards will increase motivation since "nothing succeeds like success." It is best to start with activities that the amputee can readily master. If more difficult activities are performed unsuccessfully, the amputee will profit from reverting to simpler activities temporarily to maintain a successful experience. Attention should be paid to the competition which may develop between amputees working together. If competition is to be utilized as an incentive, the amputees need to have similar levels of amputation, function and skill and be inclined to be motivated by competition to avoid discouragement. Nevertheless, amputees often help each other with humor and practical advice.

The progress of the amputee is evaluated on the basis of efficiency, that is elimination of errors and reduction of time necessary for a specific activity, as well as spontaneous use of the prosthesis. This is done on an individual level and the amputee is encouraged to improve his/her own performance rather than to compete against standards set by other amputees.

For the bilateral amputee, independence in self-care is of major importance and considerable thought should be given to supplying any attachments or adaptations that will aid in achieving a greater degree of independence. These may include a limb and sock holder, bathing and drying devices, eating utensils, clothes adaptations, telephone adaptations, rubber doorknob extensions and driving aids. The amputee also should be encouraged to use other parts of the body—mouth, knees, feet—to assist, where possible. The amputee should be supplied with wrist flexion units to allow him/her to reach the midline of the body. Hooks are more functional and are usually preferred, but a hand on one side may be used for social events. The training concentrates primarily on the bilateral control and its characteristics, as well as on self-care tasks. Each activity is a challenge. Careful selection and progression of activities is required if the amputee is to have a sense of accomplishment and is to experience success. He/she often requires considerable emotional support and encouragement to persevere and to cope with the frustrations that are encountered in the basic daily tasks. The degree of independence finally achieved will depend on the level of amputation and to a large measure on the amputee's personality, character and attitude toward the amputations.

Amputees vary in their dexterity, mechanical aptitude, motivation, experience and age and this affects their ability to learn to use a prosthesis. Some may require greater assistance in their learning process or in dealing with the frustrations that occur in using a mechanical device offering only limited compensation.

If the amputee encounters difficulty in accepting the prosthesis or working with it the possible causes for this have to be found and rectified by taking appropriate measures. During the training period, the stump is checked regularly to avoid any breakdowns from socket pressure or skin irritation caused by the harness. Ninety percent of stump problems arise from the prosthesis and, therefore, this always should be checked carefully for fit and function first. Neuromas, stump pain due to pressure or tenderness, require modification of the prosthesis. In case of weakness of the stump, the use of a lightweight hook, fewer tension bands on the hook, adjustments to the harness, as well as the use of tricks to cope with limited prehension force (*e.g.* while pulling a knot tight, the string can be wrapped around the hook finger once to prevent it from slipping through (Fig. 9.A-14)) will improve function. If the amputee has feelings of insecurity or fear or a sense of being disabled and incomplete, he/she will benefit from clarification of feelings, encouragement and from a careful choice of activities that are stimulating, can be readily mastered and improve his/her self-esteem. The healthy part of the amputee's psyche can be mobilized this way. If he/she lacks motivation and interest, a discussion may reveal emotional problems, family problems, nonacceptance of the amputation, etc., that need to be dealt with.

During the training, amputees are given the opportunity to try various terminal devices available in order to select the suitable ones for vocational and recreational needs. They also may require minor modifications of equipment they handle or it may be necessary to adapt tools to fit into the wrist unit. A more realistic appraisal of the vocational needs can be made if the therapist can visit the work place with the amputee. Also, the employer often does not know what work the amputee employee is capable of doing and is unfamiliar with prostheses and may appreciate receiving some feedback.

EVALUATION

The therapist observes the amputee and evaluates his/her use of the prosthesis in regard to efficiency, coordination, tolerance, appropriate and spontaneous use. If possible, the ability to perform the physical components of the job is assessed. This evaluation and additional information about interests, work habits, motivation and ability to learn new skills will be of assistance in vocational planning.

When the amputee is able to carry out a full day's program with complete comfort wearing the prosthesis and can demonstrate functional use of the prosthesis, the therapist performs a final evaluation of the device to ensure maximum prosthetic efficiency. The result of the training program is then reported to the team.

The length of the prosthetic training varies for each amputee, depending on level of amputation, length of stump, physical condition, age and aptitude. An average period for below-elbow amputees is approximately 2–3 weeks; for above-elbow amputees it is usually 3–4 weeks including training with temporary and permanent prosthesis. An upper extremity amputee who received proper pre- and postoperative care with no medical complications and benefitted from successful fitting and training with a prosthesis can return to work within 3–4 months after his/her amputation.

The prosthesis can be used by many amputees successfully for precision tasks (Figs. 9.A-16–9.A-19) as well as for heavy, stressful work (Figs. 9.A-20–9.A-24). However, not all amputees tolerate the latter and may need retraining for lighter work. The amputee's ability to use the prosthesis will vary according to a number of factors: level of amputation, condition of stump,

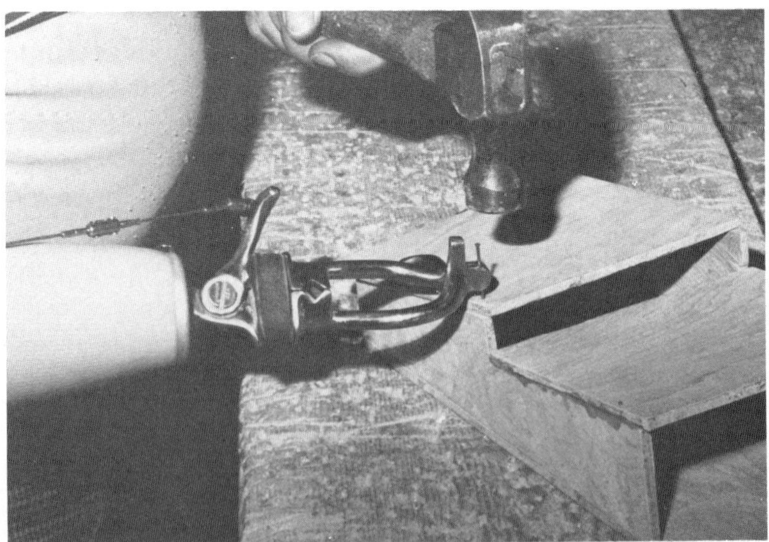

Fig. 9.A-16. The groove in the protuberance of the Dorrance No. 7 hook is used for setting nails.

Fig. 9.A-17. The cutout at the base of the hook fingers in the Dorrance No. 7 hook is used to hold tools such as chisels, nail set, etc.

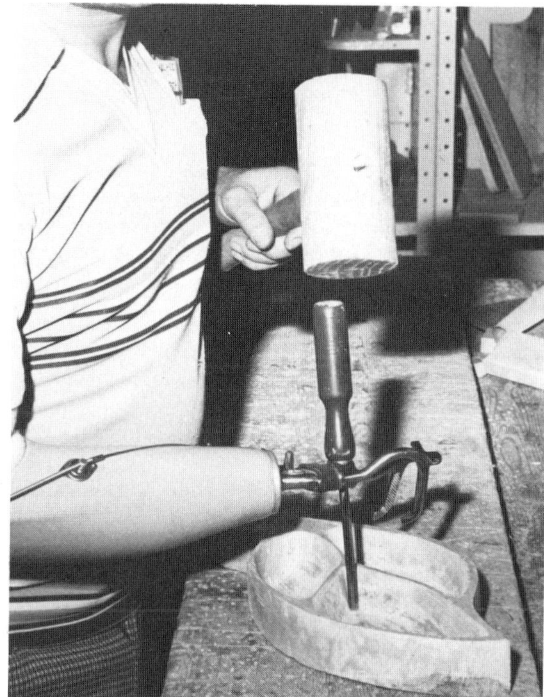

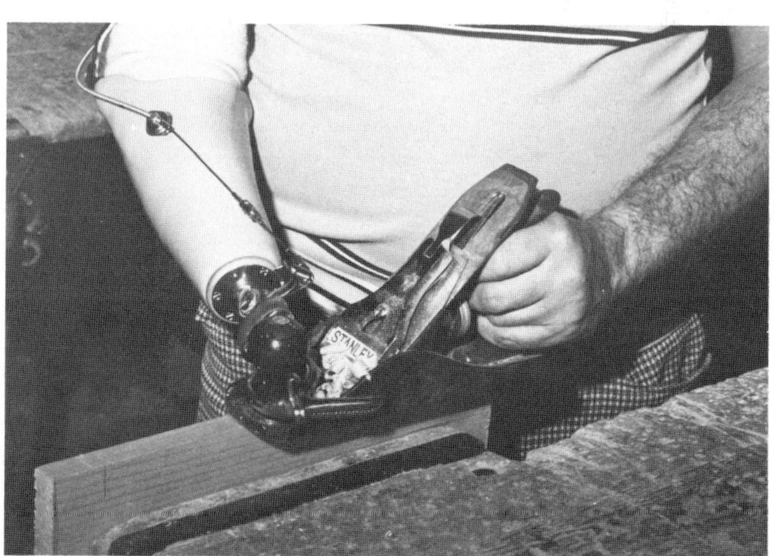

Fig. 9.A-18. The Dorrance No. 7 hook is used to stabilize the plane.

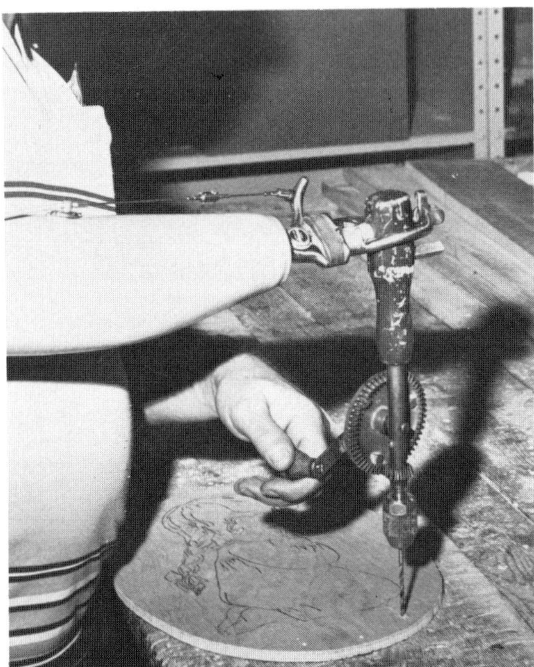

Fig. 9.A-19. The handle of a hand drill has been adapted with a short piece of keystock which fits into the cutout at the base of the fingers. This provides a better grip of the tool and allows a downward force with the hook.

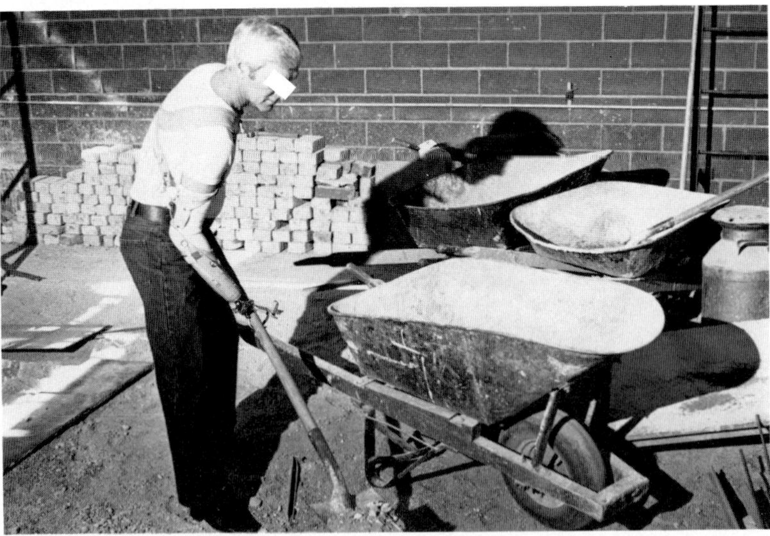

Fig. 9.A-20. The Dorrance No. 6 or 7 hook is used at the pivot point on the lower part of the handle on tools such as shovel, rake, hoe etc. In a quick change wrist unit, the hook is placed in the free rotation position. This prevents the transmission of torque to the stump and subsequent discomfort.

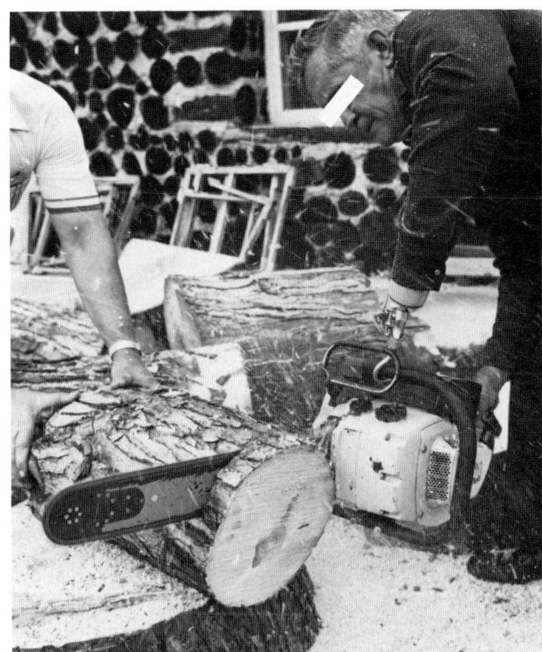

Fig. 9.A-21. The Dorrance No. 6 or 7 hook can be used to stabilize a chain saw.

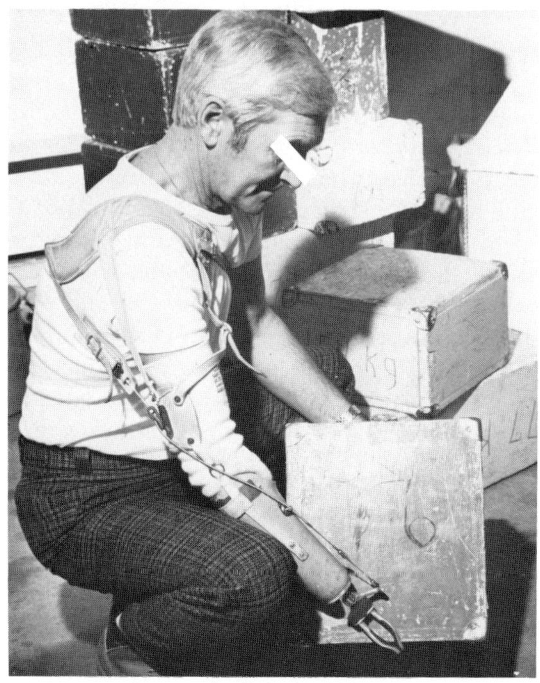

Fig. 9.A-22. The hook is used to support the object while lifting and carrying. Care has to be taken that the object does not press on the release button of the quick change wrist unit. The shoulder pad harness is more comfortable for handling weights.

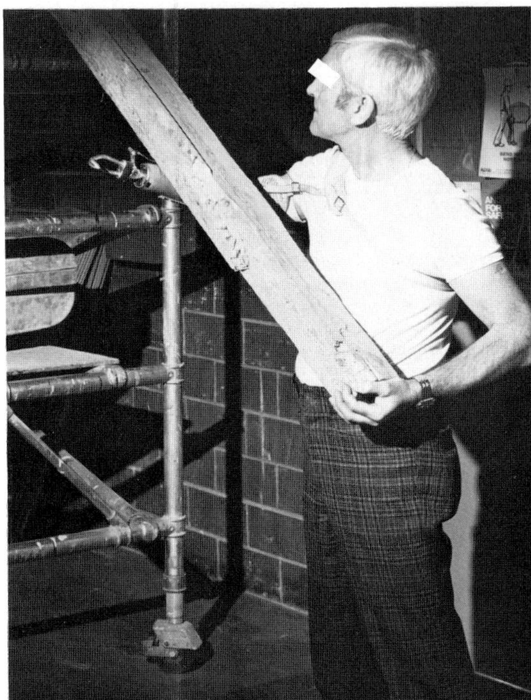

Fig. 9.A-23. Objects also can be supported on the socket.

accompanying injuries, general health, education, manual dexterity and motivation. Generally, the higher the level of amputation, the lower the level of functional activity that can be achieved with a conventional prosthesis. Unilateral below-elbow amputees are likely to be able to perform most activities that they did before the amputation, although this depends on length and strength of the stump. Above-elbow amputees will be limited in performing low level work, and in many cases will not be able to work above shoulder level. Their ability to lift objects with the forearm flexed is considerably limited. They also should be cautioned not to perform work that requires repetitive use of the remaining arm over long periods of time as this may result in straining and weakening of the arm through overuse; even with the use of a prosthesis it is not possible to give the remaining arm a complete rest as nonamputees are able to do. Shoulder disarticulation amputees will be further limited because they have to rely on the excursion and strength of the shoulder girdle and opposite shoulder to operate the prosthesis and can only be fitted with a passive shoulder joint. If they are not able to operate a conventional prosthesis due to lack of strength they may be fitted with a cosmetic prosthesis or a shoulder cap if so desired. However, in recent years electrically powered prostheses have become available for high level amputees using microswitch control for shoulder disarticulation prostheses and myoelectric control for forequarter prosthe-

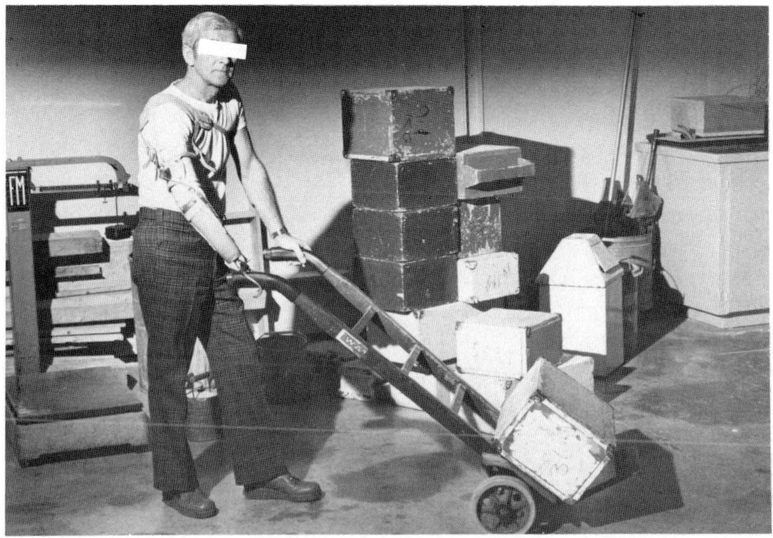

Fig. 9.A-24. The hook is used for stabilizing the cart.

ses. These controls allow the amputees full use of the grip span and force of the hand and full range of elbow movement. In a shoulder disarticulation prosthesis a wrist rotator can be added as well. The passive shoulder joint also is more useful in this prosthesis since, unlike the conventional prosthesis, the arm is not pulled back to the neutral position by a control cable. However, the three-state myoelectric control units used for forequarter prostheses require considerable specific training.

Training with the Myoelectric Prosthesis

To assist the amputee in his/her decision to get a myoelectric prosthesis, and to promote realistic expectations rather than the bionic myth, he/she needs to receive complete information about its mechanism, function and potential advantages and disadvantages.

One of its advantages is the more natural control through the use of the remaining, although not active, muscles of the stump. The myoelectric hand has superior prehension force over the hook. The grip force can be graded from light to strong without requiring greater effort and can be maintained indefinitely by shutting the hand switch off. The grip span of the hand is greater than that of the cable-operated hand. In addition, the cosmesis of the myoelectric hand is unquestionably better, making it socially more acceptable. This, in turn, favors the acceptance of the prosthesis by the amputee. Whereas for most amputees the hook is merely a tool, the myoelectric prosthesis is more often seen as a part of the body. Due to the closer fit of the socket, it further seems to provide a greater feedback. Since the self-suspended socket of the below-elbow prosthesis contains all the components, thereby eliminating the constricting harness, which is disliked by all amputees to a varying degree, it is more comfortable. Amputees with short stumps or high level amputations can be fitted successfully and provided with full use of the prosthetic hand and elbow.

The myoelectric prosthesis is, however, more expensive as well as less robust than the conventional prosthesis. The fit of the socket is crucial in maintaining good electrode contact; fluctuation in weight and excess perspiration can cause problems in suspension and control. In the below-elbow prosthesis, the range of elbow movement is restricted in the end range due to the Muenster type socket. The tightly fitting socket also may cause discomfort, particularly initially, on the areas of suspension. In addition to this, the weight of the prosthesis is usually somewhat greater than a conventional limb and has to be carried by the stump alone. The cosmetic glove is stained easily by ball point pen, ink, news print, carbon paper, dye, etc., and it is cut or torn easily. The grip and position of the hand can be awkward for holding some objects, particularly small ones; although there is a special pinch device available for this purpose. Battery power is reduced in very cold weather. The prosthesis is usually not suitable for heavy or dirty work or for handling weights due to the suspension and susceptibility to damage, however, some amputees are able to use it successfully in industrial jobs. The prosthesis requires greater care and conscientious use. Due to the latter reasons, many amputees continue to use their standard prosthesis for heavy work or for handling materials that stain or damage the glove. They seem to have no difficulty alternating between the different controls of the limbs. There are at present only a few centers that fit and service myoelectric prostheses. Relative proximity to a center may be an important factor in the decision of myoelectric fitting. Although, servicing of components does not always necessitate the presence of the amputee.

To determine the amputee's suitability for fitting with a myoelectric prosthesis she/he is assessed for a number of factors: the ability to learn new skills, to generate good myoelectric signals, the condition and maturity of the stump, the amputee's general motivation, goals, social needs and vocational suitability. She/he must want the prosthesis and be motivated to perform the myoelectric control and use training. This is essential even if she/he has had a conventional prosthesis before and knows how to use an artificial limb.

The selection of suitable control sites and the ability to generate the necessary muscle signals are crucial for the success of a myoelectric prosthesis.

TESTING AND TRAINING IN CONTROL OF MYOELECTRIC SIGNAL

The amputee is first tested on the myoelectric tester to assess his/her ability to generate sufficiently strong and independent contractions of suitable muscles, *e.g.* flexor and extensor muscles in below-elbow or above-elbow stumps, and upper and lower trapezius or latissimus in forequarter amputations. An adequate signal strength to operate the hand, using 2-state control units, is 20–30 μV although the ability to generate stronger signals will ensure that the muscles are not used at maximum capacity and the control of the prosthesis will therefore be less tiring. If a three-state control unit is to be used, the amputee has to be able to reach and hold the required level of muscle tension—relaxation, weak contraction, strong contraction.

First the skin is cleansed with alcohol or water to decrease skin resistance. The therapist then palpates one muscle group for the strongest site of contraction while the amputee repeatedly contracts and relaxes the muscles. The signal potential of the prospective site is checked by placing the test electrode on it and observing the result of the contractions on the test meter. If the signal is weak the test electrode is moved on the stump a little at a time to find a stronger site while the result is observed on the meter. After the site of maximum potential has been found the procedure is repeated with the opposite muscle group.

The amputee then has to learn to contract the muscles independently of each other, to alternate the contractions, to produce accurate signals with the arm in various positions and without visual feedback. The best result for accurate independent muscle contraction in below-elbow amputations is obtained through movements of the phantom hand, preferably through wrist extension and flexion. Sometimes, however, other movements have to be found, if the wrist cannot be felt or the phantom feels tight. The instant feedback of the tester facilitates the search for control movements.

If two muscles are to be used with the 3-state control system, as in the case of a forequarter amputee, then each muscle must be trained independently. Only after a high degree of accurate control is achieved can the amputee be progressed to alternate between the two muscle sites, contracting one without contracting the other simultaneously.

The training sessions must be kept short, to about $\frac{1}{2}$ hr, to avoid fatigue and soreness in the muscles. Although the training time varies and depends on the amputee's state of relaxation and neuromuscular control, most amputees are able to generate and isolate the signals accurately. Success in this seems to bear no relation to the time elapsed since the amputation. Even though the training in the control of the signal may require a short period only, it is most essential as it builds the basis for the effective use of the prosthesis.

The control sites must be chosen so that they are suitably located in the socket, *i.e.* not too close to the edge of the socket or to bony prominences. The stump should be mature, as a tight fit is essential. Short stumps can be fitted, but these need a special fitting technique.

TRAINING IN CONTROL OF MYOELECTRIC PROSTHESIS

When the amputee receives his/her prosthesis it is evaluated for comfort, efficient function and cosmesis. If it proves satisfactory in all aspects then the training is begun.

TABLE 9.A-2. *Patient Instruction Manual*[a]

Care of Your Myoelectric Prosthesis—Do's and Don'ts

Donning the prosthesis

Because of the intimate fit of your prosthetic socket, entry into the same may be difficult in the beginning. To facilitate entry of the stump apply baby powder, baby oil or surgical lubricant as desired.

The use of powder tends to delay the full control over the prosthesis somewhat because of its drying qualities. If you use powder, make sure that it does not cover the sites of the electrodes. Baby oil should not be used for long periods of time as it will increase the electrical resistance of the skin to the point where control over the prosthesis can be totally lost. For the same reason, the use of vaseline is not recommended.

Surgical lubricant (MUKO) will provide smooth entry and give instant control. It is available from most pharmacies.

If there is an initial delay in the operation of the hand when you put the prosthesis on you can moisten the skin at the sites of the electrodes with a bit of water to decrease the resistance between skin and electrodes.

Wearing time should be gradually increased as the stump becomes accustomed to the prosthesis. Do not try to be tough with yourself. Wear the prostheses for 3–4 hours only the first day. If you overdo it, your stump will be sore the day after.

Stump and socket hygiene

Before retiring wash your stump with warm water and mild soap. Dry thoroughly. Then wipe the socket of your prosthesis with a *damp* but not dripping wet face cloth and remove all residues of body perspiration and lubricants used. Neglect of stump and socket hygiene may cause skin irritations and odorous sockets. Any cuts or bruises on the stump should receive immediate attention and be allowed to heal. If necessary, leave your prosthesis off for a couple of days and check with your prosthetist, therapist or doctor.

If you have any odour problems with your socket because of perspiration you might try to use a cologne to wipe out the socket periodically. If perspiration proves to be a problem you might want to try the use of an astringent; this means treating your stump with a solution of 50% water and 50% rubbing alcohol once or twice a day. Some amputees have used antiperspirant sprays with success.

Care of cosmetic glove

Your glove is made from polyvinyl chloride (PVC). This plastic composition is easily stained by ball point pen, ink, carbon paper, fresh newsprint and leather dye. New clothing when wet will also stain or discolour your glove. These stains can be removed only with great difficulties and only when the stain is fresh

To keep your glove clean and supple, apply Nivea cream or Nivea hand lotion very generously once a week. Massage the Nivea cream into the glove and remove the excess with a soft white cloth.

You can use normal toilet soap or Tide for washing your glove. See Spray, a lens cleaner from Amway, is helpful for removing stains; it works best when applied immediately.

Your glove is waterproof and allows you to do dishes or laundry. *Never ever immerse*

[a] Reproduced with permission of the Ontario Crippled Children Centre/Workmen's Compensation Board Rehabilitation Centre, Toronto, Ontario

TABLE 9.A-2. (*continued*)

the prosthesis into water when the glove has been cut or torn. Torn gloves can not be repaired and should be replaced as soon as possible. To work on cars or in the garden, a light colored mitten or playtex rubber glove can be worn over the cosmetic glove for added protection.

Battery charging

Your prosthesis is powered by rechargeable nickel-cadmium batteries. The normal life span of these batteries is 2½–3 years. These batteries are likely to suffer premature damage from overcharging but especially from total discharge.

When you notice that your artificial hand opens very slowly, does not open fully or operates erratically, batteries must be exchanged (6-volt Bock System) or recharged immediately (U.N.B., R.I.M. and V.A.N.U. Systems.) Under no circumstances ever connect prosthesis and charger while you are still wearing the prosthesis. *Always take the prosthesis off and then proceed to recharge the batteries inside.* If your prosthesis for some reason is not worn (sickness, etc.) the batteries should be charged every 2 weeks.

Normal recharging time for any battery system is 12 hours. Do not exceed 14 hours ever. Keep your charger away from children. Leave the charger plugged in, insert batteries and switch on the white switch on the left side of the charger housing. Control lights indicate recharging process is on. These lights do not indicate the need for charging however. Batteries which are only partly used should be charged proportionally less. You might find it useful to use a timer to avoid overcharging since there is no automatic cutout in the charger.

At the underside of the charger is a selector switch which allows switching from 110 volts to 220 volt systems for travel abroad (Bock Systems only).

It is normal for the charger to warm up during the charging process.

Before you take your prosthesis off, remove your battery (6 volt system). When putting your prosthesis on, apply the prosthesis first, then insert the battery. This practice protects the electronic circuit from high signal loads which can damage the system.

Batteries left inserted (6 volt system) in the prosthesis are slowly being drained even if the prosthesis is not worn, as the electronic circuitry draws a standby current. Turning off the switch in the hand does not turn off the current to the electrodes. When batteries are drained totally, irreversible damage may be inflicted.

Internal hand switch

Inside your hand is a push type switch that allows shutting the hand off. This allows you to grasp an object and carry it without your muscles having to contract. It is also useful to use this switch if you have to hold on to an object for a longer time while you move your arm a lot, (*e.g.* using garden tools).

This switch may also be used to switch the hand off in areas of high power circuit interference. (Interference can be caused by some high powered colour TVs or ham radio sets.)

It is good practice (and looks more normal) to keep the fingers of the hand approximately ½″ open. This prevents the fingertips from being pressed flat under constant load. It also prevents you from sending "Close" signals when the hand is already fully closed. Sending a "Close" signal with the hand fully closed is comparable to "riding the clutch" in a car and will lead to mechanical problems.

Do not run the motor longer after the hand is closed or fully open as this not only drains the battery unnecessarily but will also eventually burn out the motor.

TABLE 9.A-2. (*continued*)

Avoid activities that cause jarring or strong vibrations (*i.e.* using a hammer, with the myoelectric hand).

If you have electrical problems with your prosthesis bring your batteries, fully charged if possible, and your charger along with your prosthesis.

If you have any problems or questions, remember we are only as far away as the phone. We are always glad to help.

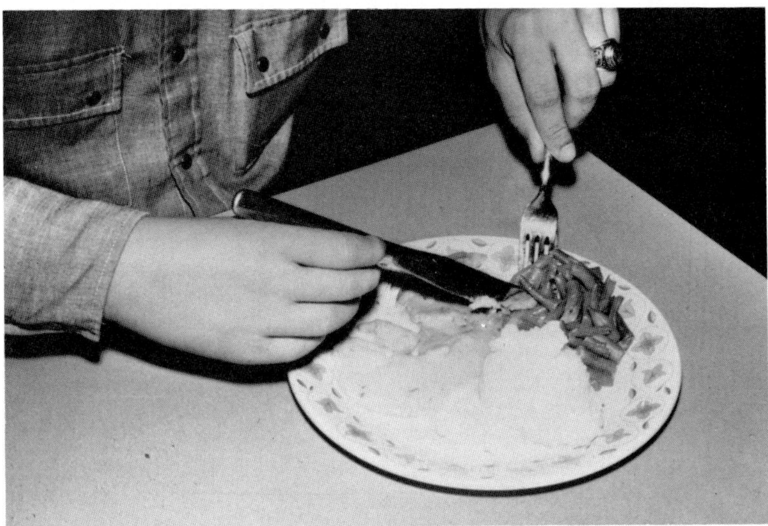

Fig. 9.A-25. The myoelectric hand provides a strong grip for holding the knife. The hand switch can be pushed into the OFF position to prevent inadvertent activation of the hand or release of the mechanical joint through the pressure exerted on the knife.

The amputee is instructed in the care and maintenance of the device (Table 9.A-2). When he/she puts the prosthesis on he/she is reminded not to rotate the stump in the socket since this might change the site of contact with the electrodes.

The amputee first practices opening and closing of the hand while holding the arm in various positions, using the full range of arm movement. She/he then practices gripping objects of different sizes and forms and stacking blocks, progressing from larger to smaller ones. This is performed both in standing and sitting positions. The tasks are kept simple so that the amputee can concentrate on smooth control, correct grasp and energy conservation. The goal is to acquire a less conscious, more automatic control of the hand.

The frequency and length of the training periods have to be geared to the amputee's tolerance. Initially, frequent rest periods are essential to avoid fatigue of the muscles.

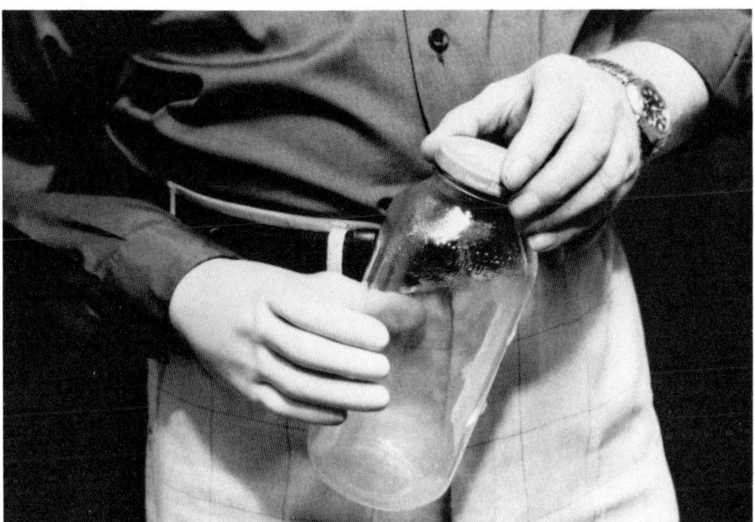

Fig. 9.A-26. The myoelectric hand provides sufficient grip and friction to open most jars.

If the amputee has any problems controlling the hand accurately it will be useful to check his/her phantom movement, his/her state of relaxation, the sensitivity of the electrodes, or the electrode contact. At this time, it is particularly important that the amputee does not compete with another amputee since this may produce anxiety and could delay progress by causing a sense of failure.

The amputee progresses to gripping soft objects such as paper cups and sponges to learn accurate control of grip force. He/she also practices quick release of objects as may be necessary in the case of an emergency. This may be achieved by using a paper cup and deciding on specific cues to signal release of the object. When the amputee can perform the gripping of the various objects smoothly and accurately, he/she progresses to simple games, *e.g.* checkers, tic-tac-toe, which adds a new dimension of concentration and leads into activities requiring focus on the task rather than the control of the device.

If the amputee has to learn to operate two control systems, such as hand and elbow for above-elbow and forequarter amputees, he/she will benefit from first activating one without the other, and only subsequently attempt to combine the controls and practice alternate functions repeatedly.

TRAINING IN FUNCTIONAL USE OF PROSTHESIS

When the amputee demonstrates good control of the prosthesis he/she is introduced to a variety of activities which will incorporate the prosthesis into his/her daily activities (Figs. 9.A-25–9.A-30). The basic principles as

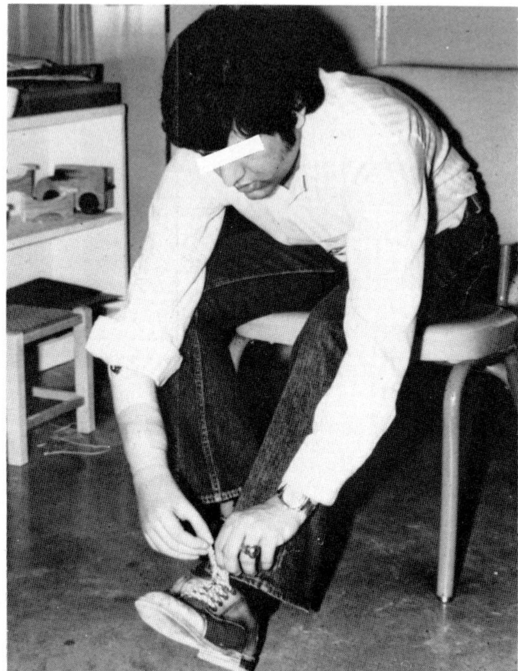

Fig. 9.A-27. Full control of the hand is possible in all planes of movement.

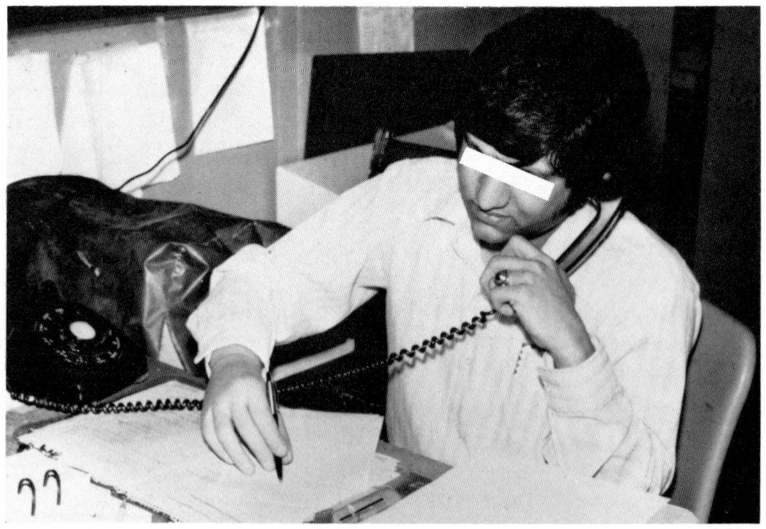

Fig. 9.A-28. The myoelectric hand can be used satisfactorily for writing.

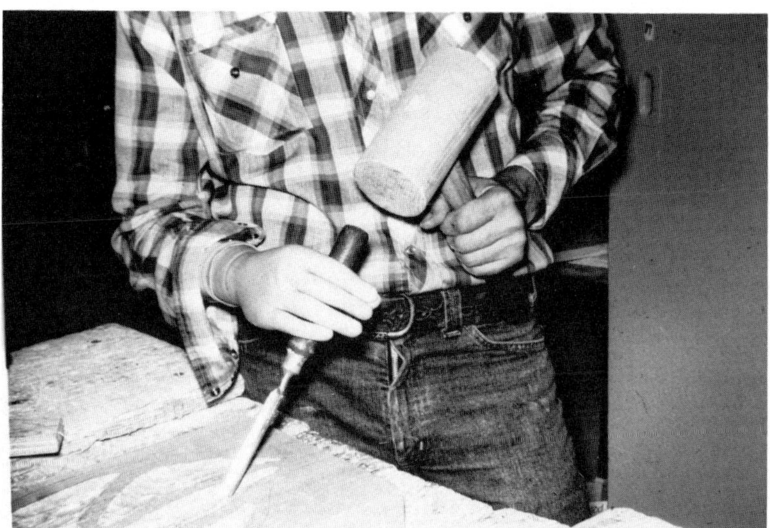

Fig. 9.A-29. The myoelectric prosthesis can be used for handling a variety of tools. The hand switch may be used to prevent inadvertent activation of the hand. The myoelectric hand never should be used to hold a hammer or other tools that cause a strong jarring motion in order to avoid damaging the hand.

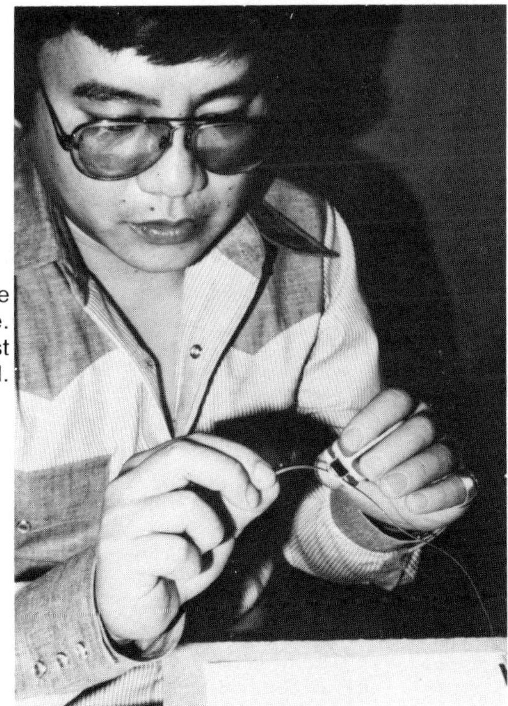

Fig. 9.A-30. For fine manipulative tasks, a special pincher is available. It is shaped to fit between the first three fingers of the myoelectric hand.

well as the general progression in the training are similar to those for the training with a conventional prosthesis. The emphasis is placed on practical and efficient use of the device, on good work habits, on preplanning of activities and on conscientious use. This is achieved by assigning selected activities which are appropriate to the amputee's interest and occupation and give him/her a sense of success. The amputee learns to make use of the special feature of the hand: *i.e.* the OFF switch is utilized to maintain a strong grip as in holding a knife to cut meat, in carrying objects, or to sustain the grip while moving the arm, *e.g.* in handling garden tools.

The amputee is given advice in "trouble shooting" in case the prosthesis does not function correctly: to check if the OFF switch is activated unintentionally, if the battery is charged, if there is excessive perspiration or dryness of the skin, and if the electrode contact is adequate. If none of these reveal the cause of the failure, the prosthetist has to be contacted.

The training periods are gradually increased and the stump is checked regularly for signs of irritation. The prosthesis is again evaluated at the end of the training program to ensure maximum function and fit. A follow-up at set intervals, *e.g.*, 1 month, then 6 months, is advisable to ensure good function of the prosthesis.

REFERENCES

1. DANZIG, A. *Handbook for One-Handers*, Federation of the Handicapped, 211 West 14th Street, New York, N.Y. 10011
2. GARDNER, W. *Left Handed Writing, Instruction Manual*, The Interstate, 19 North Jackson Street, Danville, Ill., 1958.
3. HROMEK, C., AND KING P. *Bilateral Upper Extremity Valet, Am. J. Occup. Ther., 25:* 433, 1971.
4. RICHARDSON, N. *Type with One Hand*, South-Western Publishing Company, Cinncinnati, 1959.
5. SAMMONS, F. *A Bathing Device for Bilateral Above Elbow Amputees*, Northwestern University, Prosthetic Research Center, Illinois, 1965

ADDITIONAL READING

1. COLBURN, J., *Myo-electric controls—a challenge to occupational therapists?, Can. J. Occup. Ther., 44:* 31–39, 1977.
2. FRIEDMANN, L. W. *The Psychological Rehabilitation of the Amputee*, Charles C Thomas, Springfield, Ill., 1978.
3. KLOPSTEG, P. E., AND WILSON, P. D. *Human Limbs and Their Substitutes*, Hafner, New York, 1968.
4. LEAVY, J. D. *It Can Be Done, An Upper Extremity Amputee Training Handbook*, P.O. Box 515, Lake Almanor Peninsula, Ca. 96137.
5. MITAL, M. A. AND PIERCE, D. S. *Amputees and Their Prostheses*, Little, Brown, Boston, 1971.
6. NORTHMORE-BALL, M. D., HEGER, H., AND HUNTER, G. A. *The Below-elbow Myo-electric Prosthesis, J. Bone Jt. Surg., 62B:* 363–367, 1980.
7. O'SHEA, B. Lecture on Myo-electric Training given at the Bio-Engineering Institute, University of New Brunswick, Federicton, Canada 1977.

8. Santschi, W. *Manual of Upper Extremity Prosthetics*, Dept. of Engineering, University of California, Los Angeles, 1958.
9. Tromblay, C. and Scott, A. *Occupational Therapy for Physical Dysfunction*, Williams & Wilkins, Baltimore, 1977.
10. Vargo, J. W. *Some Psychological Effects of Physical Disability, Am. J. Occup. Therapy., 32:* 31–34, 1978.
11. Wellerson, T. *A Manual for Occupational Therapists on the Rehabilitation of Upper Extremity Amputees*, Wm. C. Brown Book Company, Dubuque, 1958.
12. Willard, H. S. and Spackman, C. S. *Occupational Therapy*, Philadelphia, J.B. Lippincott, 1978.

B. Prosthetic Checkout of Upper Extremity Amputees

HANNA HEGER, O.T. (C)

The prosthesis is evaluated prior to commencing training as well as under working conditions during the functional training and before the final discharge to assure comfortable fit and maximum function. Any necessary adjustments are done before the training is continued. The evaluation procedure familiarizes the therapist with all the components of the prosthesis in detail. It also serves to give the amputee a functional analysis of the limb.

The initial and final evaluation procedure may follow the evaluation forms for below-elbow and above-elbow prostheses as shown in Tables 9.B-1 and 9.B-2. Items required for the evaluation procedure are a goniometer, a 50 lb spring scale with a loop of string big enough to put the foot in, a 30 lb spring scale with a stop, a ½″ block of wood, an adaptor to provide the link between the cable hanger and the spring scale, a cable adaptor, a tape measure, a piece of paper, and a ruler. For the purpose of convenience and efficiency it is advisable to carry out all relevant test items first with the prosthesis on and then complete the procedure with the test items requiring the prosthesis off.

Evaluation of Below-Elbow Prosthesis

RANGE OF MOTION

Only the range of motion that is affected by the prosthesis is measured. Standard procedures with a goniometer are followed. In a properly fitting socket, the lateral hinge should be centered over the lateral epicondyle. For measurement of flexion, therefore, center the goniometer over the center of the lateral elbow hinge. The arms of the goniometer are lined up with the prosthesis and the arm (not with the hinge, as the proximal part of the hinge tends to tilt back). Rotation with the prosthesis on is measured by aligning the goniometer with the hook fingers; if necessary, a pencil can be placed in the hook to assist in the alignment of the goniometer. Measurement of rotation of the stump is facilitated by marking the line of midprone position at the tip of the stump.

If the range of elbow flexion does not meet performance standards the cause may be due to an improper trim of the socket causing impingement

TABLE 9.B-1a. *Prosthetic Checkout Form: Below Elbow*[a]

Date ____________________

Name of Patient ____

Initial Checkout ( ) Final Checkout ( )
Pass ( ) Provisional Pass ( ) Fail ( )

If the patient needs further attention, please indicate the area in which treatment is required:

Medical-Surgical ______________ ( ) Training ____________________ ( )

Prosthetic ______________ ( ) Other ____________________ ( )
(Vocational, Psychological, etc.)

Comments and Recommendations:

____
____
____
____

____
Clinic Chief

Prosthetics and Orthotics
New York University
Postgraduate Medical School

[a] Table 9.B-1 reprinted with permission of Prosthetics and Orthotics Department, New York University, Post-Graduate Medical School.

of the biceps tendon. Rotation may be impeded by a too tightly fitting socket or improper trim of the socket.

TERMINAL DEVICE OPENING AND CLOSING

The opening measurement is taken with a ruler between the tips of the hook fingers with the fingers pointing medially. Mechanical range is the potential opening of the hook permitted by the design of the hook. Active range is measured with the elbow flexed at 90° and at the greatest range of elbow flexion and extension.

The possible causes for lack of full opening are excessive length of the cable housing, loose adjustment of the cable, improper adjustments of the harness or limitation of the control motions. If the hook cannot be fully closed with the fingers pronated 90°, the cable is adjusted too tightly.

CONTROL SYSTEM EFFICIENCY

This test determines how much of the force that is exerted to open the terminal device (TD) is lost through friction in the cable housing. The first measurement is taken at the hook through a spring scale attached *via* an adaptor fitting into the thumb of the hook. The hook fingers point medially, the elbow is flexed at 90°. The spring scale is lined up correctly in the

TABLE 9.B-1b. *Prosthetic Checkout Form: Below-Elbow (continued)*

	PROSTHESIS OFF	PROSTHESIS ON	PERFORMANCE STANDARDS
RANGE OF MOTION			
1. Stump Rotation (Total Range)	____°	____°	Total rotation with prosthesis on should be half that with prosthesis off.[1] (For Muenster prosthesis, see Footnote 2)
2. Elbow Flexion			Active flexion with prosthesis on should be within 10 degrees of range with prosthesis off.[2]
Maximum Extension Angle (Initial Flexion)	____°	____°	
Maximum Flexion Angle	____°	____°	
Range	____°	____°	
TERMINAL DEVICE OPENING AND CLOSING[3]	HOOK	HAND	
1. Mechanical Range	____ in.	____ in.	
2. Active Range (Forearm at 90 degrees)	____ in.	____ in.	Full opening and closing should be obtained in all test positions.
3. Active Range (at Waist)	____ in.	____ in.	
4. Active Range (at Mouth)	____ in.	____ in.	
CONTROL SYSTEM EFFICIENCY[3]			
1. Force Applied at Terminal Device	____ lbs.	____	
2. Force Applied at Harness	____ lbs.	____	
3. Efficiency = Force at Terminal Device / Force at Harness	____ %	____ %	Should be 80% or greater for single control.
STABILITY			
1. Displacement of Socket on Stump with 50 pounds Axial Load (one-third body weight for children)		____ in.	Prosthesis should not slip on stump more than 1 inch.[4] Harness should not tear.

[1] This standard applies to medium, well-formed stumps, but is often exceeded with wrist disarticulation and long below-elbow stumps. Short or fleshy stumps may not be able to attain the 50% standard.

[2] In Muenster sockets, forearm rotation is eliminated and maximum elbow flexion is considerably limited (average 105 to 110 degrees). Furthermore, because of decreased elbow flexion, the measurement of terminal device opening at the mouth may not apply. However, the terminal device should open fully at maximum elbow flexion.

[3] Fingers directed medially.

[4] Because of the intimate fit of the Muenster socket, the slippage should not be more than ½".

direction of the cable. A small block of wood is placed between the hook fingers and held by the therapist with one hand (Fig. 9.B-1). (Note: make sure that the movement of the hook finger is not impeded or assisted by the therapist's fingers.) The force required to just lift the hook finger off the

TABLE 9.B-1c. *Prosthetic Checkout Form: Below-Elbow (continued)*

CONFORMANCE WITH PRESCRIPTION

______ 1. Is the prosthesis as prescribed? If a recheck, have previous recommendations been accomplished?

DIMENSION

______ 2. Is the prosthesis the correct length?

TERMINAL DEVICE AND WRIST UNIT

______ 3. Do the terminal device and wrist mechanism function properly?

______ 4. If a cosmetic glove is used, is it undamaged, properly color-matched, and pulled completely onto the fingers?

______ 5. If a length adapter is used, is a fairing for the hand or hook installed?

ELBOW HINGE

______ 6. Does the elbow hinge function properly without pinching flesh or otherwise causing discomfort?

CUFF

______ 7. Does the cuff fit snugly without gapping during forearm flexion and terminal device operation?

HARNESS

______ 8. Is the axilla loop small enough to keep the cross of the Figure 8 harness well below the seventh cervical vertebra and slightly to the unamputated side?

______ 9. Is the axilla loop properly covered and is it comfortable?

______ 10. Is the control attachment strap below midscapular level and does it remain low enough to give adequate cable travel?

______ 11. If there are additional harness straps, can their use be justified?

______ 12. Does the front support strap pass through the delto-pectoral groove?

______ 13. If a chest strap harness is used, is the saddle of proper size and placement, and is the chest strap comfortable?

CABLE SYSTEM

______ 14. If a hook is to be interchanged with a hand, is the hook-to-cable adapter the proper length?

______ 15. Is the control cable free from sharp bends?

______ 16. Is the housing on the control cable long enough to prevent contact of the cable with the patient or with the prosthetic forearm, but short enough so it does not interfere with function?

______ 17. Is the cable housing the proper length between the housing cross bar and the retainer on the forearm, neither too loose nor too tight?

SOCKET

______ 18. Is the socket comfortable, especially when compression force and torque are applied?

______ 19. Is the stump free from abrasions, discolorations, and other signs of irritation immediately after the prosthesis is removed?

WORKMANSHIP

______ 20. Is the general workmanship satisfactory?

PATIENT'S PERFORMANCE AND OPINION

______ 21. Can the patient demonstrate effective use of the terminal device and wrist mechanism?

______ 22. Does the patient consider the prosthesis satisfactory as to comfort, function, and appearance?

TABLE 9.B-2a. *Prosthetic Checkout Form: Above-Elbow and Shoulder-Disarticulation*[a]

Date ____________

Name of Patient ______________________________

Initial Checkout ( )   Final Checkout ( )
Pass ( )   Provisional Pass ( )   Fail ( )

If the patient needs further attention, please indicate the area in which treatment is required:

Medical-Surgical __________ ( )   Training __________ ( )

Prosthetic __________ ( )   Other __________ ( )
(Vocational, Psychological, etc.)

Comments and Recommendations:

____

____

____

____

____
Clinic Chief

Prosthetics and Orthotics
New York University
PostGraduate Medical School

[a] Table 9.B-2 reprinted with permission of Prosthetics and Orthotics Department, New York University, PostGraduate Medical School.

block is recorded. Since this is a somewhat subjective measurement the test is repeated three times and the average reading is recorded.

The second measurement is taken with the spring scale connected to the proximal end of the cable on the hanger of the control strap attachment. This is done with another adaptor consisting of a flat hook which fits over the hanger. The spring scale is positioned in a continuing line with the cable (Fig. 9.B-2). Three readings are taken, as before. (To connect the control strap attachment properly following the test, it is useful to mark the position of the buckle before starting the test.) The efficiency is determined as a percentage as follows:

$$\frac{\text{Force at TD}}{\text{Force at harness}} \times 100 = \text{efficiency}$$

If the efficiency does not reach the performance standard, the cause may be sharp bends in the cable or housing, a frayed cable or improper location of the cable retainers, creating sharp angles in the line of pull.

STABILITY

This test measures the displacement of the socket on the stump when a downward force is exerted on the terminal device. The spring scale is hooked

TABLE 9.B-2b. *Prosthetic Checkout Form: Above-Elbow and Shoulder-Disarticulation (continued)*

	Prosthesis OFF	Prosthesis ON	PERFORMANCE STANDARDS
RANGE OF MOTION			
1. Shoulder Flexion	____ °	____ °	90 degrees
2. Shoulder Abduction	____ °	____ °	90 degrees
3. Shoulder Extension	____ °	____ °	30 degrees
4. Prosthetic Elbow: Mechanical Range		____ °	135 degrees
5. Prosthetic Elbow: Active Range		____ °	135 degrees
6. Humeral Flexion Required to Flex Elbow Fully		____ °	Should not exceed 45 degrees.
TERMINAL DEVICE OPENING AND CLOSING[1]	HOOK	HAND	
1. Mechanical Range	____ in.	____ in.	
2. Active Range (Forearm at 90 degrees)	____ in.	____ in.	Full opening and closing should be obtained with the forearm at 90 degrees
3. Active Range (at Waist)	____ in.	____ in.	50% or greater opening and closing should be obtained at waist and mouth.
4. Active Range (at Mouth)	____ in.	____ in.	
CONTROL SYSTEM EFFICIENCY[1]			
1. Force Applied at Terminal Device	____ lbs.	____ lbs.	
2. Force Applied at Harness	____ lbs.	____ lbs.	Should be 70% or greater.
3. Efficiency $= \frac{\text{Force at Terminal Device}}{\text{Force at Harness}}$	____ %	____ %	
4. Force Required to Flex Elbow from Position of 90 degrees	____ lbs.	____ lbs.	Should not exceed 10 pounds. Should not cause inadvertent terminal device operation.
STABILITY			
1. Displacement of Socket on Stump with 50 pounds Axial Load (one-third body weight for children)		____ in.	Prosthesis should not slip on stump more than 1 inch. Harness should not tear.

into the fingers of the terminal device and is pulled down until a maximum of 50 lb is reached. The force can be applied by hand or by attaching a loop of rope or webbing on the scale and pushing down with one foot in the loop. The amputee is instructed to resist the force. The displacement is measured

TABLE 9.B-2c. *Prosthetic Checkout Form: Above-Elbow and Shoulder-Disarticulation (continued)*

CONFORMANCE WITH PRESCRIPTION

____ 1. Is the prosthesis as prescribed? If a recheck, have previous recommendations been accomplished?

DIMENSIONS

____ 2. Is the prosthesis the correct length and do elbow levels coincide?

TERMINAL DEVICE AND WRIST UNIT

____ 3. Do the terminal device and wrist mechanism function properly?

____ 4. If a cosmetic glove is used, is it undamaged, properly color-matched, and pulled completely onto the fingers?

____ 5. If a length adapter is used, is a fairing for the hand or hook installed?

ELBOW UNIT

____ 6. Does the elbow function properly?

____ 7. Is the forearm set in adequate initial flexion?

____ 8. Can the amputee swing his arms while walking and raise his elbow 60 degrees to the side without the elbow locking involuntarily?

____ 9. Can the patient use the turntable to position the forearm satisfactorily?

HARNESS

____ 10. Is the axilla loop small enough to keep the cross of the Figure-8 harness well below the seventh cervical vertebra and slightly to the unamputated side?

____ 11. Is the axilla loop properly covered and is it comfortable?

____ 12. Is the control-attachment strap below midscapular level and does it remain low enough to give adequate cable travel?

____ 13. Is the lateral support strap properly positioned?

____ 14. If there are additional harness straps, can their use be justified?

____ 15. Does the front support strap pass through the delto-pectoral groove?

____ 16. Is the elastic front suspensor of adequate length and properly located?

____ 17. If a chest strap harness is used, is the saddle of proper size and placement, and is the chest strap comfortable?

CABLE SYSTEM

____ 18. If a hook is to be interchanged with a hand, is the hook-to-cable adapter the proper length?

____ 19. Is the control cable free from sharp bends?

____ 20. Is the housing on the control cable long enough to prevent contact of the cable with the patient or with the prosthetic forearm, but short enough so it does not interfere with function?

____ 21. Does cable housing cover the cable adequately without restricting forearm flexion?

____ 22. Is the leather lift loop the proper length and is it positioned to allow adequate terminal device operation after full forearm flexion and heavy enough to withstand buckling during use?

____ 23. Does the leather lift loop pivot on the screw and grip the cable housing tightly enough to prevent slipping?

____ 24. Does the elbow lock cable lead directly from the access hole to the deltopectoral groove?

SOCKET

____ 25. Is the socket comfortable, especially when compression force and torque are applied?

____ 26. Is the stump free from abrasions, discolorations, and other signs of irritation immediately after the prosthesis is removed?

WORKMANSHIP

____ 27. Is the general workmanship satisfactory?

PATIENT'S PERFORMANCE AND OPINION

____ 28. Can the patient demonstrate effective use of the terminal device, wrist mechanism, and elbow unit?

____ 29. Does the patient consider the prosthesis satisfactory as to comfort, function, and appearance?

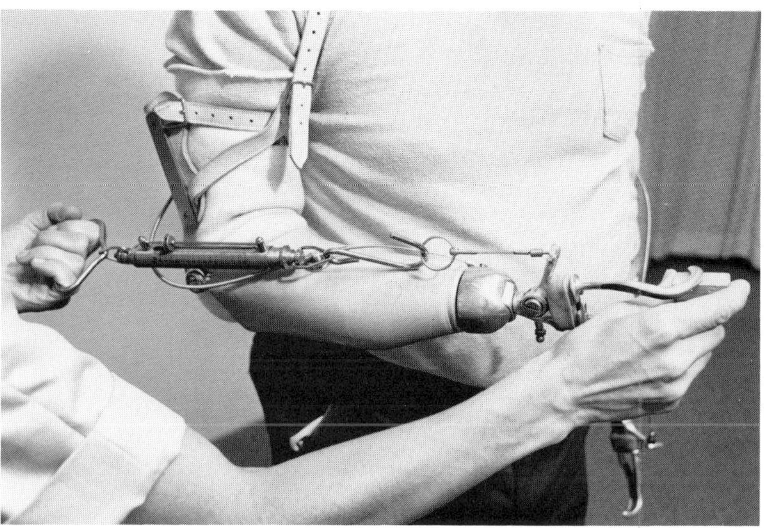

Fig. 9.B-1. First test of control system efficiency.

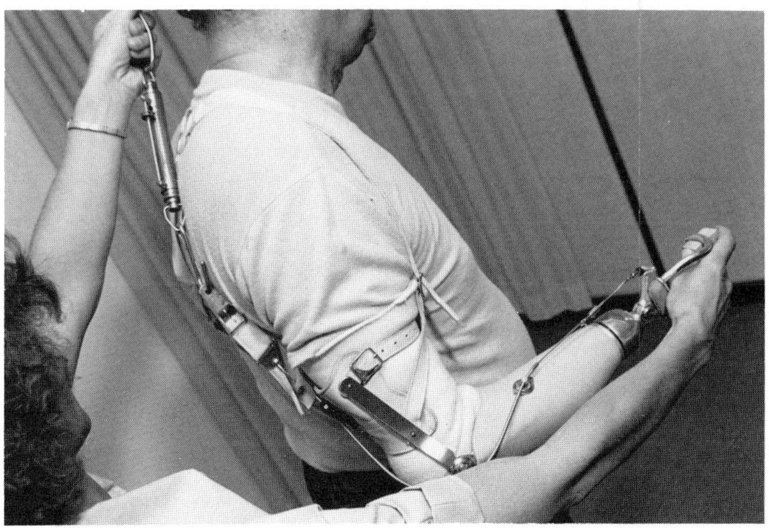

Fig. 9.B-2. Second test of control system efficiency.

by holding a measuring tape on the stump above the socket rim and marking the line of the rim on the tape before the test and when full force is applied. (It is not practical to mark the position of the socket on the stump sock because the sock may slide down as well.)

Possible causes of excessive displacement are improper socket fit, weak leather components and poor harness stitching.

To determine if the triceps pad fits tightly enough, the therapist exerts an axial pull on the hook with the elbow flexed at 90°. The socket should not slip more than ½″ on the stump. A slack fit is caused by weak leather.

The remainder of the evaluation focuses in more detail on the specific components of the prosthesis in terms of comfort, function, cosmesis and workmanship. Some practical points are worth mentioning here. For measuring the correct length of the prosthesis, the end of the hook fingers should be level with the tip of the thumb on the sound hand while both arms are held extended by the side. The level of the shoulders should be checked to ensure that they are even. The length of the stump may make it impossible to obtain the same overall length.

The grip of the terminal device is checked by attempting to slide a piece of paper between the closed hook fingers or by holding the hook against the light to determine if a line of light can be seen which indicates that the hook fingers do not close completely.

If the patient has a figure 8 harness, the cross of the harness should be located below the seventh cervical vertebra and slightly to the unamputated side. If it is too far to either side, the axilla loop will be too small or too narrow and cause discomfort. Incorrect placement of the cross also may cause the harness strap to slide off the shoulder on the amputated side. If, however, the cross does not seem correctly located but the amputee is comfortable and able to operate the prosthesis without difficulty then the cross may remain in its position.

If the figure 8 harness needs to be tightened, an equal adjustment of both the anterior and the posterior strap is necessary to maintain proper location of the cross.

After the patient takes the prosthesis off, the therapist checks the stump for signs of pressure. The impressions that the stump sock leaves on the skin will indicate the fit of the socket.

Evaluation of Above-Elbow and Shoulder Disarticulation Prosthesis

RANGE OF MOTION

This is measured with a goniometer using standard procedures. If the mechanical range of the elbow is limited, the cause may be improper trim of the forearm section or an incorrectly adjusted elbow unit. Possible causes of restriction in the active range are improper adjustment of the harness, improper positioning of the cable housing or limitations of the control motions. If more than 45° of humeral flexion are required to flex the elbow, the harness is adjusted improperly.

TERMINAL DEVICE OPENING AND CLOSING

If the opening of the terminal device is restricted the causes may be the same as for the below elbow prosthesis.

CONTROL SYSTEM EFFICIENCY

The measurements are determined in the same way as for the below-elbow prosthesis. If the efficiency is below the performance standards, possible causes are improper location of the cable retainers, sharp bends in the cable or housing, or a frayed cable.

The force required to flex the elbow from a position of 90° flexion is measured by attaching the spring scale to the hanger of the cable and pulling it in line with the cable while the elbow is supported on the table or by the amputee. The therapist stabilizes the upper part of the socket. If this force exceeds the standard of 10 lb, the possible reasons are incorrect length or location of the lever loop or improper alignment of the cable.

STABILITY

Stability measurements is made in the same way as for the below-elbow prosthesis with the measuring tape placed on the acromion. Possible causes of unsatisfactory stability are improper socket fit, improper harness stitching or weak leather components.

The correct level of the elbow is determined by looking at the amputee from behind while he or she flexes both elbows and keeps the shoulders level. The length of the stump may make it impossible for the elbow levels to be even.

The function of the elbow unit is checked by operating the elbow cable throughout the range of elbow movement to determine if the cable sticks at any point. If the adjustment of the elbow lock cable is too tight the cable can be damaged easily when objects are lifted with the elbow locked in flexion because the elbow lock cable takes then part of the load.

The initial flexion of the forearm should be at least 15°.

The elbow lock cable should be adjusted so that the amputee has enough freedom of movement to swing his/her arms while walking and to abduct the prosthesis 60° without the elbow locking unexpectedly.

The friction of the turntable should be adequate. It should resist at least 2 lb of pull to exclude inadvertent turning, but it should not be too tight to prevent rotation. It can be measured by attaching the spring scale to the hook with the elbow locked at 90° flexion; the therapist stabilizes the upper part of the socket while pulling on the spring scale.

To avoid creating pressure areas, the shoulder pad of the harness should not rest on the acromion. The harness is tightened by adjusting the chest strap.

At the end of the evaluation procedure it is useful to take an overall view of the prosthesis to get a general impression of the comfort and fit.

During the functionl training, the prosthesis is continually evaluated in terms of fit, function and comfort with active use. Adjustments are performed whenever necessary.

TABLE 9.B-3a. *Prosthetic Evaluation of Below-Elbow Myoelectric Prosthesis*

Date ____________
Name of Patient ____________ Claim ____________
Type of Prosthesis ____________
____________ Date received ____________
Initial Evaluation ____________ Final Evaluation ____________
Pass ________ Provisional Pass ________ Fail ________

RANGE OF MOTION	Prosthesis	on	off
1) Elbow flexion		______°	______°
Elbow extension		______°	______°
2) Stump rotation (if applicable)	Pronation	______°	______°
	Supination	______°	______°

TERMINAL DEVICE OPENING AND CLOSING
1) Range of grip span Norm ________ cm Actual ________ cm
2) Maximal prehension of hand Norm ________ kg Actual ________ kg
Sound hand ________ kg

SUSPENSION OF SOCKET
1) Axial load (elbow extended) ________ kg
Displacement of socket on stump ________ cm
Discomfort experienced ____________
2) Retention of socket with resistive elbow extension from 90° elbow flexion ________ kg
Displacement of socket on stump ________ cm
Discomfort experienced ____________
3) Is the socket retained satisfactorily after the hand has been operated in the extremes of range of arm movement (first with the hand behind the neck then with the hand at the side with elbow fully extended)? ____________

[a] Workmen's Compensation Board, Rehabilitation Centre, Downsview, Ontario.

Prosthetic Evaluation of Myoelectric Below-Elbow Prosthesis

The myoelectric prosthesis is evaluated in all aspects of function, comfort and cosmesis. There are at present no performance standards available. The data is evaluated to what can be reasonably expected depending on the length and condition of the stump. In Table 9.B-3 a tentative evaluation form is presented.

The evaluation procedure is performed prior to commencing training and before the the final discharge. Necessary adjustments to obtain maximal function and comfortable fit are done when required. The prosthesis also is tested under working conditions during the functional training.

For the sake of convenience for the amputee, all tests that require the prosthesis to be on are performed first. When the amputee takes the prosthesis off, the stump is checked for pressure areas and imprints of the electrodes, then the remainder of the test items are performed. The ease with which the amputee can put the prosthesis on and take it off also is observed.

TABLE 9.B-3b. *Prosthetic Evaluation of Below-Elbow Myoelectric Prosthesis (continued)*

COMFORMANCE WITH PRESCRIPTION

___ 1. Is the prosthesis as prescribed? If a re-evaluation, have previous recommendations been accomplished?

DIMENSION AND WEIGHT

___ 2. Is the prosthesis the correct length?

___ 3. Is the weight of the prosthesis satisfactory?

TERMINAL DEVICE AND WRIST UNIT

___ 4. Does the terminal device function properly?

___ 5. Is the cosmetic glove undamaged, pulled completely onto the fingers and not impairing grip?

___ 6. Is colour match satisfactory?

___ 7. Does the wrist mechanism function properly?

CONTROL

___ 8. Are the electrodes positioned over the site of maximum potential?

___ 9. Is there good contact between electrodes and skin?

___ 10. How long are the imprints visible on the skin?

___ 11. Can the amputee perform appropriate control of grip force?

___ 12. Can the amputee carry out motions and actions including stump rotation without accidentally opening or closing the hand?

___ 13. Can the amputee control the hand fully in various positions throughout the full range of arm movement?

___ 14. Can the amputee hold an object against some resistance applied to the arm without accidentally opening or closing the hand?

___ 15. Do other factors influence the control of the hand (perspiration, electrical interference, etc.)?

SOCKET

___ 16. Is the socket comfortable (especially when compression force and torque are applied)?

___ 17. Is the amputee's stump free from abrasion, discoloration, irritation etc., immediately after the prosthesis is taken off?

BATTERY, RECHARGER

___ 18. Is the battery secured in receptacle; can the battery be taken out easily?

___ 19. Are the batteries and battery charger in good working condition?

WORKMANSHIP

___ 20. Is the general workmanship satisfactory?

AMPUTEE'S PERFORMANCE AND OPINION

___ 21. Has the amputee completed a training program in the use of his/her prosthesis?

___ 22. Can the amputee demonstrate effective use of his/her prosthesis?

___ 23. Is the amputee satisfied with the prosthesis in regard to comfort, function, cosmesis?

Comments: ____

____

____

___ 24. Has the amputee been informed about care and maintenance of the prosthesis?

MEDICAL, SURGICAL AND PROSTHETIC STATUS

___ 25. Is the amputee free of immediate medical, surgical or prosthetic requirements?

FOLLOW-UP

___ 26. What follow-up arrangements have been made;

____

____

ADJUSTMENTS MADE:

THERAPIST'S COMMENTS AND RECOMMENDATIONS:

____

RANGE OF MOTION

The measurements are taken with a goniometer following standard procedures. Due to the Muenster type socket, maximum elbow flexion and extension is limited by approximately 20–25°.

TERMINAL DEVICE OPENING AND CLOSING

The measurement is taken with a ruler between the tips of the fingers. The opening may be impeded by the tightness of the glove in the web space between thumb and index finger. If the grip force of the myoelectric hand is below the specifications of the manufacturer, the clutch can be adjusted to reach the maximum gripforce. Amputees find it useful to compare the grip strength of the myoelectric hand with their sound hand.

SUSPENSION OF SOCKET

For this measurement a spring scale is fitted with a wooden handle of approximately $\frac{3}{4}''$ diameter, because the wire handle might slip through the fingers when the full load is applied. A loop may be attached to the other end of the spring scale to apply a downward force with the foot. The spring scale is suspended from the myoelectric hand which is shut off at maximum prehension force. A measuring tape is held against the stump and the level of the socket rim is marked on the tape before and at full application of a downward force. The pull is terminated when the amputee experiences more than tolerable discomfort or when the socket starts to slip off.

The next measurement determines how much force will result in the socket slipping off at 90° of elbow flexion. This can be done with a spring scale suspended on a wall at the appropriate height or by pressing the arm down on a weighing scale. Again, the test is performed with the hand shut off after obtaining maximum grip and it is terminated as above.

DIMENSION

To determine the correct length of the prosthesis, the amputee places both elbows close together on a table and brings both hands together.

CONTROL

The contact of the electrodes on the stump needs to be firm to ensure good control. After taking the prosthesis off, the electrode imprints should be clearly visible but not so deep as to cause skin irritation or breakdown.

Control of the myoelectric hand may be impeded at certain positions of the arm. One reason may be due to the tendency of the amputee to tense all muscles in the forearm inappropriately. This is caused by an effort to hold the prosthesis in order to cope with its greater weight. The amputee has to learn to relax the forearm muscles. Another reason may be due to loss of contact with the electrodes which may occur when the elbow is fully extended and the stump is lifted off the electrode. This requires adjustment to electrode or socket.

The ability to obtain the appropriate grip force is tested by gripping a solid and then a crushable object like a block of wood and a paper cup. The free and resisted movements are performed while holding a paper cup to indicate inadvertent control. The performance of these tests depends on the skill and general relaxation of the amputee as well as on the setting of the sensitivity level on the gain control of the electrodes.

C. Special Devices for Upper Extremity Amputees

HANNA HEGER O.T.(C)

Many tasks can be accomplished satisfactorily with a hook. In some situations, however, the grip or action of the hook is not sufficient or the pressure that can be applied with the prosthesis is not adequate. To rectify these problems a specific tool or object can be adapted with a threaded stud, as is used on the hook, in order to fit directly into the wrist unit. A suitable

TABLE 9.C-1. *Commercial Suppliers and Products for Amputees*

Hugh Steeper Co., Rochampton, England Adapted tools Fishing rod holder
M & W Handicapped Enterprises, Inc., P.O. Box 121, Trenton, Tenn. 38382. ACCRU-Hook System for power tools, household appliances and sports equipment
Hosmer Dorrance Corp., Campbell, Calif. Baseball glove attachment Bowling ball attachment
Warmey, Ltd., 375 Milton Road, Cambridge, CB4 1SS, England. After Bath Body Drier
T. C. Dunlop, Coinamatic Laundry Equipment Ltd., 4 Exmoor Street, London, W10 6DW, England. Luxaire After-Bath Dryer

device also may be designed to meet the need. These modifications may be made, even if the function of the hook is adequate, when the use of the device represents a gain in function. One of the basic requirements for any device is, however, that it is practical and that it justifies the time needed to exchange the terminal device with the special device. The gadget tolerance of the amputee should not be exceeded.

Some devices are commercially available while others have been developed by prosthetists, therapists or by an amputee who has struggled with the limitations of the hook. At times, a device may have to go through several changes until the most functional version is found.

Commercially Available Devices

The following tool adaptations and devices for recreational activities are commercially available (Table 9.C-1).

TABLE 9.C-2. *Devices Designed and Manufactured by Prosthetists, Therapists and Amputees*

Prosthetic Services, Sunnybrook Hospital, Toronto, Ontario, Canada:
- Release button protector (Fig. 9.C-1)
- Adapted hammer (Fig. 9.C-3)
- Gun holder (Fig. 9.C-9)

Ed Pringlemeir, Guelph, Ontario, Canada:
- Straight gripping device (Fig. 9.C-2)
- Screw driver aid (Fig. 9.C-5)
- Gear shift device (Fig. 9.C-7)
- Golf club holder (Fig. 9.C-12)

Workmen's Compensation Board, Rehabilitation Centre, Downsview, Ontario, Canada:
- Tool clamp (Fig. 9.C-4)
- Adapted knife (Fig. 9.C-17)
- Adapted crutches (Fig. 9.C-18)
- Adapted nailclippers (Fig. 9.C-19)

Larry Todd, Milton, Ontario and Ronald Brett, Prosthetics Department, Kingston General Hospital, Kingston, Ontario, Canada:
- Template holder (Fig. 9.C-6)
- Adapted shovel (Fig. 9.C-8)

William Bowman, Hamilton, Ontario, Canada:
- Adapted floor hockey stick (Fig. 9.C-10)

Prosthetic Department, Ontario Crippled Children's Centre, Toronto, Ontario, Canada:
- Hockey stick attachments (Fig. 9.C-11)
- Weight lifting device (Fig. 9.C-13)
- Guitar pick holder (Fig. 9.C-16)

Stephen Zduriencik (9):
- Bow adaptor

Lawrence Roy, Hamilton, Ontario, Canada:
- Fishing rod holder (Fig. 9.C-14)

Richard Vaughan, Haliburton, Ontario, Canada:
- Adapted trumpet (Fig. 9.C-15)

Brian Steed, Timmins, Ontario, Canada:
- Adapted canoe paddle (Fig. 9.C-20)

Fernand Riberdy, Scarborough, Ontario, Canada:
- Holder for electric screwdriver (Fig. 9C-21)

University of California at Los Angeles, Child Amputee Prosthetics Project
- Hook for playing piano

F. Sammons, Northwestern University, Prosthetics Research Center, Chicago, Ill.
- Bathing device for bilateral above-elbow amputee

Caren R. Zatlin, Else Hemmen, Thomas A. Krouskop, Mark Sklan: Guitar Capo for a Bilateral Upper Extremity Amputee (11).

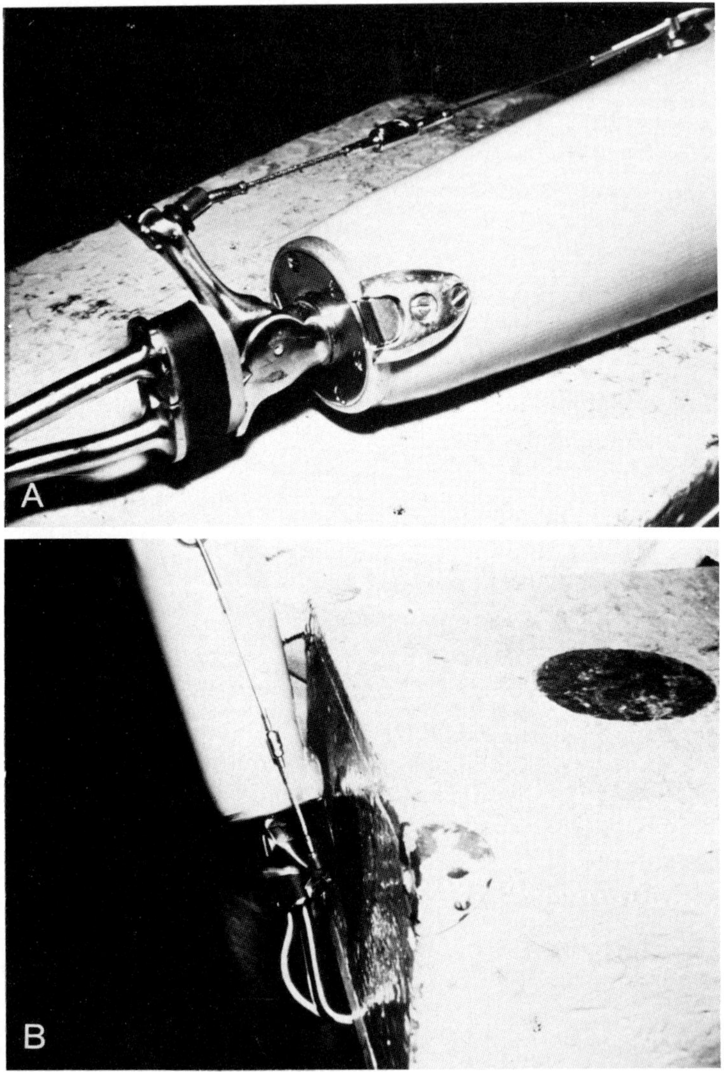

Fig. 9.C-1 *A* and *B*. Release Button Protector (Table 9.C-2). The location of the release button for the quick-change wrist unit may interfere with the carrying of an object; if the object presses on the button the hook may release and the dropping object may cause injury. *A*, a small metal plate with a cut-out for the button is mounted on the socket. The metal plate extends slightly over the button so that the carried object will press against the plate rather than the release button (*B*).

Adapted Tools. Long nosed pliers, quick grip pliers, tweezers and a universal tool holder are modified to fit into the prosthesis and are activated by the control cable. A spade grip with universal joint and clamping screw to hold the tool fits into the Steeper wrist unit (Steeper).

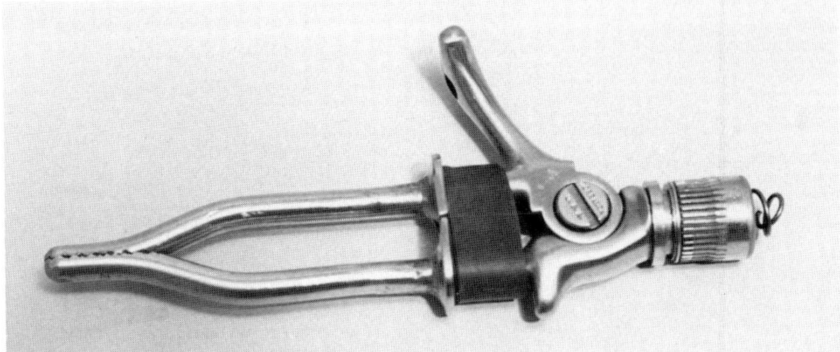

Fig. 9.C-2. Straight gripping device (Table 9.C-2). The fingers of a Dorrance No 5 hook are cut off at the base and two metal rods are welded on instead. The rods are straight with serrated surfaces to allow a plier-like grip. This device was designed by an industrial electrician to facilitate work in small confined spaces such as connector boxes.

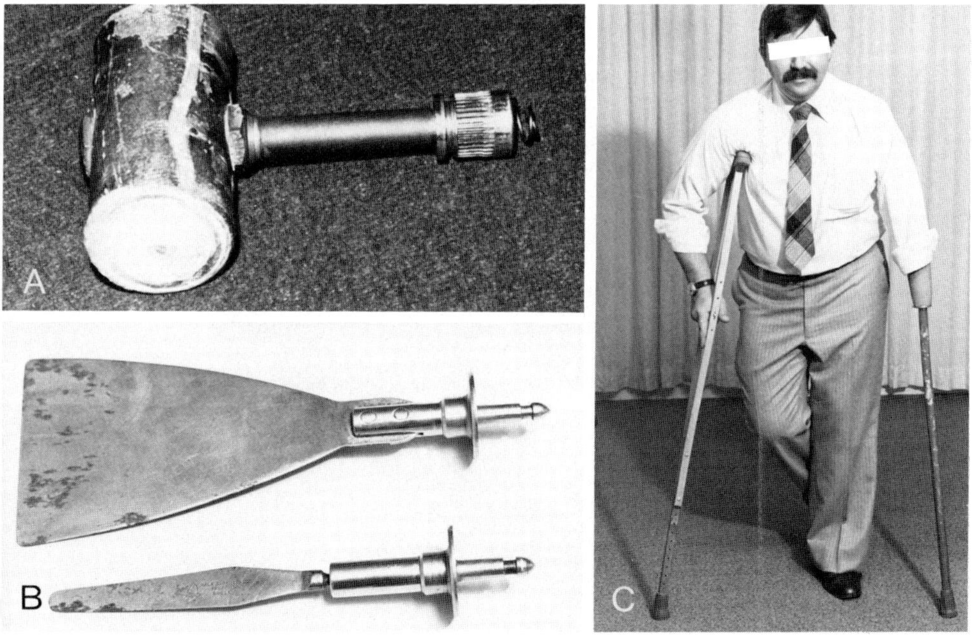

Fig. 9.C-3. Adapted hammer (Table 9.C-2). The handle of the hammer (*A*) is exchanged for a metal rod with a ½-20 thread at the end for the wrist insert. Using the hammer in the prosthesis leaves the sound hand free for fine manipulative tasks such as guiding leather tools or holding a handful of nails and feeding them one-by-one as, for example, a roofer has to do in his work. The same principle can be used for a variety of other tools such as a knife, potatoe peeler, can opener, wrench, palette knife or scraper for a mill (*B*), or a fishing rod. It also can be applied to a cane (*C*) in case of a leg injury.

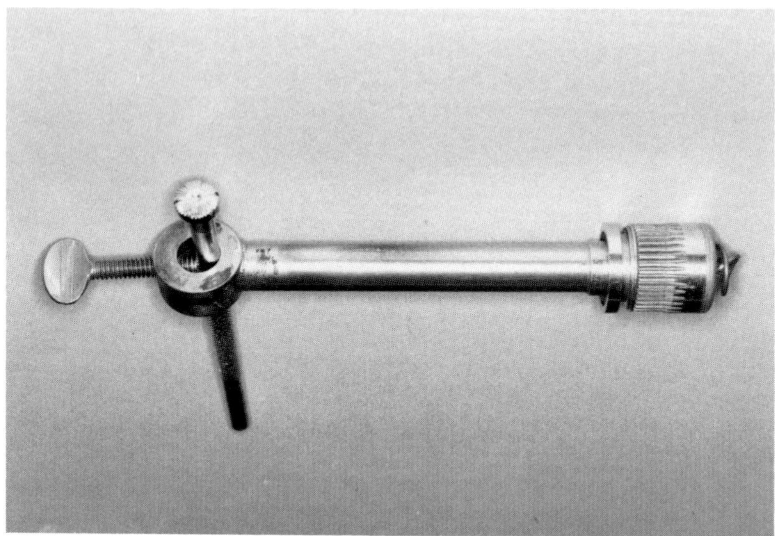

Fig. 9.C-4. Tool clamp (Table 9.C-2). Small tools such as leather carving tools can be held securely in a short metal sleeve which is brazed to a metal rod that fits into the wrist unit. The size of the hole in the sleeve is determined by the diameter of the tools to be used. A set screw is used to secure the tool in the metal sleeve.

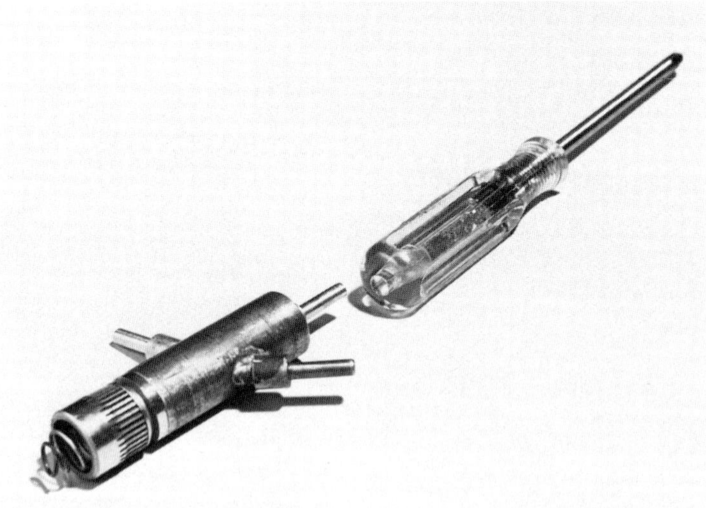

Fig. 9.C-5. Screwdriver aid (Table 9.C-2). A metal rod is fitted with a wrist insert and three thin pins with wider bases. The pins are set at different angles (0°, 45° and 90°) to allow work at different heights or in confined spaces. A slightly larger hole is drilled into the end of the screwdriver handle to fit the pins. In this way, the prosthetic side can provide the pressure while the sound hand turns the screwdriver.

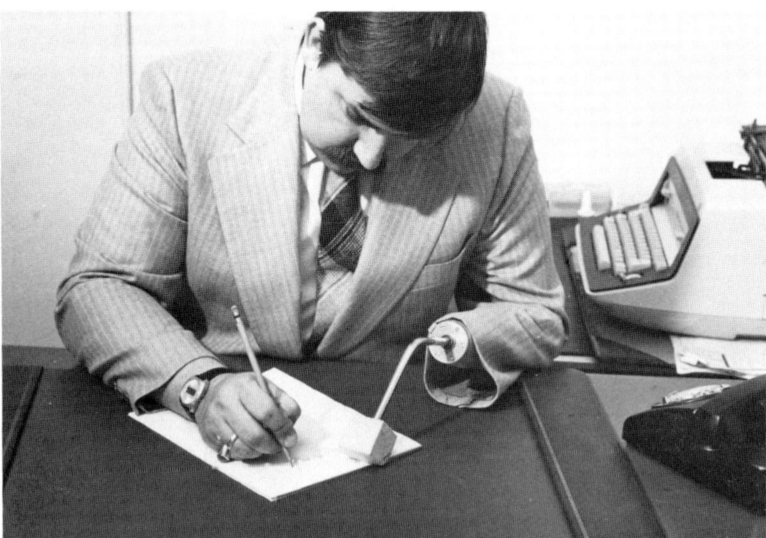

Fig. 9.C-6. Template holder (Table 9.C-2). This device was designed by an above-elbow amputee who found it difficult to hold down templates and paper at his desk because he could not reach the desk surface well with his hook and apply sufficient pressure. A felt block is glued to a metal rod. The bottom edge of the block is cut to provide a larger area for pressure. The best length and angle of the rod is determined by the position of the arm on the desk. When the device was used it became apparent that it was necessary to weld a short metal rod with a receptacle to the device similar to the thumb on the hook to allow for connection of the control cable to control forearm flexion.

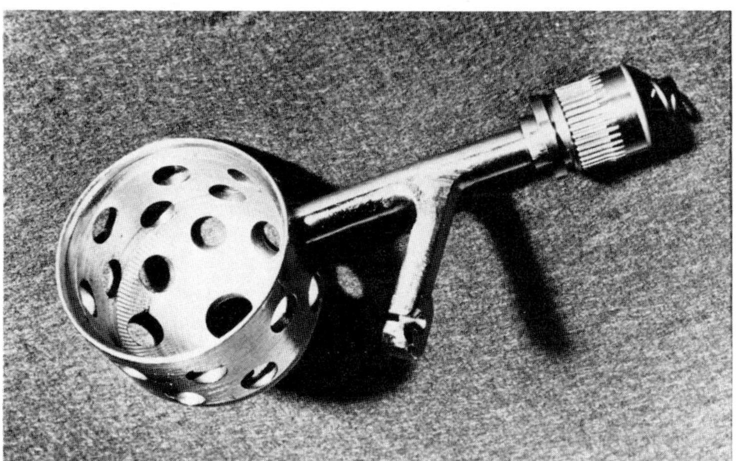

Fig. 9.C-7. Gear shift device (Table 9.C-2). This device is used for operating gear shift levers on heavy equipment such as bulldozers, or on cars with standard transmission and floor shift. The size of the lever knobs determines the size of the cup. Holes are cut into the cup to reduce the weight of the device. The thumb is added for above elbow amputees to receive the ball of the control cable to allow control of the elbow unit.

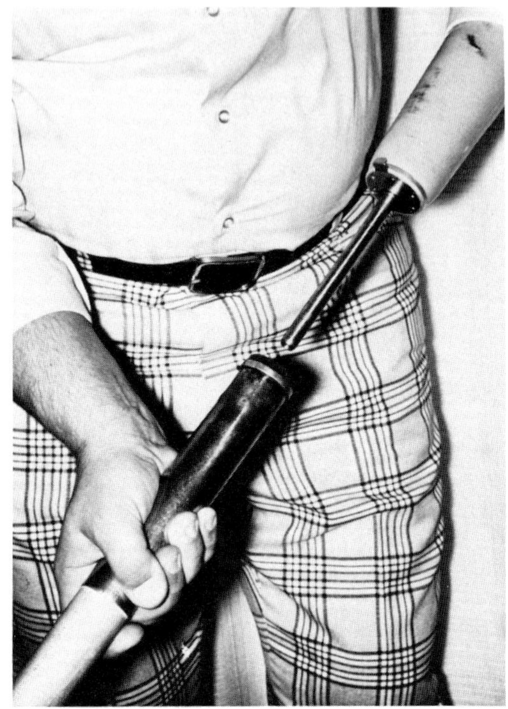

Fig. 9.C-8. Adapted shovel (Table 9.C-2). The D-handle of a snow shovel is cut off. A hole is drilled into the handle and a metal sleeve and plate are used to reinforce the handle. A metal rod, that is fitted with a wrist insert at one end, slides into the hole. A ring of neoprene is glued to the top of the metal plate. The hole in the neoprene is slightly smaller than the diameter of the metal rod and a few small cuts are placed radially around the hole. The friction of the neoprene prevents the rod from sliding out too easily. The neoprene needs to be replaced periodically to assure good friction. The advantage of this adaptation is that the shovel can be easily rotated by the sound hand to throw off the snow while the prosthetic side assists in pushing the shovel through the snow. A similar design of a rotating metal sleeve, fitted below the D-handle, was used to allow rotation of a shovel and a pitch fork. This enabled a forequarter amputee with a myoelectric prosthesis to use the tools. While the prosthetic hand remained stationary on the handle he could turn the lower end of the shovel with the hand and unload it at all levels up to shoulder height.

The *ACCRU-hook system* consists of a triangular post which is mounted on the tool or appliance and corresponds with an opening in the stationary finger of a modified hook (like Dorrance No. 5XA). The post is locked in place by a small lever on the dorsal side of the hook. This combination provides a firm control of the tool and leaves the movable finger of the hook free to activate switches; if necessary, a lever-type adaptor is added for the latter action. The system can be used for power tools, household appliances and sports equipment (M. & W. Handicapped Enterprises).

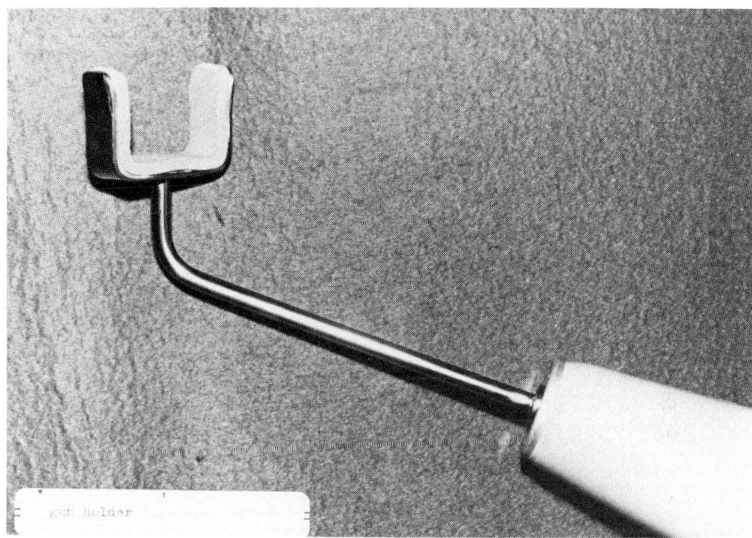

Fig. 9.C-9. Gun holder (Table 9.C-2). The gun rests on a U-shaped metal bar which is lined with neoprene to protect the barrel. This support is welded to a metal rod that is fitted with a wrist insert. The device is made-to-measure, with the length and angle of the rod and the shape of the support corresponding to the size and shape of the gun. This device prevents the gun barrel from being scratched by the hook.

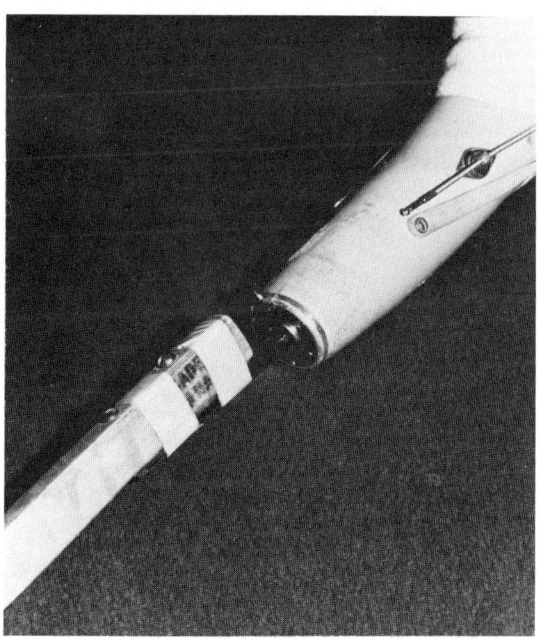

Fig. 9.C-10. Adapted floor hockey stick (Table 9.C-2). A metal rod is mounted on the end of the floor hockey stick with screws and secured with fiberglass tape. The end of the metal rod is threaded with a ½-20 thread and fitted with a wrist insert.

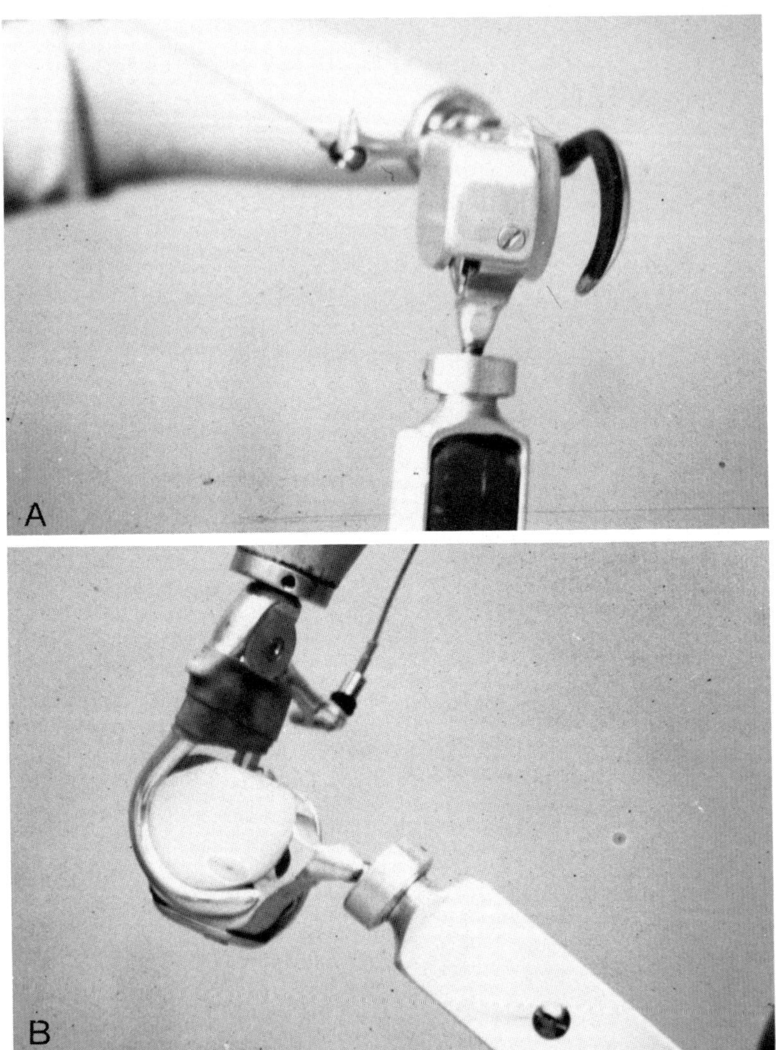

Fig. 9.C-11. Hockey stick attachment (Table 9.C-2). Various methods have been used to hold a hockey stick. Some amputees use the hook and protect the hockey stick with tape to prevent damage to the handle; however, using the hook is not accepted in organized hockey due to the danger of possible injury to other players by the hook. The prosthetic hand is used occasionally, but it is not robust enough and can cause injury as well. *A* and *B*, A special hockey stick attachment has been designed. It consists of a machined receptacle that contains a groove for the movable hook finger. The stationary hook finger closes in at the side and rests on a plastic plate shaped to the curve of the hook finger. This receptacle is connected through a ball joint with a U-shaped metal plate that is mounted to the end of the hockey stick. This combination allows great freedom for handling the hockey stick. For protection, the hockey glove is pulled over this attachment; the glove is cut on the inside to the center of the palm to give room for the device. The design of the device can be modified to meet individual needs. *C*, a device for holding a hockey stick at midshaft consists of a metal ring and a nylon disc. The disc has a square cut-out which allows a sliding movement along the shaft of the stick. *D*, the metal ring fits into a groove of the disc and can rotate easily. It is equipped with a single swivel unit which further increases mobility. *E*, the metal ring has a hinge and springloaded locking mechanism to allow easy attachment and removal of the device.

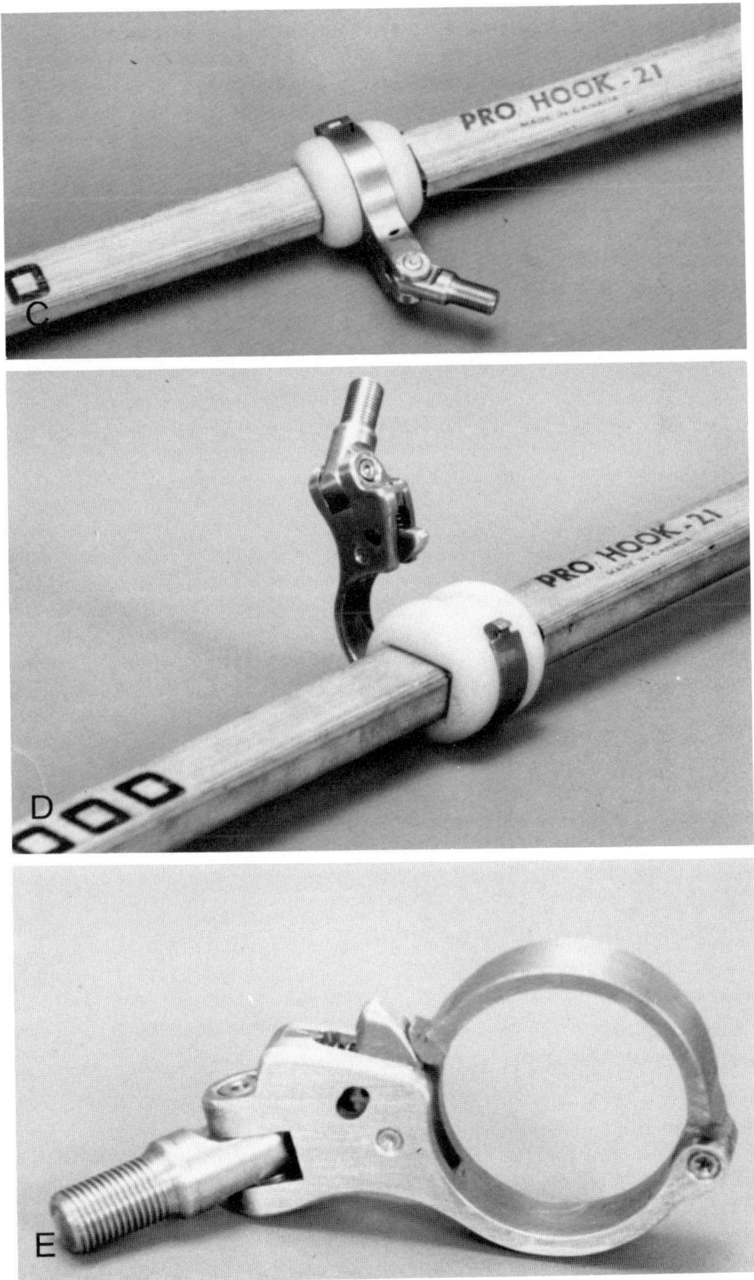

Fig. 9.C-11. *C–E.*

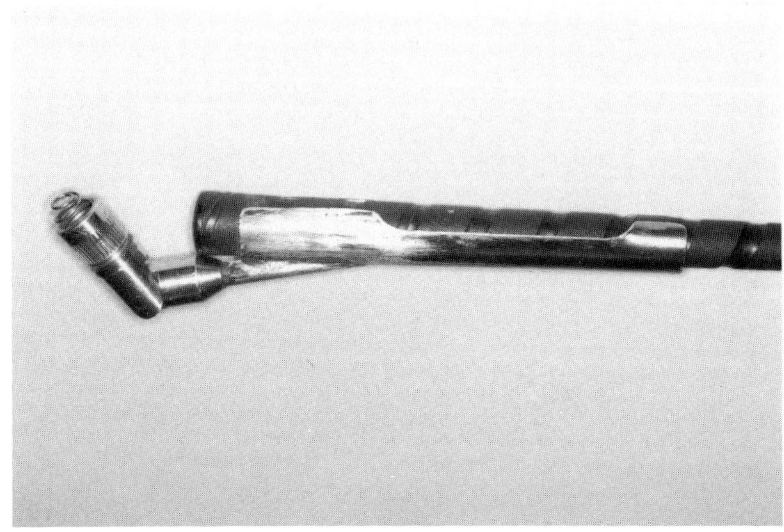

Fig. 9.C-12. Golf club holder (Table 9.C-2). The ways in which amputees handle golf clubs vary greatly. Some amputees have become adept in a one-handed swing, while others use the prosthetic hand, and a few use the hook. Some below-elbow amputees have found this device useful in assisting with a bilateral swing. The trough is approx. 6.½" long, slightly tapered to fit the club handle, and covers half of its circumference. Both ends of the trough extend further around the handle, leaving an opening large enough to slide the thin part of the golf club through when placing the device on the club handle. A short metal rod which extends approximately ½" from the edge of the trough, is welded to the back of the trough at an angle of approximately 15°. The rod is fitted with a single swivel unit, allowing 180° of movement. A wrist insert is attached at the other end of the swivel unit. Some friction tape can be glued to the inside of the trough to prevent rotation of the club. The sound hand holds the club by gripping over the device.

Baseball Glove Attachment. This device is shaped to fit into a standard baseball glove and provides the gripping action in the thumb and forefingers of the glove (Dorrance).

Bowling Attachment. A neoprene expansion sleeve at the end of the device fits firmly into a hole in a tenpin bowling ball. It is released by the same action which is used to open a conventional hook and which resembles the natural action in bowling (Dorrance).

Fishing Rod Holder. The fishing rod is held in a C-shaped hook with a V-shaped support for balance (Steeper).

Other Devices

Table 9.C-2 lists devices which have been designed and manufactured by prosthetists, therapists or amputees. Most of these aids are shown in Figures 9.C-1–9.C-20.

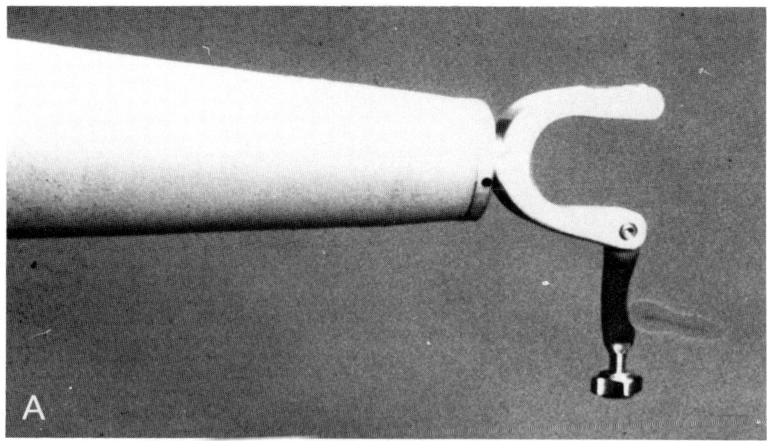

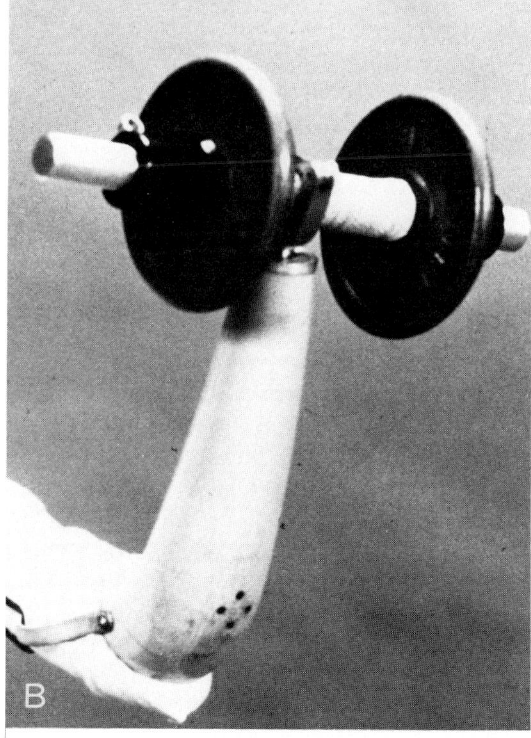

Fig. 9.C-13. Weight lifting device (Table 9.C-2). The handle of a bar bell fits into the U-shaped metal piece. A metal bar across the top of the U locks the handle into the device. The metal bar is held by a pin at one end and fits into a cut-out at the other end of the U; it is tightened by a wing nut. The inner side of the metal bar is concave to fit the handle of the bar bell.

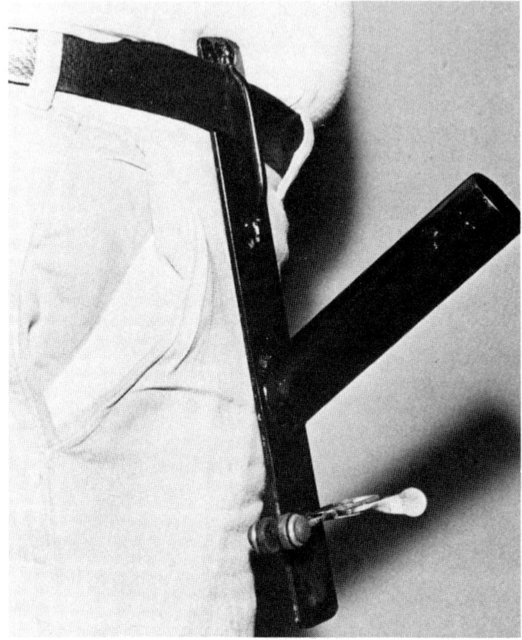

Fig. 9.C-14. Fishing rod holder (Table 9.C-2). This device was designed by an amputee with a shoulder disarticulation who could wear his prosthesis only for limited periods. It consists of a flat piece of metal with a metal pipe welded on, at an angle of 60°, to hold the fishing rod. A thin metal bracket is shaped and welded to the upper end so that the holder can be fastened to the belt. A harness clamp, welded to the lower end, is used to hold the fishing hook when the bait is put on.

A hook for playing piano is shown in the film "Musical Instruments for the Limb Deficient Child" (University of California at Los Angeles (Table 9.C-2). A guitar capo has been developed for a bilateral upper extremity amputee (10). Further information regarding music instruments for amputees can be found in the following articles: "Musical Instruments for Upper-Limb Amputees" by Carole Kral (5). A chart of instruments that can be played by upper limb amputees has been published by Alice Mailhot (6) in the article "Musical Instruments for Upper-Limb Amputees." There is also "Music for One-Handed Pianists" (8) is available from the Disabled Living Foundation, based on their 1976 report "Access to Music for the Physically Handicapped Schoolchild and School Leaver". The "Left Handed Guitar" (1) is an instruction book by Nicholas Clarke, published by The Bold Strummer Ltd., 1416 York Avenue, New York, N.Y. 10021.

Activities of Daily Living Devices

Activities of daily living (ADL) devices are available from medical supply companies or local stores. Some can be made in the occupational therapy department.

Useful devices for unilateral amputees are the following: Poyet knife or rocker knife, Velcro fasteners, elastic shoe laces, suction hand brush, nail clippers mounted on wood or with a C clamp to the table, jar opener, octopus suction holders, DYCEM nonslip matting, cutting board with corrugated nails and corner guard, clip-on apron and card holder.

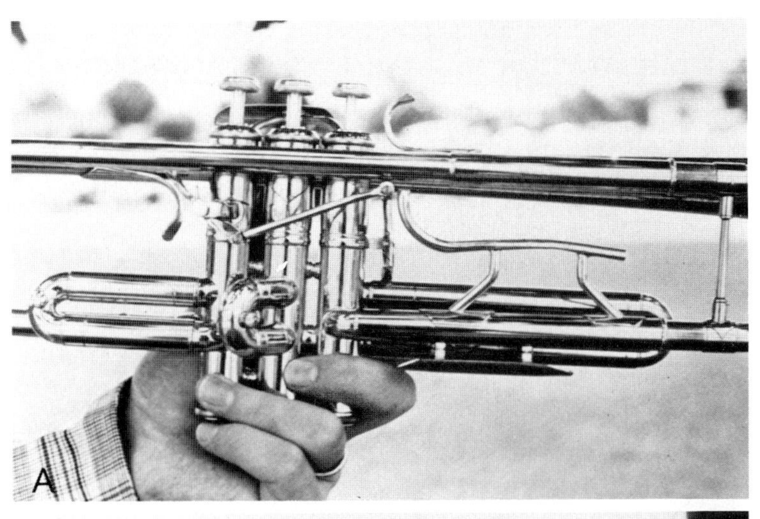

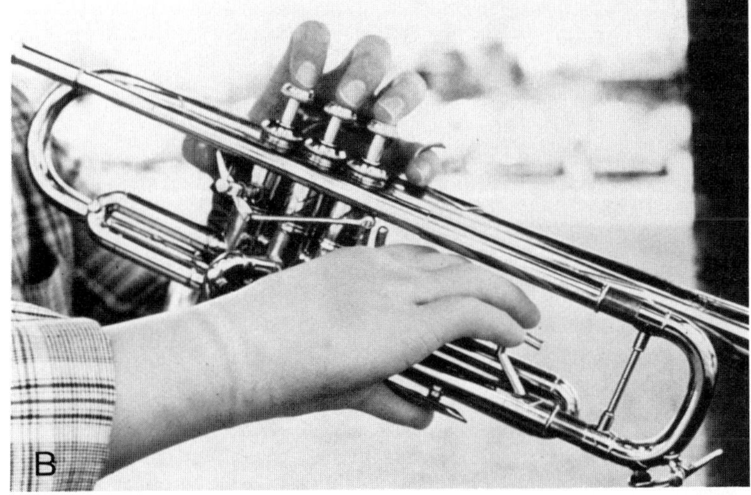

Fig. 9.C-15. Adapted Trumpet (Table 9.C-2). Normally, the left hand holds the trumpet with the fingers wrapped around the valve casings. The left ring finger controls the third valve tuning slide by a ring through which the finger passes. This slide must be moved while playing certain notes to insure good tuning. The first three fingers of the right hand play the three valves while the small finger wraps around a small hook to position the hand. For a right below-elbow (RBE) amputee to play the trumpet, everything must be reversed, *A*. By the addition of two specially designed bars, the prosthesis can hold and secure the trumpet, *B*. The left hand plays the valves and the left thumb, by means of a specially designed system of rods and levers, controls the movement of the third valve tuning slide. The small finger hook is placed so that the left small finger can use it to position the hand. It was found that the prosthesis could not quite hold the trumpet steady, so a further support was added to fit under the palm of the left hand. This helps to counter the slight rotational movement of the trumpet when the valves are quickly pushed down (this is something the left hand would normally do). The result is a trumpet that can be played quite well by a RBE amputee (assuming the player has the necessary skill). The only problem is a situation where the trumpet is muted by placing one of the hands over the bell while playing. This is impossible unless the notes to be played are those which are "open" *i.e.* no valves are pushed down. Then the left hand can mute while the prosthesis holds the trumpet. This, however, is a minor problem.

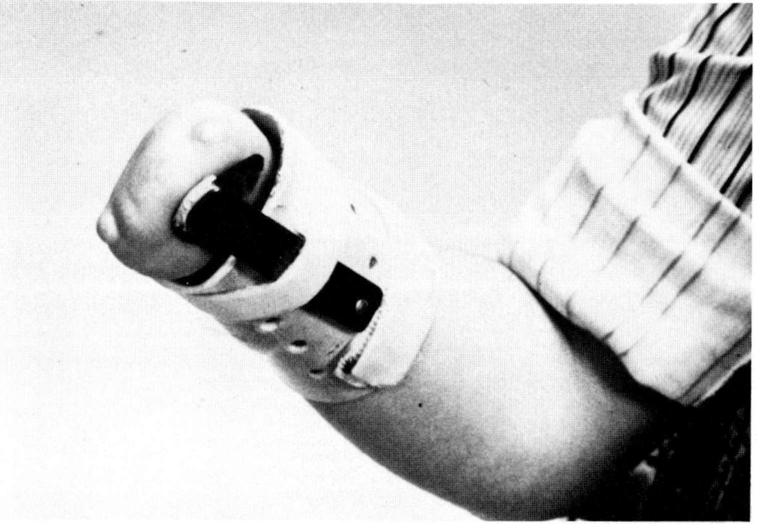

Fig. 9.C-16. Guitar pick holder (Table 9.C-2). The guitar pick holder is suitable for wrist disarticulation or transcarpal amputations. A metal bar is mounted on the medial side of a Sansplint cuff which is closed with Velcro. The end of the metal bar is covered with a nonslip surface such as neoprene. The pick is held against it with the stump. This allows the amputee to vary the pressure on the pick.

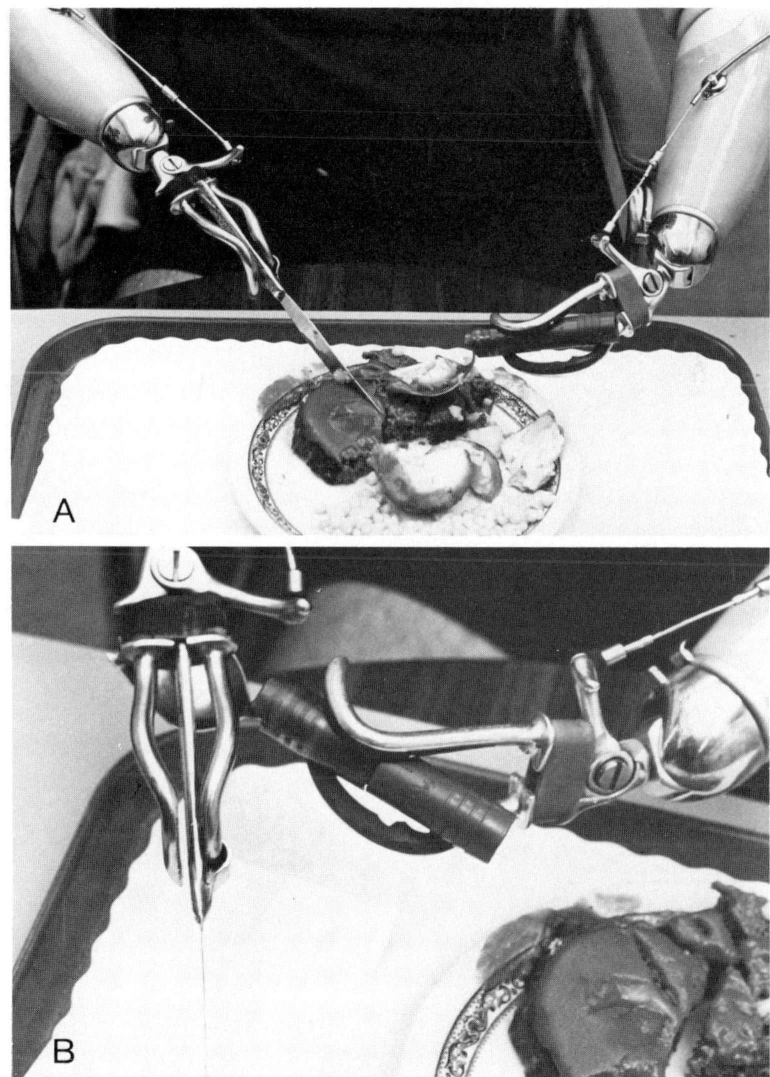

Fig. 9.C-17. *A* and *B*, Adapted knife (Table 9.C-2). A few bilateral amputees found an adapted knife useful. The knife handle is fitted with a metal band that is formed around one hook finger and riveted or brazed to the handle. The end of the knife rests against the base of the fingers. This allows normal sawing motion and prevents the knife from sliding through the hook fingers when pressure is applied or drop from the hook if inadvertent tension is applied.

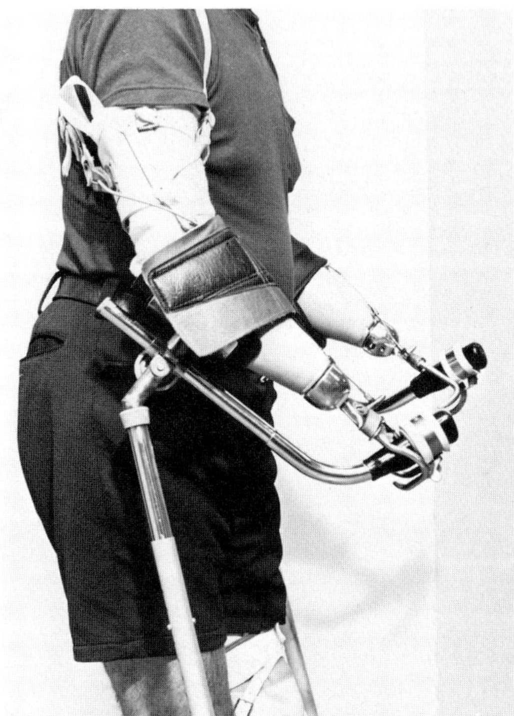

Fig. 9.C-18. Adapted crutches (Table 9.C-2). A bilateral below-elbow amputee with a below-knee amputation was supplied with modified gutter-type elbow crutches. The gutter arms, instead of being horizontal, are welded on at a 45° angle. The arm rests are fitted with wide leather straps with Velcro closure. Foam rubber is tightened by hose clamps to the ends of the handles to prevent the hooks from slipping off the handles.

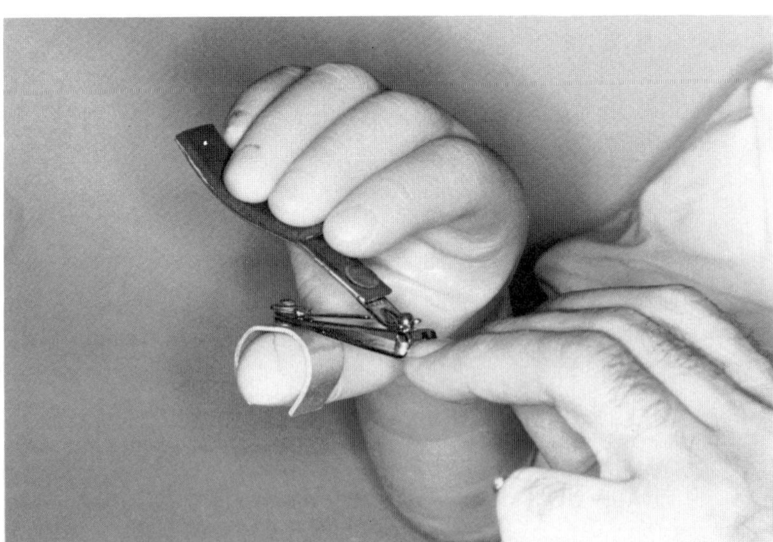

Fig. 9.C-19. Adapted nail clippers (Table 9.C-2). Nail clippers are adapted for use with a myoelectric prosthesis. A small metal bar, shaped to fit over the thumb, is riveted to the end of the clippers. A second metal bar, slightly curved to align with the fingers, is riveted to the lever and lined with neoprene.

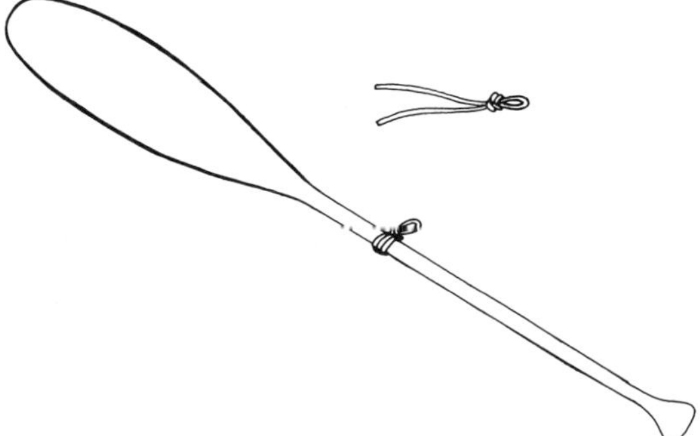

Fig. 9.C-20. Adapted canoe paddle. (Table 9.C-2). A small loop is tied in the middle of a thin rope. The ends of the rope are tied tightly around the lower end of the canoe handle. Some waterproof tape can be put over the rope to protect it, if desired. The hook holds the loop rather than the canoe handle. This protects the handle from damage by the hook fingers and allows steering maneuvers in the stern of the canoe. The elbow lock cable in an above-elbow prosthesis needs to be adjusted loosely to allow greater freedom of movement to prevent disengagement of the lock during paddling.

Devices for bilateral amputees include swivel utensils, sandwich holder (2), Velcro fasteners, loops on garments, rings on zipper tabs, a button hook, bath mitts, adapted towels, rubber door knob extensions, phone adaptations, sock and prosthesis donners (4) (*see* Figs. 9.A-8 and A-9).

Special devices have been developed for amputees with high bilateral amputations such as the "Bathing Device for Bilateral Above-Elbow Amputees" (Table 9.C-2), ADL aids for bilateral shoulder disarticulation (7, 9, and 10) and toiletting self-care methods for bilateral high level upper limb amputees (3). Electric body dryers are commercially available (Warmey, and Dunlop, Table 9.C-1).

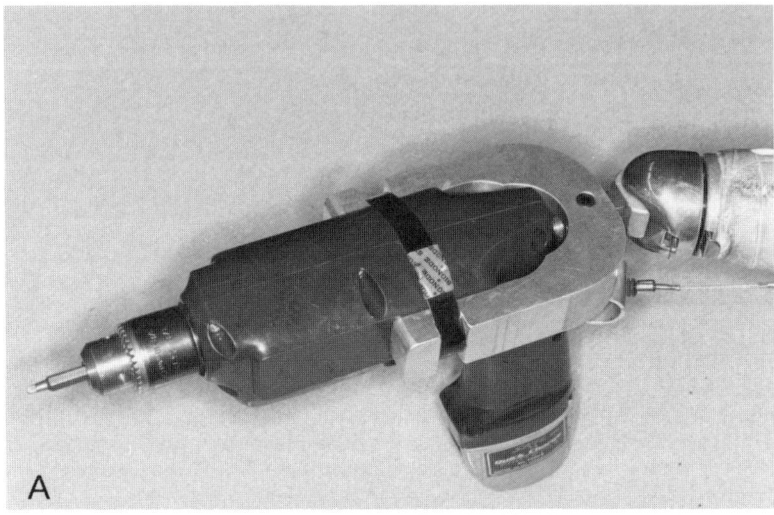

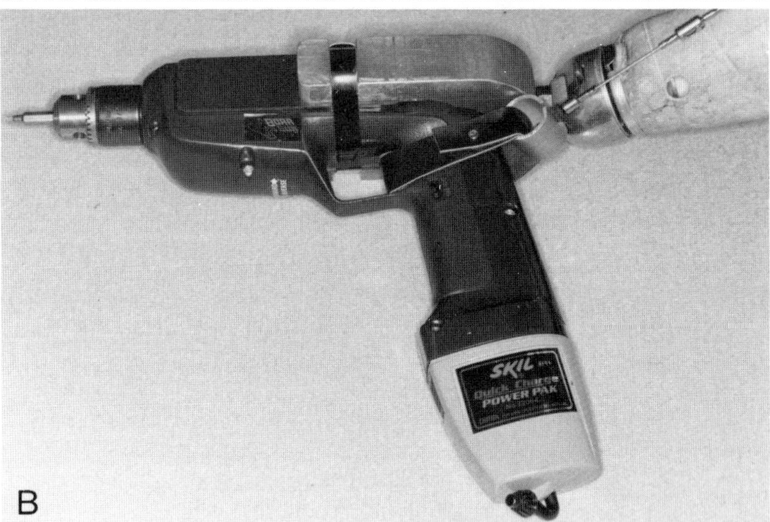

Fig. 9.C-21. Holder for electric screw driver (Table 9.C-2). *A*, U-shaped aluminum bracket, with a threaded stud for the wrist unit, is mounted on a battery operated screw driver with a metal band. *B*, a leather loop for operation of the speed control button is attached to the cable by means of a ½″ wide aluminum ring which has a cut-out for the ball end of the cable.

REFERENCES

1. Clarke, N. *Left-Handed Guitar*, The Bold Strummer, New York.
2. Friedman, L. Bilateral Upper Extremity Amputee Sandwich Holder *Am J. Occup. Ther. 28:* 358, 1974.
3. Friedman, L., *Prosthet. Orthot. Int.*, 4: 23–36, 1980.

4. Hromek, C., King, P. M. Bilateral Upper Extremity Valet, Am. J. Occup. Ther. *25:* 433, 1971.
5. Kral, C. Musical Instruments for Upper-Limb Amputees. *Inter-Clin. Infor. Bull., 12:* No. 3:13–26, 1972.
6. Mailhot, A. Musical Instruments for Upper-Limb Amputees. *Inter-Clin. Infor Bull. 13:* No. 10:9–15, 1974.
7. Marker, M. A. Adaptive Living Aids for a Bilateral Shoulder Disarticulation, *Am. J. Occup. Ther. 31:* 584, 1977.
8. Music for One-Handed Pianists. In *Access to Music for the Physically Handicapped School child and School-Leaver*. Disabled Living Foundation, London, 1976.
9. Poole, J., and Parkinson, M. Bilateral Shoulder Disarticulation: Equipment Used to Facilitate Independence, *Am. J. Occup. Ther. 34:* 397–399, 1980.
10. Rottgen, H. Aids to Daily Living Dressing Machine, *Proceedings of the Sixth International Congress of the World Federation of Occupational Therapists*, Vancouver, B.C., Canada, 1974.
11. Zatlin, C. R., Hemmen, E., Krouskop, T. A., Sklan, M., Guitar Capo for a Bilateral Upper Extremity Amputee. *Am. J. Occup. Ther.* 35: 736, 1981.
12. Zduriencik, S. *Am. J. Occup. Ther. 20:* 99–100, 1966.

D. Driving Aids for Amputees

HANNA HEGER O.T.(C)

Being able to drive increases independence and self-sufficiency for the handicapped person and may enhance vocational opportunities as well. Adequate safe equipment and proper training is needed to operate a car effectively. Hand controls and assistive devices such as steering devices and control extensions for upper and lower extremity amputees are often commercially available (*see* item 1 in Table 9.D-1). These devices have been standardized and tested to meet the safety criteria determined by the government. Some devices are specific for the year, make and model of a car in terms of handles, mounting brackets and throttle connections. If devices are custom made to meet individual needs they should be designed for optimum function and maximum driving safety. They also should be well built and not affect the conventional use of the standard controls by nonhandicapped drivers.

The mechanical hand control systems consist of rods and fasteners connecting manually operated levers to the accelerator and brake pedals and are mounted near the steering wheel. They are classified into three types: pull-push, right angle-push and twist-push. The brakes are activated by applying a pushing force to the control handle—away from the driver and parallel to the steering column. The accelerator is controlled by the remaining motion of either pulling toward the driver, a downward movement at a right angle to the push, or a twisting movement. Each type has certain advantages and disadvantages. The hand controls are attached in such a way that they do not impede the use of the car by a nonhandicapped person (*see* item 2 in Table 9.D-1).

It is essential for a safe driving performance to select the appropriate adaptive equipment. Driver Education Centers are able to assess the driving ability of a disabled person and recommend the most suitable effective type of adaptive equipment (*see* item 3 in Table 9.D-1). They also can locate training facilities and give information on proper maintenance and precautions against problems encountered outside the car. The assistive devices should be installed by competent personnel and tested for maximum driving safety.

The following is a general guide for assistive devices and hand controls for various levels of amputations.

TABLE 9.D-1. *Driving Aids: Information and Suppliers*

1. Distributors of therapy equipment often supply adaptive devices and hand controls.

   Information on manufacturers of hand controls and adaptive devices is available through American Automobile Association.

   A monograph, "Driving Systems for Independent Mobility" is available from Elise Brown, ADL, Inc., 6 Hurlow Court, Rockville, Md. 20850.

   A manual, "Hand Controls and Assistive Devices for the Physically Disabled Driver" is available from Mr. E. C. Colverd, Director of Driver Education, Human Resources Center, I. U. Willets Road, Albertson, N.Y. 11507.
2. "Teaching Driver Education to the Physically Disabled", Human Resources Center, Albertson, N.Y. 11507.
3. "The Handicapped Driver's Mobility Guide", published by the American Automobile Association

   For information about Driver's Training Program, or for the manuals "Evaluating Driving Potential of Persons with Physical Disabilities" and "Teacher's Preparation Course in Driver Education for the Physically Disabled" contact Director of Driver Education, Human Resources Center, I. U. Willets Road, Albertson, N.Y. 11507

   Guide for Disabled Drivers in Ontario, publ. by the Ontario Advisory Council on the Physically Handicapped, 700 Bay St. 3rd Floor, Toronto, Ont.
4. Custom driving aids are available from: Cameron Enns Co. 13637 S. Madsen Ave. Kingsburg Cal. 93631

   Die-A-Matic Inc. 4004 Fifth Road N, Arlington, VA 22202
5. *Rehabilitation Brief*, Vol. III No. 9, June 1980, Physically Disabled Driver, Rehabilitation Research Institute, College of Health Related Professions, University of Florida, Gainesville, Florida 32610.
6. T. E. Sensky, A simple and versatile driving appliance for upper limb amputees, *Prosth. Orth. 4:* No. 1:47–49, 1980.

Upper Extremity Amputees

An arm amputee will benefit from a spinner knob mounted on the steering wheel. This permits safe operation of the steering wheel with one hand. The spinner has either a knob grip for use with the sound hand or prosthetic hand, or a ring-type grip (Fig. 9.D-1) for use with the prosthetic hook. The spinner knob receptacle should be attached to the steering wheel at the 4 o'clock position for right-hand operation and at the 8 o'clock position for left-hand operation.

The levers mounted on the steering column will require extensions for operation with the sound hand. A left arm amputee will need a right-hand extension for the directional signal. The device can be attached over or under the steering column and is usually located in close proximity to the spinner knob at the 4 o'clock position. A right arm amputee will require a left-hand extension of the gearshift lever.

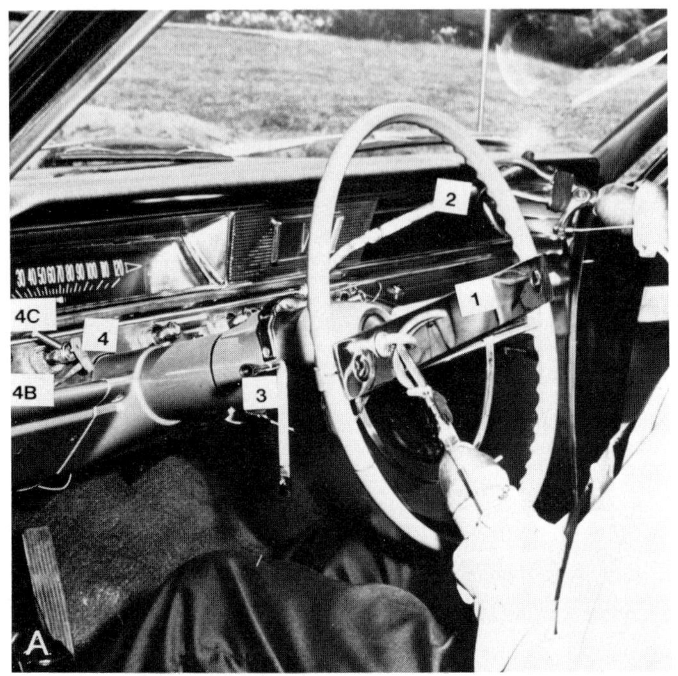

Fig. 9.D-1. *A–C*. Adaptations to a car for a bilateral above-elbow amputee. *1*, steering wheel bar. A bar made of stainless steel is mounted across the center of the steering wheel. The bar is equipped with a ring placed about one-quarter of the distance from the left hand side. The amputee operates the steering wheel entirely with the left prosthesis—the left terminal device is placed through the ring. *2*, gearshift lever. The lever is extended beyond the side of the steering wheel. The amputee operates it with the right terminal device. *3*, turn signal lever. A bar projecting downwards from the turn signal lever has been added. The amputee operates it with the left knee. *4*, window wipers and washers. *4A*, the washers and wipers are started by a bar operated by the left foot (*see* Fig. 9.D-1*B*). *4B*, The bar is connected to a rod which presses on the switch to turn it on. *4C*, To stop the wipers the amputee must reach forward with his left prosthesis and operate a projecting bar. *5*, headlight switch. A loop of heavy wire is attached to the headlight switch. The amputee operates it with his right prosthesis by pulling on the loop of wire. *6*, Key. The ignition key and trunk key have been attached to opposite ends of a twisted metal plate. *7*, Horn. The horn is operated by pushing a knob on the floor with the left foot. The above adaptations are made on a General Motors Pontiac. Some of them would not be suitable for another make of car, *i.e. number 4* adaptation is possible because of the particular design of the windshield wiper system.

A simple driving appliance in the form of a fixed V-shaped stainless-steel hook also has proven useful (Table 9.D-1 item 6).

If a car is equipped with a standard gearshift on the floor, a special gearshift device can be made for the right arm amputee (*see* Fig. 9.D-1 *C*).

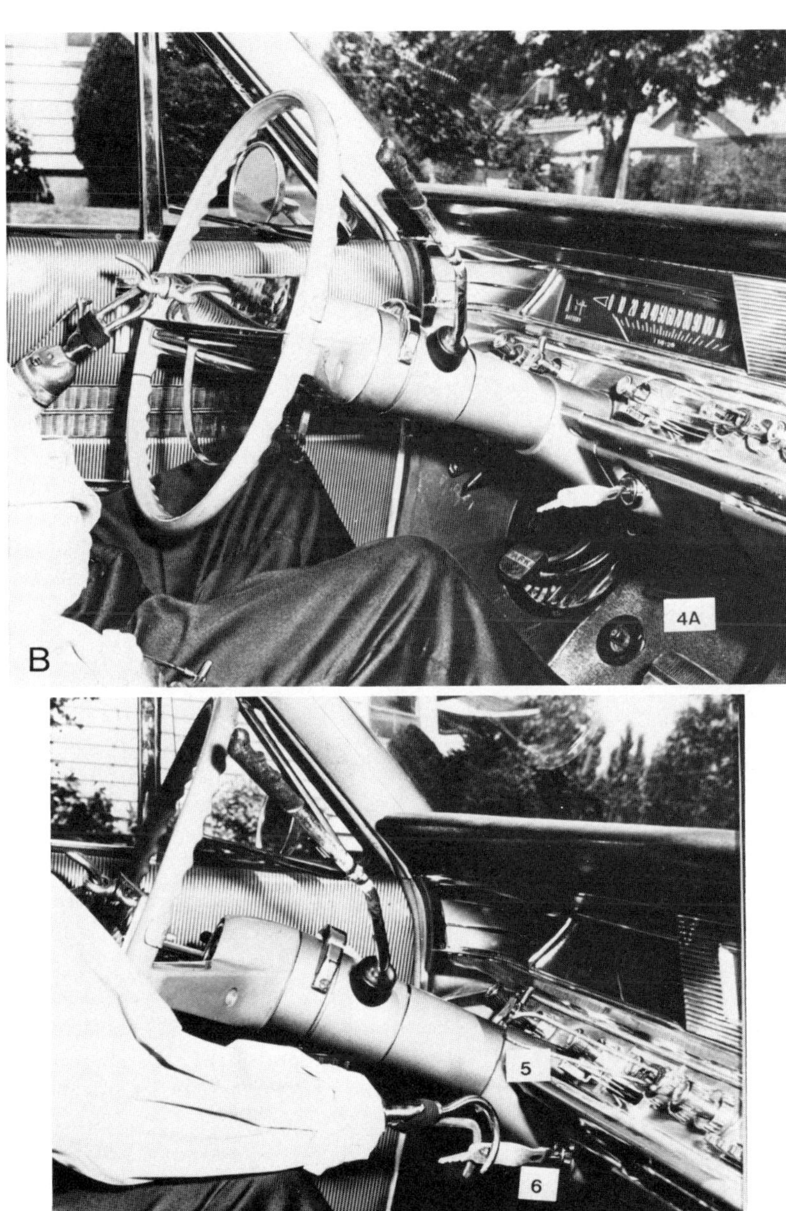

Fig. 9.D-1. *B* and *C*.

It provides a better hold on the gearshift knob than is possible with a prosthetic hand or hook.

A bilateral below-elbow amputee needs a car with automatic transmission, power steering and a Sierra driving ring. For bilateral above-elbow amputees, further modifications are required. Examples of custom made driving aids are shown in Figure 9.D-1. For high bilateral amputees, some cars can be equipped with foot-steering controls and modifications to all other levers and switches for operation with the feet or legs (*see* item 4 in Table 9.D-1).

Lower Extremity Amputees

A left below-knee amputee may receive sufficient feedback through the prosthesis to be able to operate the dimmer switch and parking brake and possibly the clutch in a car with standard transmission. If the feedback is not satisfactory, or if the amputation is above the knee, a car with automatic transmission has to be equipped with a hand parking brake and a hand-operated dimmer switch. A car with standard transmission can be adapted with a left-hand operated clutch, a hand dimmer switch with horn button, a hand parking brake, and a spinner knob for the steering wheel.

A right below- or above-knee amputee will require a left foot accelerator and a hand dimmer switch for a car with automatic transmission. (Some right below-knee amputees have enough kinesthetic awareness to use the gas pedal.) This left pedal can be folded back and disengaged when not in use, this leaves the right pedal free for use by a nonhandicapped person. A safety note should be placed in the car advising drivers that the car is equipped with a left-foot gas pedal.

For a car with standard transmission, a left-hand operated brake and throttle control, a hand dimmer switch with horn button and a spinner knob for the steering wheel are available. However, these modifications are not recommended for safety reasons.

A bilateral leg amputee can drive a car with automatic transmission if the car is equipped with a left-hand operated brake and throttle control, a hand dimmer switch with horn button, a hand parking brake, and a spinner knob for the steering wheel. (The hand control is preferred on the left side unless the right hand is too weak for steering.) Power brakes are recommended, because they require less movement of the control arm and provide quicker control of the car. Power steering is recommended as well.

The driving aids usually are designed to fit a variety of cars but some cars are better suited to meet individual needs. A two-door sedan model with its wider doors allows greater ease of access to the front seat. This is particularly important when transfer from a wheelchair is necessary. The chair also can be stored more easily in the rear seat. Automatic transmission, power steering and power brakes are highly recommended options. An adjustable (tilt) steering wheel allows more space when entering, exiting and when operating the controls. Power seats are more convenient for correct positioning.

REFERENCE

1. Physically Disabled Driver. *Rehabil. Brief*, 3: 1980.

E. Assistive Devices for Lower Extremity Amputees

PAT BOLTON O.T.(C)

Many lower extremity amputees become independent in all routine activities once they have been fitted with a satisfactory prosthesis and may not require any other device for independent functioning at home. However, many elderly dysvascular amputees and patients with multiple amputations will require assistive devices for independent living. The assessment of these needs can be carried out in hospital and through home visits.

Transfers

Transfers for the lower extremity amputee usually only pose a problem when the prosthesis is removed.

BED-TO-CHAIR: BILATERAL ABOVE-KNEE AMPUTEE

A sliding or transfer board is invaluable in aiding bilateral above-knee (AK) amputees to transfer from either wheelchair or chair to bed. The board is placed on the bed, the chair is drawn up parallel and the sides are removed. The free end of the board is placed under the patient's thigh nearest the bed and he/she slides over using his/her arms to stabilize.

BED-TO-CHAIR: UNILATERAL BELOW-KNEE AMPUTEE

The chair is placed either parallel or 90° to the bed. With brakes on and footrests swung back the patient stands on his foot and pivots around to sit on the bed (Fig. 9.E-1).

TOILET: BILATERAL ABOVE-KNEE AMPUTEE

Using a zipper back on the wheelchair, the patient reverses in, opens the back and, with brakes on, slides backward onto the toilet. If there is room, the chair can be brought parallel to the toilet. With one wheelchair arm removed, the patient slides horizontally onto the toilet.

BATH

The patient sits on the edge of the bench, swings his legs into the tub and slides over to the center of the bench.

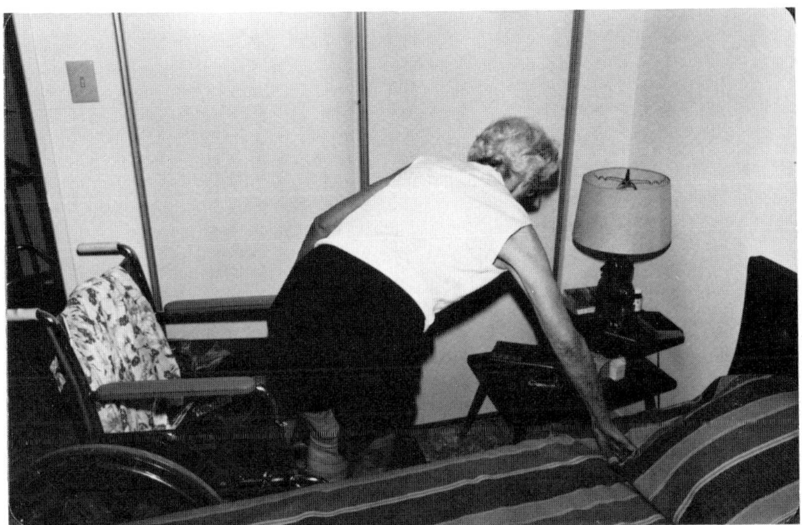

Fig. 9.E-1. Amputee transferring from wheelchair to bed.

Wheelchairs

Wheelchairs are often recommended for unilateral or bilateral lower extremity amputees for either permanent use in the absence of prostheses or as a back-up for conventional walking aids.

In selecting an appropriate chair, consideration should be given to the patient's size, weight and the eventual use of the chair. If the chair is custom ordered, two basic types are given consideration, however, if a standard wheelchair is to be used, an amputee adapter can be attached to the chair adapting it sufficiently.

LIGHTWEIGHT MODEL

A younger amputee, likely to be more active outdoors, may prefer this model as it is easier to lift in and out of cars and requires less energy to propel and maneuver. The rear wheels are set back 2½″ to maintain proper chair balance. Pneumatic tires can be substituted for use on soft, sandy or rough ground. This model comes with detachable desk length arms and swinging detachable foot rests for those patients with prosthesis. The latter two features allow for close approach to bed, tub, table, car, etc. As an alternate, fixed, full length, arms can be attached for those without artificial limbs.

STANDARD AMPUTEE WHEELCHAIR

This model is most suitable for the older, less active, amputee. It is similar to the lightweight model in all features and alternatives, with the exception of the rear wheels being set back 1½″ to compensate for transfer of weight due to limb loss (Figs. 9.E-2–9.E-3).

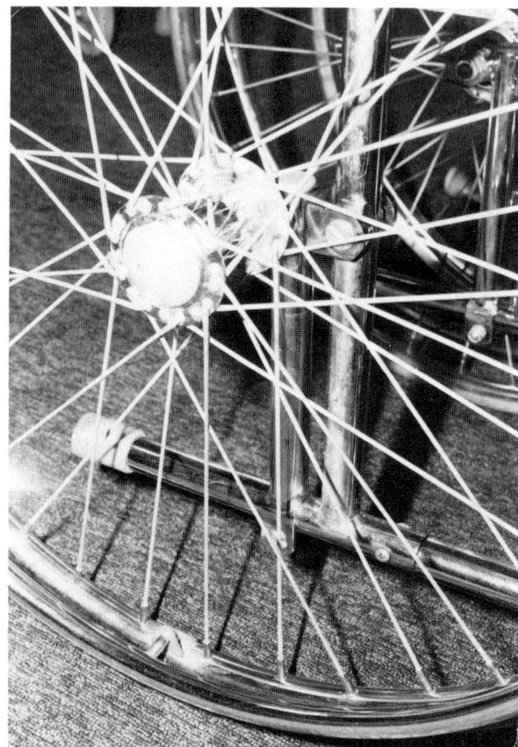

Fig. 9.E-2. Center of rear wheels on wheelchair set back 1½" to compensate for transfer of weight due to limb loss.

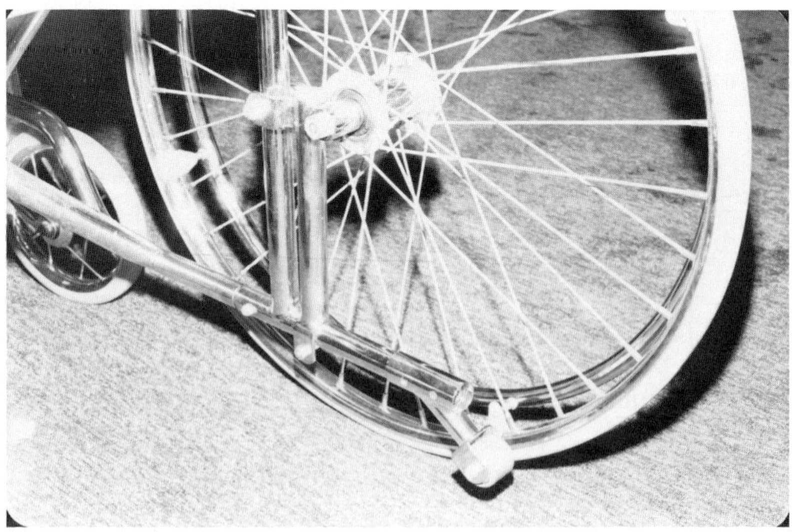

Fig. 9.E-3. Standard amputee wheelchair, adapted to prevent tipping backward.

Accessories

Zipper back permits entering or leaving the chair from the rear, a technique used by bilateral above-knee amputees in transferring to the toilet when space is limited.

Reduce-A-Width reduces wheelchair width as much as 4″ permitting unassisted passage through narrow doorways (Fig. 9.E-4).

Seat Cushion. Various types are available ranging from synthetic lambs wool to foam or gel and air-filled interiors. These are designed to distribute weight away from pressure points for long periods of sitting. A homemade model found to work well is constructed of 1.5 density foam for average weights and 2.3 density for those over 200 lbs. The surface is cut in 1″ squares to within 1″ of the base. This is an economical pressure cushion (Fig. 9.E-5).

Structural Adaptations

In the home, the occupational therapist may be called upon to suggest structural changes to accommodate wheelchair users in particular. The following are some measurements for the most common areas requiring alteration.

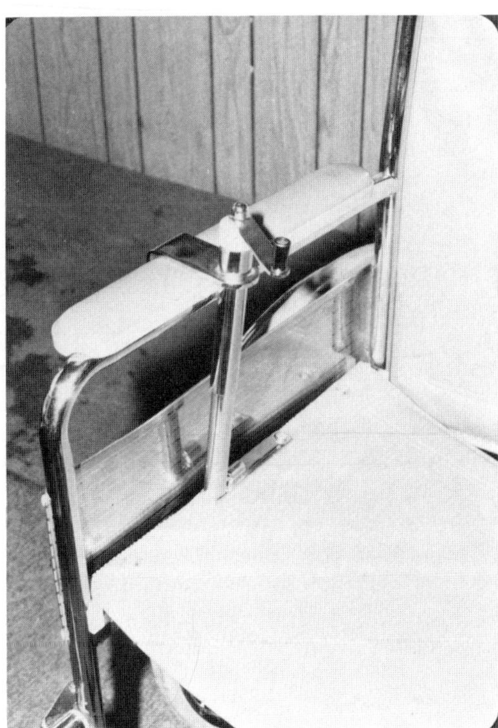

Fig. 9.E-4. Reduce-A-Width feature on wheelchair.

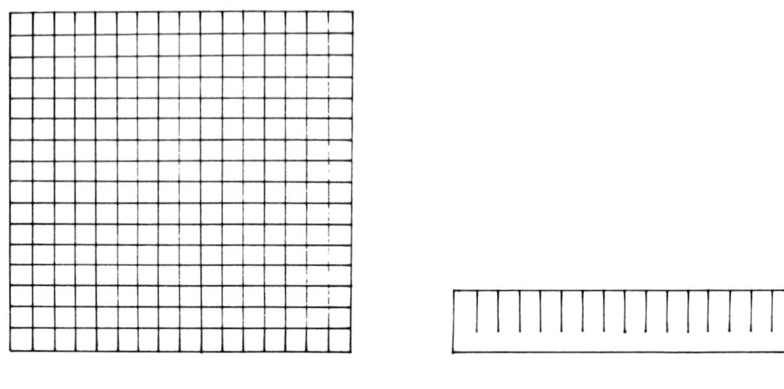

Fig. 9.E-5. Seat cushion (homemade model).

RAMPING

Where stairs render the home inaccessible a ramp may be considered. If it is being custom built it is usually of wood with a nonslip surface. The preferred gradient is 1:20 but 1:12 can be used for a maximum length of 30 ft. A curb 6″ high or a guardrail 8″ above the deck should be installed to prevent wheelchairs from slipping off the ramp. The unobstructed width of the ramp should be 2′10″–3′2″, to allow easy maneuvering of the chair. Upper ramp landings should leave an area of 2′ × 5′ free to accommodate swing doors, etc. Handrails also should be installed for both wheelchair users and ambulatory patients at a height of 3′ and 2′6″ (Fig. 9.E-6).

INDOOR STAIRS

In two-story homes where the bedrooms and washrooms are on the second floor many people consider the installation of a stair lift or chair glide. This electric track and chair combination can be operated independently and is available from major medical supply houses.

TOILET

There should be an area measuring 2′6″ in width at one side of the toilet to allow for side transfer from a wheelchair to the toilet seat. Similarly, the space in front of the toilet should measure 3′6″ to accommodate frontal approach to the toilet. The ideal height for toilet seats for most disabled persons is 1′6″ to 1′8″. As these are difficult to alter it is sometimes recommended that the person use a removable raised toilet seat as an alternative.

WASHBASIN

Normal heights are 2′7″ and are adequate for wheelchair users. However, ambulatory patients may prefer basins a little higher at 2′9″. The mounts should be able to withstand a minimum edge load of 250 lb as ambulatory patients lean on the basin for support. For wheelchair users the space under the basin should be 2′6″ wide by 2′2″ high. This area is also recommended under kitchen sinks and counter tops.

DOORS

The minimum clearance of 2′6″ is required for wheelchairs to pass through doorways. Corridors should be a minimum of 3′2″ wide, and up to 3′6″ wide to accommodate hand rails. All doors that are hinged should open outwards to save space in smaller rooms such as washrooms. If space remains a problem, replacing the conventional door with louver or sliding doors may be required or the door may be removed entirely. Fire doors in apartments are heavy to handle but should not be tampered with without permission.

All of the above measurements have been taken from the Central Mortgage and Housing Corporation's publication "Housing the Handicapped".

Activities of Daily Living Equipment

Activities of daily living (ADL) includes tasks such as eating, bathing, grooming, dressing, and home management, including food preparation and cleaning. In the case of amputees, it is often necessary to introduce aids and equipment to facilitate return to independent functioning. In conjunction with these, energy conservation techniques are taught along with work simplification methods.

BEDROOM

As with the rest of the home, the bedroom should be kept free of clutter to allow free access to bed, closet, *etc.*, for those persons using either walking aids or a wheelchair.

Scatter rugs likely to precipitate unwanted falls should be removed and any curling edges of rugs should be secured, using double-sided carpet tape.

Casters should be removed from furniture to improve the stability of transfers.

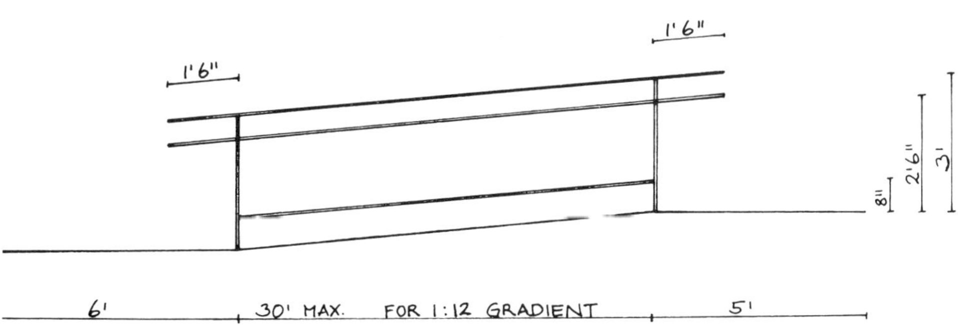

Fig. 9.E-6. Ramp with a 1:12 gradient.

Bed height and chair height should be such to allow easy transfer, either independently or from wheelchair using a transfer board.

Bed or chair blocks can be made to increase height. These should be approximately 3″ square, recessed 2″ and the height according to the patient's needs (Fig. 9.E-7).

Rope Ladders attached to the lower end of the bed are used to pull up to a sitting position. Similarly a *trapeze bar* overhead can serve this purpose.

BATHROOM

Most lower extremity amputees find showering using a bath bench, hand shower and safety mat a safer method of bathing than an emmersion tub bath.

Benches. These can be bought commercially and are preferable to shower stools for easy transfer and overall safety (Fig. 9.E-8). A homemade wooden adjustable bath bench is equally effective made of 1″ plywood with blocks and grooves allowing free movement of blocks to adjust to the width of the tub (Fig. 9.E-9). This model is unsuitable when there is less than 1″ of tub available on the wall side or where the outer sides of the tub are unusually rounded.

It should be noted that sliding shower doors tend to hinder transfers, and many benches have difficulty fitting over the rails of the door on the outer edge of the tub. It is therefore recommended these be removed.

Hand Showers. Many varieties are available commercially. For best value and endurance the sturdier chrome models are preferred with at least 6′ of tubing to reach as far as the bath bench.

Grab Bars. These can be affixed to walls or clamped on to the sides of tubs. It should be reinforced that use of soap dishes and towel racks for support can be dangerous due to their easy detachment from the walls (Figs. 9.E-10–9.E-12).

TOILET

Lower extremity amputees often benefit from toilet aids such as: 1) a *raised toilet seat* which raises the level from 4″ to 8″; and 2) a *Versa frame* which attaches around the toilet and offers support while rising from seat and adjusting clothing (Fig. 9.E-13).

Commodes are often installed in rooms other than bathrooms where access to the toilet is difficult due to area space or the inaccessability of stairs. Commodes range in design from the basic tubular frame model to more deluxe armchair styles (Fig. 9.E-14).

WASHING AIDS

These are used in particular for upper extremity amputees without prosthesis, although not exclusively: 1) long handled sponge, 2) bath mitt, and 3) suction brush (Fig. 9.E-15).

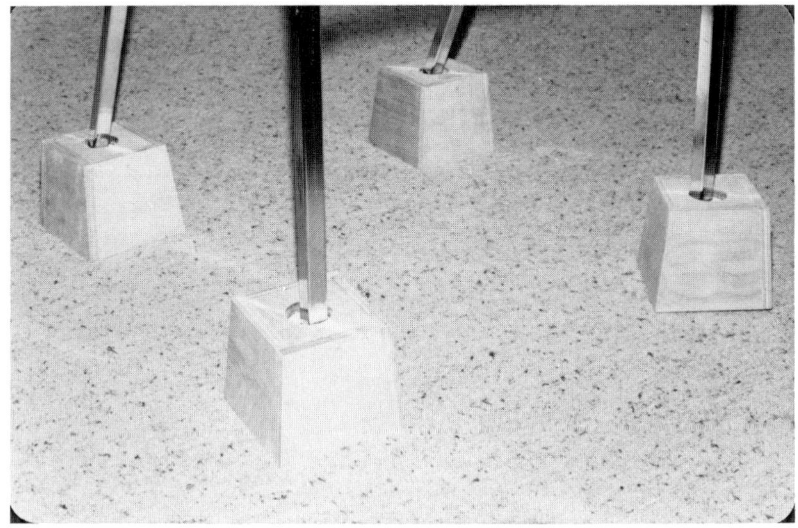

Fig. 9.E-7. Bed or chair blocks.

Fig. 9.E-8. Commercially available bath benches.

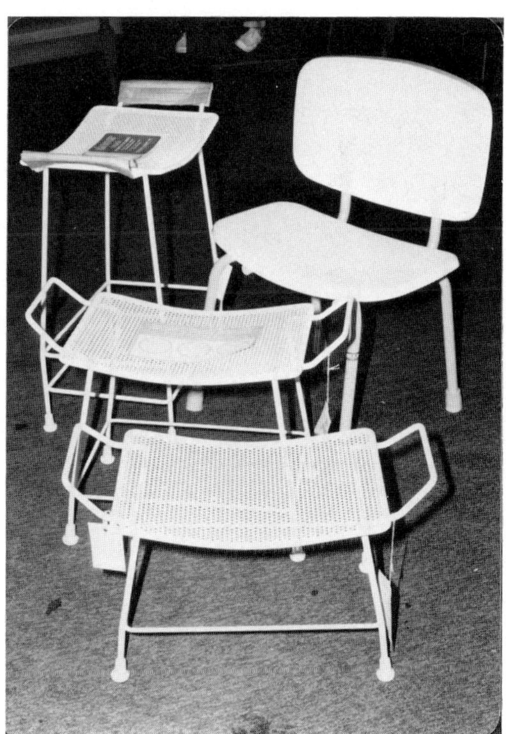

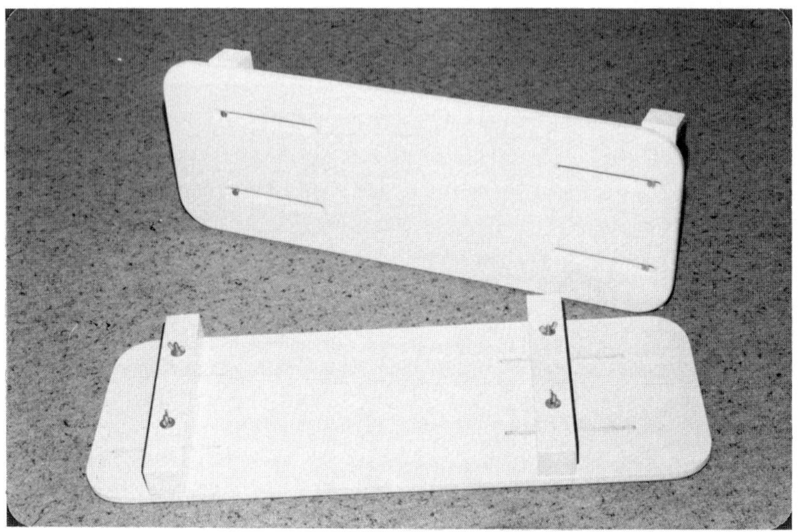

Fig. 9.E-9. Homemade wooden adjustable bath bench.

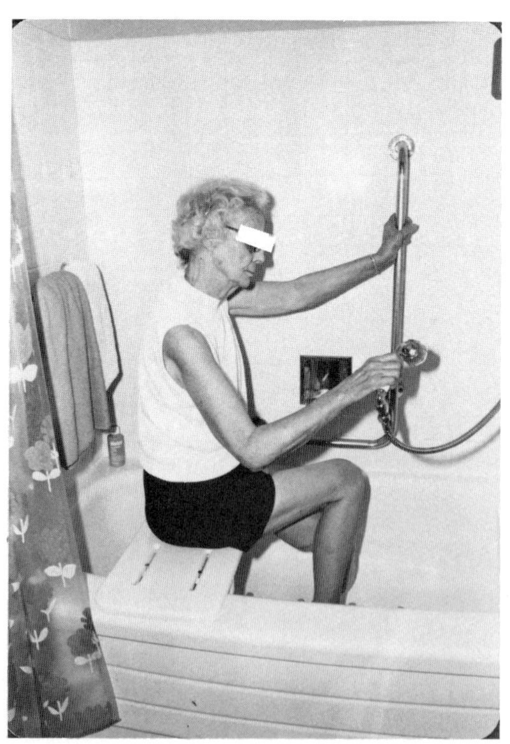

Fig. 9.E-10. Amputee using hand shower, homemade bath bench and grab bar.

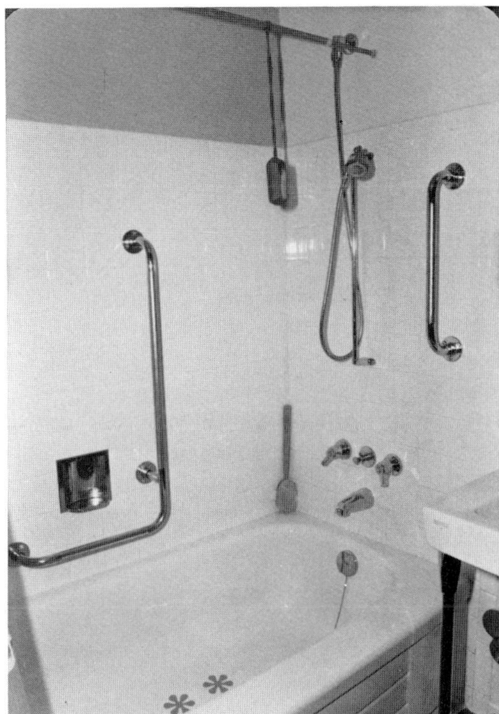

Fig. 9.E-11. Grab bars fixed to the wall.

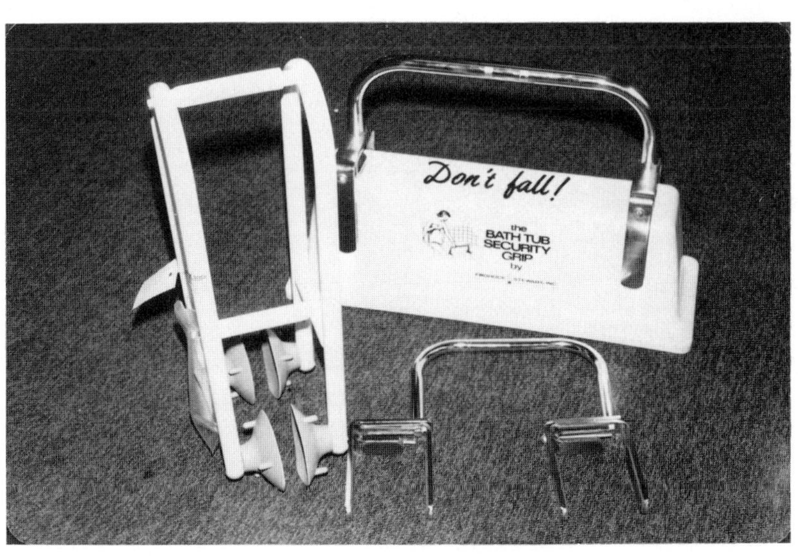

Fig. 9.E-12. Clamp-on grab bars.

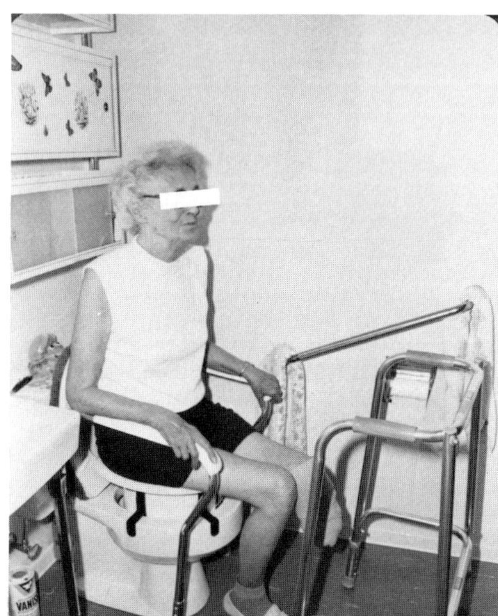

Fig. 9.E-13. Amputee using raised toilet seat, and the Versa Frame around the toilet.

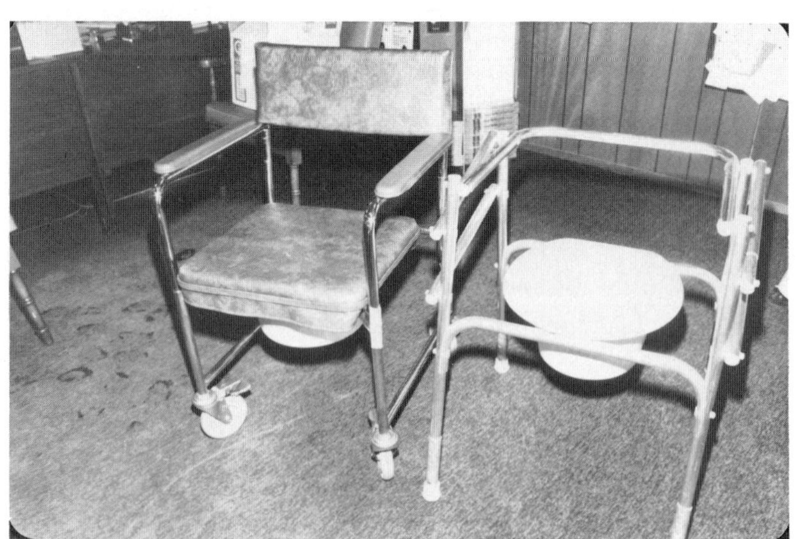

Fig. 9.E-14. Two designs of commodes.

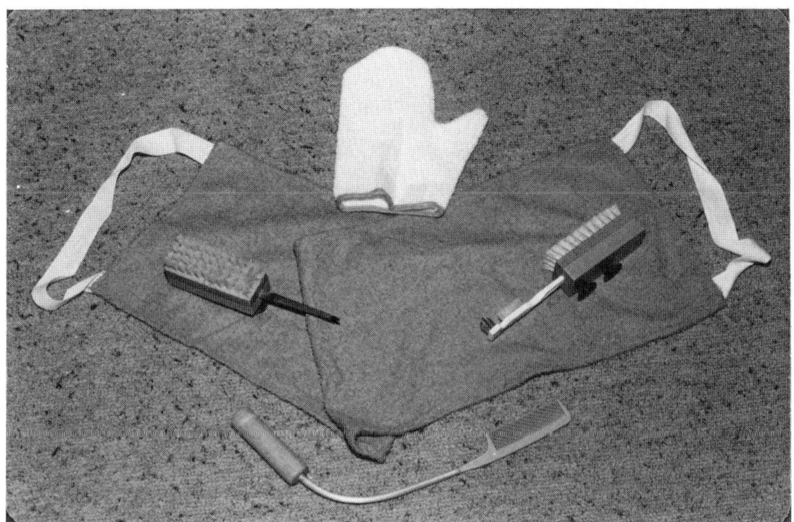

Fig. 9.E-15. Self-care aids: bath mitt, bath towel, suction brushes, and long handled comb.

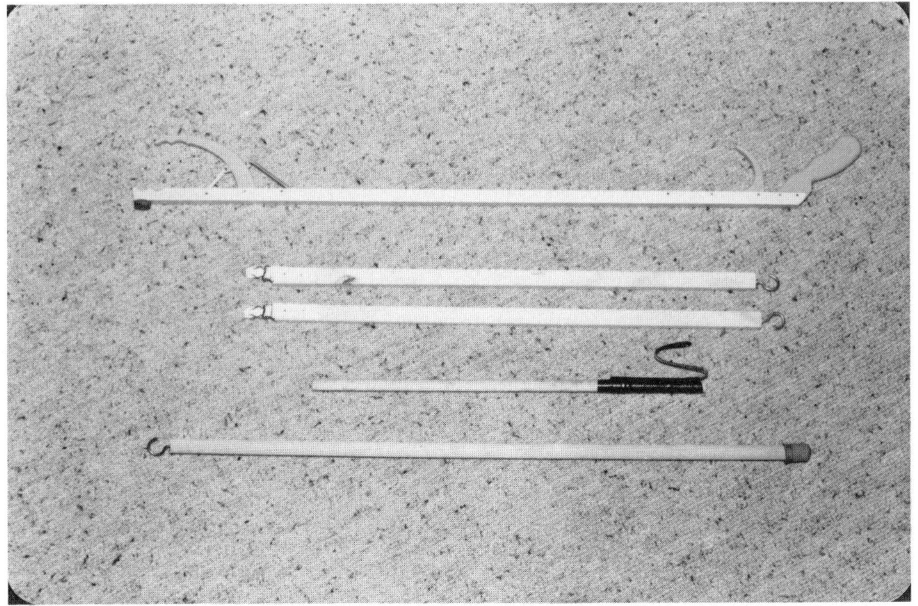

Fig. 9.E-16. Various types of dressing sticks.

DRESSING

Velcro closures are excellent substitutes for buttons, hooks and zippers and can be purchased in strips or dots from fabric stores.

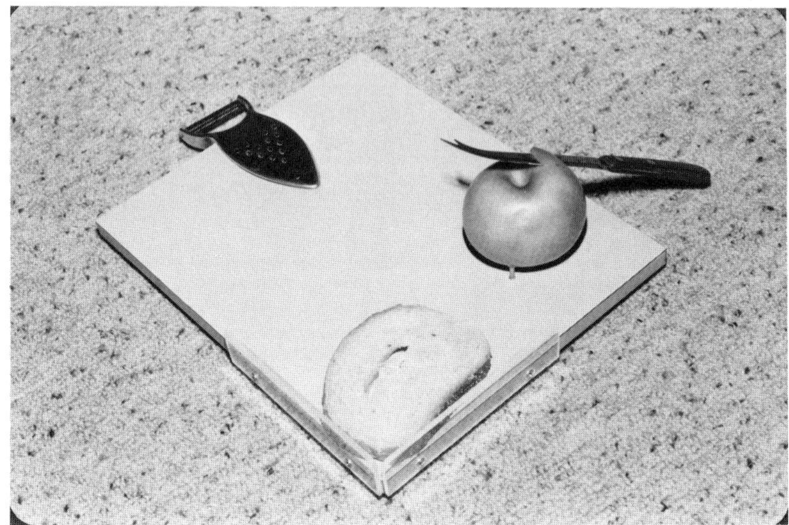

Fig. 9.E-17. Cutting board with mounted potatoe peeler, corrugated nails for holding vegetables, and plastic corner.

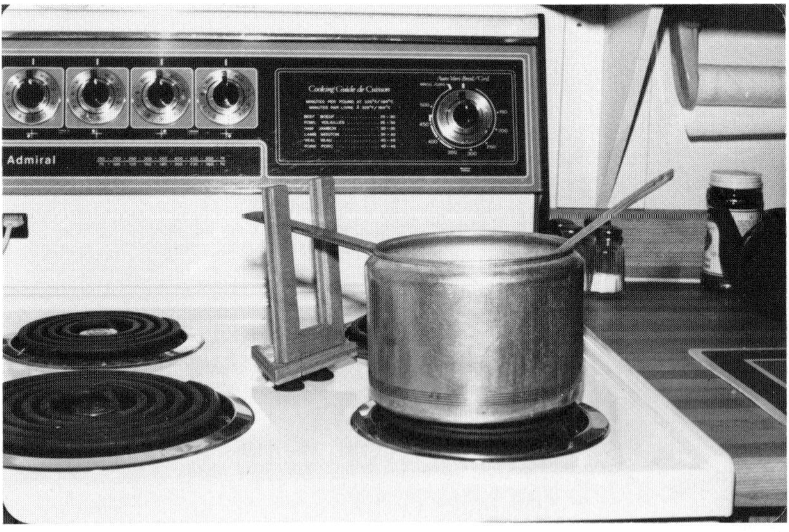

Fig. 9.E-18. Pot holder.

Dressing sticks are used to pull up trousers and underclothes over the legs, and blouses etc. over the shoulders. These can be homemade from ½″ dowel rod with either a cup hook or rubber thimble at one end and a shaped coat hanger at the other (Fig. 9.E-16).

KITCHEN

The key to success in the kitchen is energy conservation and work simplification for both upper and lower extremity amputees. Some points to consider for lower extremity amputees in particular are:

1. Access to sink for wheelchair users. Below-sink cupboards prevent close contact to the working area and therefore should be eliminated.
2. Long handled lever taps for easier reach, or use of tap turners for conventional taps to extend reach.
3. Rearrangement of cupboards to make frequently used items more accessable by lowering their shelf position.
4. Use of Lazy Susan turntables and other stacking devices to reduce stretching.
5. Long-handled dustpans and mops.
6. Long-handled reachers such as Superarm to use in cupboards or for retrieving items on the floor.
7. A tea trolly is beneficial for transporting items across a wider expanse of floor. Many varieties can be bought commercially.

Cutting Board. For upper extremity amputees a cutting board is of particular value. These can be made inexpensively from melamine or Arborite or unvarnished wood. (Fig. 9.E-17).

Pot Holder. To prevent pots from rotating while stirring on the stove top a homemade pot holder is invaluable for upper extremity amputees (Fig. 9.E-18).

Dycem Mat. This nonslip rubber matting comes in plate sizes or in rolls. It renders surfaces nonslip and is used under plates, mixing bowls etc.

10

Psychosocial Assessment and Management of the Amputee

DIANNE KINDON, M.S.W.
TERRY PEARCE, M.S.W.

When a person undergoes an amputation to remove a limb, they of course, lose a part of their body but, more importantly, they lose forever that sense of wholeness or that sense of being an intact person. He/she feels mutilated. In order to physically function again as an active person, the amputee must relearn almost every activity necessary to their life style. The healing of the emotional wounds, however, takes longer and is often more difficult to accomplish. The amputee has lost along with the limb, all hopes and plans for the future that would have involved that limb. As Parkes and Napier (7) have stated "The amputee has not just lost a limb, he has lost a slice of his world and a large part of his future."

To effectively rehabilitate a person who has undergone an amputation, it is important to understand his/her emotional reaction to the amputation. With such an understanding, persons involved with the amputee's physical rehabilitation can help him/her cope and adjust more effectively to his/her altered physical state. Foort (3) surveyed a group of amputees, asking them how they felt about their amputation and subsequent rehabilitation. All stated that "... of paramount importance was the need for psychological insight on the part of the people treating them, including the doctor, therapists, prosthetists and nurses."

This chapter will discuss the issues involved in the psychological adjustment of the amputee from the time preceding surgery to the completion of his/her physical rehabilitation and reentry into the community. The most common reactions to amputation will be described as well as techniques of effectively managing the psychosocial rehabilitation of the amputee. The techniques described will include the use of a multidisciplinary team, psychosocial assessment, peer support group, patient coordinator, family meetings and patient education group.

Reactions to Amputation

Reactions to amputation vary depending on a number of factors including the age at the time of amputation, the sex of the amputee, personality traits of the amputee, his lifelong pattern of coping with stress and loss, the type of amputation sustained, the amputee's expectations for his rehabilitation, his perception of problems arising from his amputation, and the human resources available to the amputee through family, friends and his community. It is important for professionals working with an amputee to examine these factors in order to understand the reaction they will see. Each amputee will vary in his reaction because of these factors. For example: A man who loses a limb as a result of an injury sustained in combat might not display feelings of depression and anger but, in fact, of relief and gratitude because, indeed, he could have lost his life and not just a limb. On the other hand, a young healthy person who loses a limb as a result of a motor vehicle accident or an industrial accident may be devastated by the loss. His loss was not anticipated and he may be very depressed and bitter under the circumstances. Both reactions could be considered normal and in fact could be anticipated, given knowledge and information surrounding the reasons for each amputation. Nevertheless, in general, there would seem to be two reactions experienced by all amputees: 1) a feeling of alarm or anxiety which is the normal emotional reaction to stress and danger, and 2) a grief reaction in response to feelings of loss.

ANXIETY

A feeling of internal alarm or anxiety is usually the initial reaction that a person experiences when faced with an impending amputation. It is the response to stress caused by hospitalization and the removal of the person from his normal living environment which temporarily deprives him of the support of his family and friends. This is usually a temporary situation and most persons can cope with a short-term change in environment. However, sometimes this anxiety starts even before the amputation is sustained. When this occurs it is often because the individual is fearful of real and/or imagined changes in his life as a result of the amputation. Therefore, thoughtful preparation of the amputee prior to surgery can help reduce and/or alleviate this anxiety. This point will be discussed later in this chapter.

GRIEF

The process of grieving is a universal reaction to a loss, such as the loss of a limb. Parkes and Napier (7) state that the grieving process experienced by an amputee is comparable to that of a person grieving a lost loved one. In both situations, there is initially a feeling of numbness experienced by the person, which may last a few minutes to a few hours. This feeling is followed by severe pain and distress produced by any reminder of the lost object. Tearfulness and extreme anxiety usually occur. The individual focuses attention on the lost functions of the limb and longs for them intensely. He finds it extremely difficult to keep his/her mind off his/her loss, as reminders are constantly present and cannot be avoided.

Depression usually occurs as part of the grieving process and can be recognized in a person by the symptoms of tension, restlessness, insomnia, loss of concentration and appetite, irritability, tearfulness and withdrawal from social contact. Feelings of guilt are often experienced by the amputee if he/she blames himself/herself for any actions or omissions he/she might feel led to his/her amputation. Loss of self-esteem or lowered self-image are common reactions to an altered physical state.

Stages of Adjustment

PREOPERATIVE PHASE

Adjustment to an amputation begins prior to the actual surgery to remove the limb. The reason for the amputation will determine the length of time a person has to adjust to the idea of losing a limb. Most persons with severe chronic occlusive arterial disease, have a lengthy period of time to adjust to the fact that they will eventually undergo amputation. Someone with chronic occlusive arterial disease will endure a long period of illness, increased disability and often pain before the amputation. This is in contrast to those persons with a malignant tumor who usually have less time prior to surgery to adjust to the idea of losing a limb. Their amputation is to alleviate a life-threatening situation and usually must be done quickly.

When gangrene sets in, the possibility of surgery to remove the limb is most probable. Friedmann (5), in his book *The Psychological Rehabilitation of the Amputee*, recommends that when gangrene is present the person should be told that an amputation is probably in order to stop the spread of the gangrene. He feels that introducing the probability of amputation at an early stage helps the person adjust to the idea of amputation. In the case of elective surgery to remove a limb, Friedmann recommends an open discussion between patient and surgeon, outlining the type of surgery and the benefit of the amputation to the person's overall health. A review of the efforts that have been made to save the limb often helps the person adjust to the idea of amputation. The patient then will view amputation as the final treatment intervention. With elective surgery it is a good idea to include the physician who will be responsible for the rehabilitative care in the discussion when outlining the person's expected level of performance. This can help the person be more realistic about what he/she will be able to do with his/her prosthesis and may prevent overly optimistic expectations and the "bionic man syndrome."

Where amputation is necessary because of a malignant tumor there is usually no time to delay surgery. Often the amputation is the secondary worry, cancer is the real concern, and life and death the issues. In this situation, the amputation often is viewed as a life-saving measure and part of the treatment. However, some persons do not want to know their diagnosis and will permit an amputation without questioning why it is needed. Such situations usually indicate that the defense mechanism of denial is very strong. Denial should not be confronted directly and broken down unless the denial interferes with the treatment.

Traumatic amputation, as a result of an industrial accident or motor vehicle mishap, allows no time to prepare the person for the loss of a limb. As a result, these totally unprepared patients are often more vulnerable to severe emotional reactions following surgery to remove the limb.

In all situations, once there is agreement between surgeon and patient that an amputation is necessary, it should be carried out as quickly as possible. This waiting period, for most persons, causes agitation and anxiety and sometimes can result in stress-related illnesses.

Questions from the patient regarding aspects of the amputation should be encouraged prior to the surgery. Patients often want to know if their life expectancy will be shortened by the amputation. These persons should be reassured that an amputation itself will not shorten their life but that their life expectation is dependant on other factors such as the cause of amputation and related diseases.

Frequently, a person who is not retired worries about what effect the amputation will have on his employer, fellow workers and whether or not he will be able to do the same job as he was doing prior to the amputation. Often preliminary discussions with personnel departments at places of employment may help ease a person's worry about the future of his job. It is important to point out to the person that his psychological adjustment and ability to use the prosthesis will greatly affect his ability to work at the same job and be accepted by fellow workers.

Most persons also worry about what effect the amputation will have on family and friends. They wonder whether people will relate to them as a normal person or as an invalid. It is helpful to point out that usually the reactions of others are dependent on the amputee's degree of acceptance. If the amputee does not view himself as an invalid, etc., others will treat him as they did prior to his amputation.

The question of sexual potency and performance is often not asked but frequently wondered about by many patients and sometimes enquired about in an indirect manner. Stating in general discussion with the person that an amputation bears no direct influence on a person's sexual potency may allow the person to ask further questions or just be reassured by this information. Sexual performance may of course be influenced depending on the type and nature of the amputation.

Patients often want to know how disabled they will be after the amputation. This of course depends on their physical condition prior to the amputation. Sometimes the best way to answer and illustrate this to a person is to match them with an amputee of similar condition and age. Often a person will feel freer to ask questions of another amputee who has been through the experience themselves than to ask a professional.

Friedmann does not advise that a detailed discussion on the various types of prostheses be delivered prior to surgery. He feels that a person is so preoccupied with their emotional reaction to the amputation, that they cannot assimilate technical information such as that used to describe the types and uses of different prostheses.

POSTOPERATIVE PHASE

It is the normal expectation that anyone who undergoes an amputation will be anxious about what the future holds for him/her as an amputee. He also will be depressed and grieve over the lost limb. The circumstances of the amputation will determine the nature and degree of these reactions and give clues as to whether or not the person is experiencing an abnormal or inappropriate emotional state.

Those persons who undergo a traumatic amputation are expected to experience the most severe emotional reaction. This is because the thought of an amputation has most likely never occurred to them. Now, because of an accident, they are suddenly faced with the future of being an amputee. Feelings of shock, disbelief and denial are commonly the initial reactions. The amputee will say that they cannot believe this happened to them (denial) and they will feel that at some point they will awaken from this nightmare and find their body intact. After a few days, the shock and disbelief will be replaced by depression and anger as the amputee starts to grasp the reality of the situation.

The way in which a person reacts in hospital prior to surgery for amputation often will predict their degree of postsurgical adjustment. Patients who exhibit severe anxiety and fear, sleep disturbances, agitation, and restlessness often maintain this high level of anxiety after surgery. They often are preoccupied with the fears of helplessness and loss of control that frighten them both before and after surgery.

Some patients deal with their anxiety and fear by being overly solicitous towards staff and express gratitude in exaggerated terms. They also may be very demanding of staff and have periods of hypochondriasis. They need and demand a great deal of support and actually may be getting secondary gains from the amputation, such as increased attention, etc. from family members. These persons usually are very difficult to reassure and preoperative information regarding surgery and rehabilitation does little to lower their level of anxiety. Severe anxiety is indicative of a preexisting psychoneurosis which usually cannot be alleviated in the time allowed for rehabilitation.

Other reactions such as denial and the "stiff upper lip" stance are seen pre- and postsurgery. These persons initially may be viewed as model patients and be seen as making excellent adjustment to the amputation. However, the defense mechanism of denial may just delay the inevitable emotional reactions of anxiety and depression until the person returns home. Often depression will then set in and, at this time, unfortunately, the person usually has less resources (apart from his family) to draw upon to help him/her through this difficult phase.

Persons who lose a limb as a result of progressive vascular disease often demonstrate feelings of relief over the lost limb. This is because the amputation is viewed as a means to end the severe pain and disability that they have been experiencing over a period of many years as their condition worsened. Sometimes they feel that the removal of the limb and the addition of a new one in the form of a prosthesis will enable them to physically be more active than they have been in recent years. Usually a prosthesis does not turn someone into a "new person." For the amputee who has set unrealistic expectations on the prosthesis, the result is frustration, depression and anger when they realize that learning to use a prosthesis is not easy and takes a great deal of energy and hard work.

Persons who become amputees as a result of the removal of a malignant tumor often feel a sense of relief that the limb, or as they view it, the diseased portion of their body has been removed. These amputees are hopeful that their health will be restored through the amputation and that they will be given a greater life expectancy. Responses of anxiety, depression, etc. seen in these amputees are usually related to the life-threatening disease and not the amputation.

REHABILITATIVE PHASE

After the surgery to remove the limb is over and the stump and the psyche has begun to heal, the next major step for the amputee is limb fitting. In recent years many rehabilitation programs have tried to utilize an immediate postoperative prosthesis program because it seems to have a positive effect on the morale of the amputee. Recent studies have indicated that the earliest possible fitting is best and may even avert some of the severe depressive reactions.

The prosthesis has two components—one concerned with function and the other concerned with cosmetic effect or appearance. One component always will be more important to a person than the other. As a general rule, men are more concerned with an effective working prosthesis, while women seem to be more concerned that the appearance of the prosthesis resembles as closely as possible the amputated limb. Criticism of the prosthesis is common because of its appearance. For example, often a lower extremity amputee will hesitate to be seen in public while their prosthesis is still in the training and fitting stage. They do not like the temporary device because it "does not look like a real leg." Similarly, an upper extremity amputee may reject a hook primarily for its look although, functionally, it may be superior to an artificial hand.

The fitting of a prosthesis forces a person to face the reality of a lost limb. This event often causes an emotional breakdown where there had been initial acceptance. The amputee must now learn how to use his artificial limb proficiently, just as he had to learn the same movements and coordination once before as a child. He also must learn to accept his altered physical condition, his changed body image and physical limitations. These are all difficult tasks and the enforced helplessness and dependency will most likely cause the person to feel quite resentful. Nevertheless, a person must learn to accept these changes if he is to make a realistic adjustment to being an amputee. Persons who have placed too high expectations on the artificial limb must reevaluate and revise these expectations at this time. As stated earlier, personality traits will influence a person's ability to accept and adjust to this new learning task.

During the stage of prosthetic fitting, the question of future employment often plays a major part in determining the overall reaction to the amputation. Manual workers, of course, are more likely to experience occupational difficulties simply because their physical handicap will now interfere with their job performance. Clerical or professional workers probably will have less difficulty in their work situation. At this time, vocational counselling can play a very important role. Sometimes amputees have to be retrained for other jobs suitable to their disability and aptitude. Several factors influence the successful adjustment of a disabled person into a job situation. The attitudes of employers and co-workers play a major role toward the acceptance of a handicapped person in the work situation. However, the amputee's attitude is just as important, if not more so, in the process of his getting and keeping a job. Some amputees feel so anxious and insecure about the prospects of getting employment that they accept the first job that is offered even if they could get a better one based on their skill and qualifications. On the other hand, sometimes an amputee will deny to themselves that they have changed because of the loss of a limb. This person appears driven to convince themself and everyone else that they are not physically handicapped. They often will strive to do the same job as before, even if they are now physically unable to do the work safely. When the defense mechanism of denial breaks down and the amputee is faced with the fact that they are disabled, a severe depressive reaction usually sets in.

Then the amputee's expectations must be re-examined and more realistic goals set for their employment future. Occasionally, an amputee becomes so depressed and discouraged that they give up all hope of working or walking again. They believe that others see them only as a cripple which, of course, is how they feel about themselves. This attitude makes it extremely difficult for both the amputee and personnel working with them in the rehabilitation program. Adequate preparation and knowledge of rehabilitation possibilities often can decrease the intensity and frequency of this response.

Phantom limb pain can cause chronic disability. Phantom limb pain is often thought of as having psychogenic origins but it can be caused by physical complications with the stump and the healing process. Most amputees experience some degree of phantom limb pain but only a small number have chronic incapacitating pain. A number of studies have been done to attempt to isolate the characteristics of those amputees with chronic limb pain from those without. Some of these factors identified in a study by Morgenstern (1966–1970) (cited in Ref. 7) are as follows: over 35 years old, numerous operations prior to amputation, operations resulting from chronic osteomyelitis, and history of recurrent depressions. Parkes (1973) (cited in Ref. 7) found a higher incidence of rigidity and/or compulsively self-reliant persons among amputees with persisting phantom pain. He also identified such factors as stump complications, pain in phantom limb or stump during the first month, persisting illness with threat to life or limb after amputation, and unemployment or retirement.

Few statistical studies have been done to determine outcome of long-term adjustment once the immediate period of adjustment to loss of limb is past. Parkes and Napier (7) found that the most marked psychological reactions were in those amputees with lasting physical defects and those who were the most emotionally upset following the surgery to remove the limb. With more statistical studies of this nature, those amputees who are at greatest risk of developing chronic phantom pain of a psychogenic nature could be identified earlier. Then, a greater effort could be made to focus help and resources on these amputees to prevent this chronic disability.

DISCHARGE PHASE

When an amputee is discharged home either from a rehabilitation hospital or an outpatient amputee clinic, they often feel increased anxiety related to the perception of "being on his/her own" without the daily support of professional rehabilitative staff. They may feel a sense of let-down and abandonment as they face the day-to-day activities and problems on their own or within their family unit. Their expectations still may be too high and they may feel frustrated in their attempt to restore normality to their life style. If they are a member of a family, the family unit may still be adjusting to changed roles and expectations of a member who is now an amputee.

The amputee patient at his/her first recheck appointment at the clinic may appear to have regressed and be demonstrating signs of depression and hopelessness. For these reasons it is important that a community support system be set up prior to discharge so that the patient and his/her family do not feel that they have been abandoned by the amputee unit. Of course some feelings of anxiety are expected and are normal when an amputee is discharged. Explaining this reaction to him/her and the family ahead of time may alleviate future alarm on their part.

Special Amputee Populations

CHILD AMPUTEE

In the case of infants and young children, the parents' reaction and adjustment are often the determining factors in the child's management. Following the birth of a child with congenital amputation, or a traumatic injury to a young child, most parents react with shock. Some are completely overwhelmed and grief stricken. Parents who "adjust" too quickly and proclaim their understanding of difficulties which face their child often are masking a failure to really appreciate the full implications of the child's handicap. In the long run, those parents who seemed at first completely overwhelmed by the situation, given time, may be better equipped to involve themselves and plan for their child's future, than those parents who appear to accept the situation more quickly. The first type of parents have realized the full implication of the situation for their child and have grieved for their child's loss. Denial of the disability often can be maintained with an infant who is so very dependent anyway. It is only as the child grows, and comparisons are made with other children in the same age group, that reality may confront the parents. Their emotional reaction may be frustration and despair at a time when the child and those working with him need the parents' utmost cooperation and involvement, in order to help the child most effectively.

ADOLESCENT AMPUTEE

With the older child or adolescent, the parents again are involved with the planning of the treatment, usually to the exclusion of the child. An older child or adolescent is of the age to understand and grasp the implications of surgery, etc. and should be involved in such discussions. If they are not, reactions such as depression or anger occur and often lead to noncompliance on the part of a young person. Peer relationships at this age and stage of development are very important and, consequently, exposure to other young people with similar handicaps may be very helpful to an adolescent amputee.

ELDERLY AMPUTEE

In the case of the elderly amputee, the reaction of close relatives is usually the key to their successful rehabilitation. His/her physical resources are usually not enough if his/her relatives will not carry some responsibility for his/her maintenance. Involvement of family members prior to the surgery can facilitate the family's understanding of the process and may help them avoid a panic reaction and refusal to accept responsibilities later on. The elderly amputee usually recovers more slowly and takes longer to rehabilitate because of their diminishing physical resources. They need much encouragement and patience from those working with them to help them to return to society as an independent person. Without this, they may all too often give up, withdraw, and become physically and psychologically dependent on those persons around them.

Psychosocial Assessment

INDIVIDUAL ASSESSMENT

A psychosocial assessment usually done by a social worker on a rehabilitation team is an important aspect of the overall assessment of the patient and aids in the planning of their rehabilitation program. It includes an assessment of both the individual and their family and describes their reactions and ability to cope with the adjustments demanded by an amputation. Information gained in this assessment can help all the other team members know how to approach and work most effectively with each amputee.

When doing a psychosocial assessment, it is important that the amputee and their family understand why such an assessment is necessary and helpful to the team members. An explanation should be given, outlining the importance for the staff to understand the amputee as a person and the effect the amputation has had on them and their significant others. It also is important to add that such an understanding can assist the staff to work more effectively with the person and may prevent serious misunderstandings regarding expectations, goals, etc. between the amputee and the rehabilitation staff.

The psychosocial issues will vary depending on the stage of the rehabilitation. Prior to surgery to remove the limb, it is important to know what people are going to be affected by the surgery and how. Questions such as how do family members feel about the surgery and what are their worries about coping with an amputee should be asked. As well, it is important to find out what resources the amputee and his/her family have to help them through this time, including emotional support systems, social and financial resources. If the amputee is the breadwinner in the family it is important to ask how the family will manage financially while he/she is out of work. For example; what insurance, sick benefits, family contributions or savings are available to the individual and his family? The additional strain of financial pressures can impede the rehabilitation process by increasing the amputee's tension and anxiety and may cause him/her to be distracted and worried about financial pressures.

In the situation where the amputee will be hospitalized for most of their rehabilitation, it is often helpful to know what previous experience the person has had with hospitalization, major illness and/or surgery. It is important to know what fears, if any, the person has about hospitals, doctors, etc. Questions such as how the person has coped with previous life stresses such as the death of a loved one, should be asked. This will give you some idea of the person's ego strength and how they will most probably react to their present loss of a limb. Imagined fears and fantasies the individual and their family may have about the amputation and its long-term effects should be explored. The family should be consulted regarding their perception of what assistance is required. Communication patterns of the amputee and the family should be identified. For example, are feelings communicated directly within the family or are emotional reactions expressed behaviorly rather than verbally?

It often is helpful to interview the individual and their family members separately, as well as together. Initially, family members often will try to protect each other and not disclose fears and worries as a group. However, they may discuss these individually. Of course, at some point, these concerns will need to be dealt with within the family system.

The defense mechanisms the amputee is employing to help him cope with the stressful situation should be identified. Often denial is present and it is important to realize that denial can be an adaptive defense, allowing the person some "time out" in order to rally his inner resources to accept the loss of a limb. When denial is adaptive and is not interfering with treatment and the progress of the individual, it should not be confronted and destroyed.

The projection of anger and frustration also may be seen in an amputee. Often these feelings are directed at staff or family members. It is important that these feelings be identified and that the family understand what is happening with the individual when such a reaction is present. If this is done they may not reject the individual when he/she needs them most. A team meeting with the family is often a preventive measure to facilitate direct communication between the family and the team. Involvement of the family with treatment often can alleviate conflicts between family and team as the family can be helped to understand what is happening with the individual and his/her program.

Regression and withdrawal usually are part of a depressive stance and are normal reactions when grieving. Concern with a person's mental state should arise where prolonged and increasingly severe depressive characteristics are observed to be interfering with his treatment. At this time, psychiatric consultation and intervention with medication may be necessary and helpful.

FAMILY ASSESSMENT

As mentioned earlier it is important to include the family of the amputee in the rehabilitation plans. This will facilitate their understanding and cooperation in attaining the rehabilitation goals. In order to understand the amputee and his/her family and the effect of the amputation on the family, it is necessary to interview the family members. Included in the psychosocial family assessment will be information regarding family roles, communication patterns, affective responsiveness, goals, expectations and problem-solving ability. Usually the social worker on the rehabilitation team is the most qualified person to meet with the family and obtain this information.

Changes and shifts in family roles will automatically occur when a family member is hospitalized or physically unable to maintain the same level of functioning as he previously did. Former roles within the family need to be clarified and explored and present changes in these roles identified. Information about who made decisions in the area of finance, recreation, child care, etc., will help identify family roles. Enquiries about how this has changed, if at all, will provide insight into role changes. For example, if a young man who previously had the role of the sole breadwinner in the family is incapacitated because of an amputation, his wife may have to find a job to provide income for the family while he is being rehabilitated. The wife will have feelings about her new role in the family as well as her husband. She may unconsciously resent this added responsibility and be angry at her husband for putting her in this situation. On the other hand, the husband may feel inadequate because of his disability and be depressed because of what he views as a loss of his self-esteem and his role as a family provider. Whatever the feelings experienced by family members, they should be identified and clarified early in the process to avoid serious conflict or family crisis at a later date.

Information about patterns of communications on both an affective and instrumental level should be obtained. Questions such as how the family accomplish the tasks of daily living will elicit information related to instrumental communication. On the other hand, enquiries about how family members let each other know how they are feeling will give information regarding the affective life of the family. It is a generally accepted fact that families who do not communicate effectively on instrumental levels also will not communicate well affectively. These families tend to be highly disorganized and show more pathology than families whose greatest difficulty lies in communicating their feelings. Information about family communica-patterns will aid staff in planning the approach to take with both the patient and his/her family when meeting with them.

The family's goals and expectations regarding the amputee's rehabilitation also are important to explore. At times, family members are more unrealistic than the amputee himself, constantly telling him that he will be better than ever once he gets his prosthesis. This bionic man myth can lead to frustration, disappointment and despair later when the amputee and his family finally realize that he will not "be better than ever" or even "as good as before."

In special cases such as with congenital amputation or traumatic amputation with the young child, feelings of guilt and responsibility may be present and must be identified and explored with the family. Often parents will need help in coming to terms with these feelings, so they can relate effectively to their child. Feelings of responsibility and the degree of commitment should be explored with families of the elderly amputee. This is because family involvement and support usually is so often necessary to ensure successful rehabilitation of amputees in this age group.

COMMUNITY SUPPORT SYSTEMS

When assessing the individual and their family it also is important to obtain information regarding the community in which they live and function. Information regarding community resources and support systems such as visiting nurses, homemakers, transportation for the handicapped are essential in order to plan effectively for the amputee's reintegration into their community. Recreational facilities available to amputees should be known and identified to the families. Involvement in these clubs and organizations will help facilitate a sense of well-being and acceptance within the amputee.

INTERVENTION STRATEGIES

Individual Counselling

Based on the psychosocial assessment which will identify problems of concern to the amputee, the social worker will negotiate a contract with the individual to work on alleviating these problems and reducing stress in the patient. This contract often will involve individual counselling in the form of ego supportive case work. This process involves working through feelings of loss, anger and grief, in a supportive atmosphere. Learning new problem-solving techniques to aid in planning for the future also are involved in this process. Relaxation and assertiveness training are therapeutic modalities available to the therapist.

If a patient is experiencing a severe emotional reaction and demonstrates symptoms of clinical depression or psychosis, a psychiatric consultation is necessary and intervention with psychotrophic drugs may be used.

Access to a patient for individual counselling is much easier when the amputee is an inpatient in a rehabilitative unit. When the amputee attends an outpatient amputee clinic for treatment and rehabilitation, it is easier for him to avoid engaging in a therapeutic relationship for the purpose of helping him adjust and come to terms with this major change in his life. Transportation problems, scheduling conflicts, and so forth all lead to interference and interruption of the counselling process. Of course, commitment on the part of the patient and his/her understanding of the need to resolve feelings of loss, anger, fear, etc. in order to be totally rehabilitated are needed to ensure the patient's compliance. These factors also are dependent on the manner and skill of the therapist in a counselling situation.

Family Counselling

As well as individual counselling, and sometimes instead of individual counselling, the psychosocial assessment will indicate problems within the family unit. If the family has been functioning poorly prior to having one of its members undergo an amputation, this added stress often will throw the family into a crisis situation. At such times families are most vulnerable to change and the quick intervention on the part of the social worker can do much to change family behavior and alleviate stress in individuals within the family.

As with individual counselling, the family members must see and understand the identified problems and be committed to the idea of working together to solve the problems or the whole process will fall apart. Families often need help to identify and express feelings of guilt, anger, fear, frustration with each other before they can be resolved and plans for the future made. Families, like individuals, need time to grieve, ventilate feelings and reorganize their strengths to prepare for the future.

Strategies for Making Rehabilitation Work

INTERDISCIPLINARY TEAM MEETINGS

The physical and emotional components of an amputation always interact and successful rehabilitation is the result of the acknowledgement of this fact. Given this, the use of a multidisciplinary team in both outpatient amputee clinics and rehabilitation hospitals is an excellent method of managing an amputee's rehabilitation. Members of a multidisciplinary team working with amputees would include physician, nurses, physiotherapists, occupational therapists, prosthetists, vocational counsellors and social worker. However, with this approach, the amputee also is viewed as a team member. As a result, he/she has input into the planning of the program through his/her attendance and participation at team meetings. For most amputees, this practice gives them a greater feeling of control and responsibility for their part in the rehabilitation process.

In the case of the child amputee, the parents, of course, would attend the team meeting on behalf of the child. With the elderly amputee, close relatives would be encouraged to attend the team meetings also. Attendance at a team meeting is usually weekly or bimonthly to review the person's progress and plan for changes in his program. However, when problems arise between scheduled team meetings, discussion and problem solving will be done by team members to ensure that the person's treatment program is not interrupted. One of the advantages in using a team approach, is that all team members and the amputee himself are aware of any changes or difficulties arising in his rehabilitation program. Through open discussion, the resolution of these problems usually can be accomplished at the team meetings. Communication problems usually can be prevented or alleviated through the practice of regular meetings to review the treatment plan of each team member and the amputee's progress and expectations to date.

Team meetings can be time consuming but they are essential when a number of persons from different disciplines are working together towards a common goal. Although most persons working within a multidisciplinary team structure feel that this method is the best way to effectively rehabilitate an amputee, scientific research studies are needed to identify the strengths and weaknesses of this technique and to prove its effectiveness.

PATIENT COORDINATOR

In our practice of using a multidisciplinary team approach at Chedoke-McMaster, we also have used the concept of a *patient coordinator*. Each patient is assigned to a team member who acts as his coordinator. The coordinator's function is to be responsible for overseeing and coordinating all aspects of the patient's rehabilitation program. The patient coordinator acts as the main liaison between the patient, his family members and other team members. Sometimes the patient coordinator is assigned to a patient arbitrarily, but most often the patient coordinator is selected at a team meeting based on information from the total assessment of the patient. From this assessment the area which will probably be most problematic for the patient is identified and a coordinator selected from the discipline working within that area. For example, if it appears that the prosthetic fitting will be the major challenge in the amputee's rehabilitation, then the prosthetist will usually be assigned as the patient coordinator. On the other hand, if the amputee appears to have major psychosocial problems within the hospital or the community, then the social worker on the team would be the most appropriate coordinator for that patient. This selection and assignment process usually works well, but problems do arise when there are personality conflicts between the patient and his coordinator. However, these conflicts usually are alleviated through open discussion between the patient and coordinator, and rarely is it necessary to reassign another coordinator to the patient.

GROUP

A group is a useful modality in helping individuals through periods of readjustment and reeducation. Working with the amputee is no exception. Rogers *et al.* (8) state that the purpose of a group is to provide the patient with 1) social support, 2) factual information, and 3) an opportunity for emotional interaction. Fischer and Samelson, (2) have found that "... amputees differ sufficiently from other physically disabled people so that their placement in a group containing amputees would facilitate their adaptations to limb loss." Knowing that a group can be useful, one must still ask, "Why use a group as opposed to individual treatment?" One also must ask whether a group is useful within an individualized rehabilitation program? The following section will address these questions.

Educational Group

The amputee must have access to a wide range of information during rehabilitation. To simplify the logistics of educating the amputee, a group can be formed to satisfy these needs. Both inpatient and outpatient can be accommodated if a group is formed to meet on a weekly basis. The person in charge of the group can develop a curriculum which will cover a variety of topics and retain some flexibility to incorporate patient needs. The following topics are recommended.

1. Stump care.
2. Home exercise and fitness.
3. What is a prosthesis and how does it work?
4. Preventing further amputations through health education.
5. Occupational therapy aids and government assistance programs.

One can draw on the resources of other team members or other disciplines within one's setting to provide the specific information pertaining to each of the curriculum topics.

GROUP—A Tool for Psychological Readjustment

The promotion of an affective, problem-solving group has been demonstrated as useful when treating amputees. The interpersonal group can assist the amputee with feelings of helplessness, isolation and depression. The group that is run for psychosocial adaptation provides the patient with an opportunity to share feelings and gain support from their peers. The group leader can arrange for an amputee who has successfully completed the program to visit the group to share feelings and answer questions that the patients have. It is important for the patients to meet someone who has been successful in the rehabilitation program to encourage them and give them some hope during a time when they are feeling at a loss for direction and control over their lives. When starting a group for psychological adaptation or education, it is important to consider the following issues:

Purposes and Composition. The leader must be clear about the purposes of the group. If the leader cannot present the purposes clearly to potential members, then confusion arises. Also, attention must be paid to the composition of the group. A group cannot be too large or too small. An appropriate size is 5–10 patients. The group can be made up of both in- and outpatients, as long as outpatients make a commitment to attend. The outpatients should be encouraged to attend, since they often lack the informal contact with other amputees that the patient on a rehabilitation ward experiences. There is no reason why the group could not include both male and female patients, although it may inhibit some discussions around sexual issues and body image. Finally, all patients should be given the opportunity to be involved, but not coerced into attending. The anger of a patient forced into attending a group could be potentially destructive. One's own discretion and judgement must be used to solve any problems and resistance.

Group Leader. The role of the group leader is to help the group define its purpose and establish common issues. The leader in the early stages will need to provide both structure and control. As the group develops and goes through progressive stages, the leader will be less involved and the group members must take on more responsibility. The leader must have a good understanding of group process and stages of group development. By identifying problems with group formation, the leader can assist the group in problem solving which will facilitate group process.

Group Modality. The group modality is an important component in the total rehabilitation structure. The use of group can be both rewarding and challenging when working with the amputee patient. The response of the amputee patient to the group process has been, for the most part, very positive. The educational and psychosocial adjustment components that are so important to total rehabilitation are well served by the use of groups and anybody interested in pursuing this modality should be encouraged to do so. Some groups have been intended to serve a dual purpose. Rogers *et al.* (8) have used group education as a lead into discussing issues of psychological adjustment. In our rehabilitation setting, we have tried this but found that the dual agendas confused both patients and staff. We have found that by separating the two groups, objectives remain much clearer and there is much less chance of creating confusion around the purpose of the group.

FAMILY CONFERENCES

A family conference is usually held at two points during the rehabilitation. The first family conference is scheduled soon after the amputee has been admitted to a rehabilitation unit or referred to an amputee clinic for rehabilitation, and prior to discharge. The family conference gives the rehabilitation team, patient, and his/her family an opportunity to meet and exchange information regarding assessment findings, treatment plans, and discharge plans. The purpose of such a conference is to give a cohesive and comprehensive presentation of the patient as a whole to his family, and to give patient and family the opportunity to share information and participate in the rehabilitation program. There are several objectives of the family conference. 1) Education and orientation—this objective is very important at the first family conference. At this time assessment results are shared with the family members. These results outline the patient's level of functioning, plans for their rehabilitation program and a tentative prognosis including their expected level of performance. 2) Patient issues—a discussion of any concerns the patient may have that they have shared with team members and/or the family. 3) Family issues—a discussion of concerns that the family may have; clarification and support are offered where necessary. 4) Team issues—a discussion of any concerns the team members may have apart from those introduced by the patient and family. Issues related to discharge planning are raised with the family at this time, because it is a good idea to reinforce to the patient and his/her family that the goal of rehabilitation is to reinstate the person back into the family and community as soon as possible. Discharge planning strategies with family and patient are thus initiated and followed up during the rehabilitation process.

The patient coordinator is usually the person who arranges and sets up the family conference with the patient and family. If a patient coordinator is not used by the rehabilitation team, then the social worker on the team is the member who most often takes the responsibility for such meetings. This person would then chair the family conference and clarify the purpose of the meeting with the patient and family prior to the meeting. The agenda and objectives of the family conference must be identified by the team and clarified prior to the family conference. Any areas of conflict and disagreement should be resolved before the team meets with the family so that a cohesive and unified message is presented to the family. Open disagreement between members in the presence of the family only leads to confusion, anxiety and mistrust on the part of the family.

It is important that all team members participate at the family conference, but the chairperson must be able to control the meeting in terms of seeing that all agenda items are discussed within a reasonable time frame. One hour for family conferences is usually sufficient time to cover all issues and discuss plans and resolutions of problems.

Although family conferences are at times difficult to organize and to run smoothly, they usually aid in the rehabilitation program simply because most patients and family members appreciate the opportunity to meet with the rehabilitation team and discuss patient issues openly. Family conferences usually lead to less communication problems and frustration between the team and the patient and his family.

Strategies for Facilitating Reintegration of Amputee into Community

DISCHARGE PLANNING

Discharge planning is an issue that is related to all amputees, whether they are returning home from an acute care setting and being treated as an outpatient or leaving an inpatient rehabilitation setting following the completion of a rehabilitation program. The rehabilitation philosophy is to return the amputee to as close an approximation of previous functioning as possible. Without careful orchestration, the amputee will be faced with a painful and negative experience. The pressure resulting from this psychological trauma can isolate the individual and undermine any gains made during the rehabilitation process.

Each person on the multidisciplinary team is involved with discharge planning from the perspective of their own speciality. A person is needed to act as a patient coordinator to liaise with the patient to orchestrate these plans. The patient coordinator on the team will coordinate the assessment of the patient's needs following discharge and begin to plan and priorize as it becomes appropriate during the time of admission. When the patient is admitted to the hospital, the best way to determine the needs of the patient, as defined by him- or herself and the family, is to have an initial assessment interview with the family to discuss the problems that they may envision. The areas that should be covered during this initial meeting, in terms of instrumental needs, are as follows:

Accommodation

It will be important to understand exactly where the patient has lived in the past and whether the accommodation will be suitable for the patient to return to, or must alternate plans be made. Is there a need for modifications within the home and, if so, who will coordinate the restructuring? The occupational therapist is usually best at assessing the home accommodations and making recommendations to the family for changes.

Finances

Patients who have been supporting themselves in the past now may find themselves in need of financial support. An assessment of eligibility for both government and private assistance plans may be of great benefit to the patient. The cost of rehabilitation and the prosthesis is a major burden to people who are on a fixed income. If assistance is going to be arranged for the person, it is best to start immediately when the person is admitted.

Community Support System

The third area for investigation is the potential need for support systems within the community. Discharge support is coordinated by the Home Care Services in Ontario. There is provision for visiting nurses, physiotherapy, occupational therapy, transportation and Meals on Wheels. Understanding the patient's needs will direct you to make arrangements for appropriate services when the patient returns home.

Vocational Retraining

A fourth area to investigate is vocational retraining. Both public and private institutions may provide some assessment facility to help the patient reenter the working community and once again become independent and self-sufficient. Vocational counselling is an essential component to the rehabilitation program of the amputee who must reenter the work force. Vocational counselling involves identifying problems with the former employer, negotiating with employers regarding job change, and if necessary, arranging for aptitude testing where a new job is needed because of the disability. The vocational counsellor would arrange retraining programs and obtain financial aid for the amputee while he is learning a new trade or skill.

Having a job to return to can greatly influence the amputee's attitude towards their rehabilitation and future. Knowing that he/she can still work and earn a living for themselves and their family are essential to maintaining a person's self-esteem. Where loss of job or a decreased job status results, the amputee often will become despondent and feel inadequate. The vocational counsellor can aid in helping employers learn about the vocational ability of the amputee. This will help to ensure the acceptance of an amputee in the work setting.

Recreation

The final area to explore with the patient and his family is around recreation. Avocational issues are often overlooked as not being an issue for the amputee. It is most important for a person's outlook on life to be involved with other people and friends, as before. If the patient is going to be involved in life as a whole person, then avocational activities play a large role in maintaining both mental and physical health.

From this initial assessment with the family and patient, many problems will be identified and it will be up to the person planning discharge to help both the family and patient solve the problems prior to discharge. During the period of involvement with the patient and his family, constant reevaluation of potential problems must be made and dealt with as they become evident. It cannot be expected that all discharge plans will be finalized when the patient leaves hospital, and alternate plans must always be ready so that the person knows that there is support for them if they encounter difficulties. For the patient who is being discharged from an inpatient setting, again, the family conference is the best medium for exchanging ideas and bringing the family up-to-date about discharge plans and plans for following the patient when they return home. Discharge conferences should be held approximately 1 week prior to discharge to ensure that any difficulties that arise at the meeting can be dealt with before the person goes home. The discharge conference should include the patient and all family members that are going to be involved with the patient when he goes home. The professional staff at that meeting should include representation from all disciplines and the patient coordinator who has been arranging discharge plans. Some communication also must be made with the people who will follow-up in the community. If a visiting nurse will be taking on the main responsibility for follow-up, they should be included in the discharge conference. It also is important to document the plans for discharge and give them to the patient to help them remember who to contact in the event of difficulties. Letters can be written to other members who will be following up the patient, including the family physician to explain follow-up procedures and aid them if they are contacted by the patient, looking for assistance.

The staff also must utilize a strategy that provides the patient with coping and problem-solving skills. The amputee must be assisted to maximize strengths and overcome weaknesses by practicing daily living activities while in hospital. In the case of the juvenile amputee or the geriatric patient, these skills also must be taught to the responsible family member or the institutional staff caring for them. The strategy is to help the patient pace himself and first approach a task that is easily completed. The completion of a task builds self-confidence, increasing the feeling of control for the patient. All too often, the patient will attempt many things that are beyond his/her capabilities and fail. This approach increases the risk of physical and psychological set back. The team must reinforce strategies to build confidence in slow, gradual steps. The family or community support services must share these views, so as not to have expectations that are at too high or too low a level.

Follow-up

At Chedoke-McMaster we have found that a suitable time for follow-up is at 1-, 3- and 6-month intervals following discharge. The frequency of follow-up outside these scheduled visits will depend on the problems encountered by the patient. During this period, one can expect considerable changes in both stump volume and shape, which will require frequent adjustment to the prosthesis. Once the patient has become stable and has been fitted with a final prosthesis, the patient will be seen every 6 months from that point; this gives the patient an adequate amount of time to test himself in the home and community environment. The patient must feel that the rehabilitation team will be supportive during the short term. Both mechanical, functional and psychological difficulties can soon start a regression that will lead to the prosthesis being stored in the closet and never being worn. The patient must be prepared for the possibilities of problems and encouraged to deal with them quickly and to utilize the rehabilitation team in this process.

The professional staff has the power to help the patient shape their world so as to better cope and maintain independence. This is not a unilateral venture. The patients must draw on the expertise of the multidisciplinary team in order to develop the skills to eventually lead a productive and rewarding life. The rehabilitation staff must recognize times to reduce contact and indicate to the amputee that they are capable of managing on their own. This is the last step in achieving the ultimate goal of independent living.

Conclusions

An amputation of any nature leaves a person with both physical and emotional scars. For rehabilitation to be effective, time and attention must be given to healing the emotional wounds as well as achieving a good fit with a prosthesis. An amputee will always be "disabled" or "crippled" if he cannot make a healthy adjustment to his disability.

A multidisciplinary team that takes a holistic approach to the rehabilitation of the amputee seems to be an effective means of working with this patient population. Peer groups, individual and family counselling all appear to aid the rehabilitation process.

The rehabilitation literature has few articles dealing with the psychosocial needs of the amputee. Even fewer articles are written about intervention strategies to meet these needs. The studies that have been done are largely descriptive in nature, and for the most part present a subjective view by the authors. Evaluative research studies using control groups are needed to accurately measure the effectiveness of such intervention strategies as peer support groups, the use of multidisciplinary teams, and psychosocial counselling. At Chedoke-McMaster we feel that the above-mentioned modalities and techniques are effective but that is also based on subjective rather than objective data.

Increased interest and concern in the psychosocial aspects of the rehabilitation of amputees will lead to more evaluative research studies that will demonstrate effective intervention strategies to facilitate the emotional adjustment to an amputation. These studies are necessary to ensure the continuing improvement in the rehabilitation of the amputee patient.

REFERENCES

1. Caine, D. Psychological Considerations Affecting Rehabilitation After Amputation. *Med. J. Aust. 2:* 818–821, 1973.
2. Fischer, W. G., and Samelson, C. F. Group Psychotherapy for Selected Patients with Lower Extremity Amputation. *Arch. Phys. Med. Rehabil. 52:* 79, 1971.
3. Foort, J. How Amputees Feel about Amputation. *Orthotics Prosthet. 28:* 21–27, 1974.
4. Freeman, A. M., and Applegate, W. R. Psychiatric Consultation to a Rehabilitation Programme for Amputees. *Hosp. Community Psychiatry 27:* 40–42, 1976.
5. Friedman, L. W. *Psychological Rehabilitation of the Amputee,* Charles C Thomas, Springfield, Ill., 1978.
6. Lipp, M. R., and Malone, S. T. Group Rehabilitation of Vascular Surgery Patients. *Arch. Phys. Med. Rehabil., 57:* 180–183, 1976.
7. Parkes, C. M., and Napier, G. G. Psychiatric Sequelae of Amputation. *Br. J. Psychiatry, Special Publication No. 9,* 440–446, 1975.
8. Rogers, J., MacBride, A., Whylie, B., and Freeman, S. J. J. The Use of Groups in the Rehabilitation of Amputees. *Int. J. Psychiatry Med. 8:* 1977–1978.

11

Stump Complications and Management

V. NANDA KUMAR, M.D.

Stump complications following amputation of extremities occur because each amputee presents a complex situation stemming from variable etiologies, different anatomical levels and differing physiologic and psychologic reactions to the amputation, producing differing attitudes toward the resultant physical disfigurement. In addition, amputation stumps have been prepared by physicians from various disciplines such as general surgery, orthopedic surgery, and plastic surgery, each with his own specific abilities, attitudes, and interests in amputation surgery. (24) In recent times amputee clinics are being established in most of the large hospitals and this seems to have improved preprosthetic care, more adequate and efficient prosthetic prescription, improved training in the usage of prosthesis, and better and more sustained followup mechanisms. Stump complications may be divided into two areas—the preprosthetic and the postprosthetic phases, each of these phases being further subdivided.

Preprosthetic Complications

SKIN ULCERS

One of the early complications encountered following amputation is delayed healing of the surgical incision. Many amputations seen in an amputee clinic, especially for the lower extremity, are performed for peripheral vascular disease, and delayed incision healing may be noted in these patients. This problem naturally delays the fitting of the definitive prosthesis and any attempt at fitting a prosthesis at an early date may widen the slowly healing skin incision or produce necrosis. Any further necrosis may necessitate revision of the stump. Necrosis of the skin edges also may be seen and, if the necrotic area is less than ½″ wide, healing by secondary intention is usually sufficiently rapid to obviate the necessity for further surgical intervention. However, if the area of skin necrosis is greater than ½″ in width, surgical closure will speed the healing process and an early prosthetic fitting is a good possibility (Fig. 11.1). Sometimes it may be noted that the skin sloughing is only superficial and, in such cases, a revision of the stump should not be performed and a split thickness graft may be applied to the cleansed debrided area.

The desire to preserve stump length occasionally has encouraged the performance of extensive skin grafting in order to retain a stump length sufficient to allow use for prosthesis. If the area of split thickness graft is extensive, and certainly if the grafts are laid over exposed bone, this area may well be a problem in fitting and using a definitive prosthesis (Fig. 11.2). Adherent grafted skin or adherent scars over exposed bone surfaces usually require loosening from the underlying bone before either will stand the stress and strain of pressure and/or friction from a definitive prosthesis. Frequent use of massages each day by the therapist and by the patient will sometimes decrease the adherence of skin grafts or scars to underlying bones, promoting the development of subcutaneous fat.

CONTRACTURES

Joint contractures are one of the common preprosthetic joint problems: especially so in lower extremity amputations. Contractures may affect any of the proximal joints in the lower extremity that remain after an amputation. In an above-knee amputee with a short stump, abduction flexion joint

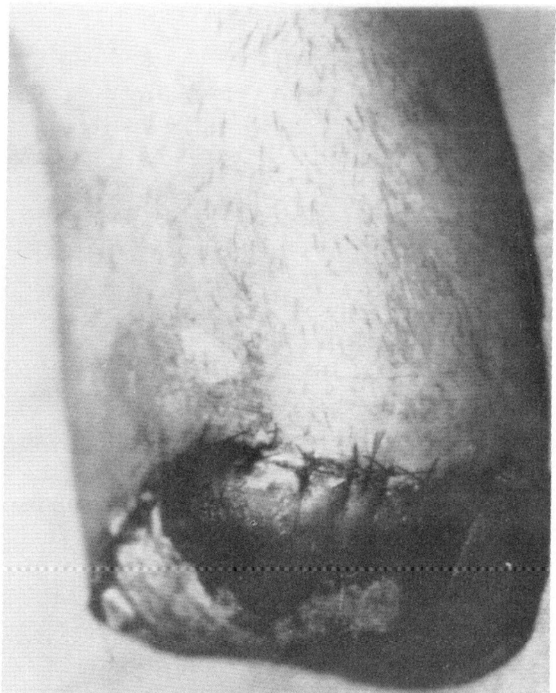

Fig. 11.1. Skin necrosis sufficient to require stump revision. (Courtesy of Dr. Thompson.)

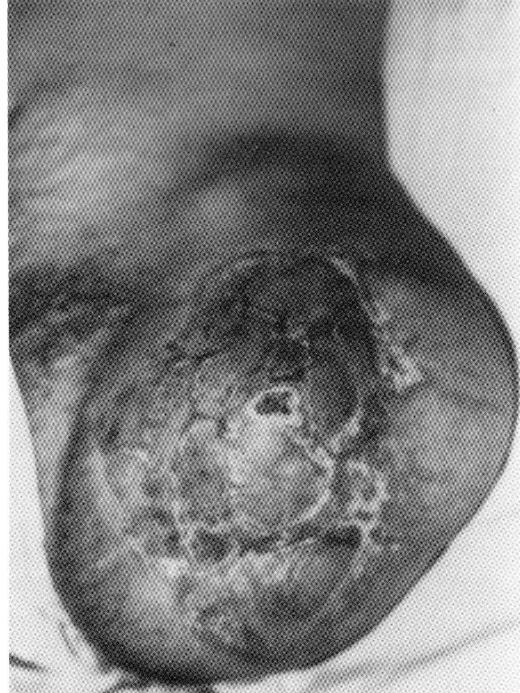

Fig. 11.2. Extensive split thickness grafting of above-knee stump that did not tolerate prosthetic usage. (Courtesy of Dr. Thompson.)

contractures are likely. To prevent such contractures, the patient should be instructed to avoid use of a stump-elevating pillow and, further, to avoid the usually more comfortable abducted externally rotated and flexed stump. The patient should be instructed to lie on his stomach 1–2 hr a day to stretch his hip flexors and decrease the possibility of hip flexion contracture, particularly in the short above-knee stump. The patient also should engage in a vigorous exercise activity to strengthen his adductors of the hip to counteract the overpull of the abductors resulting in the contracture. Excessive use of wheelchairs by amputees aids in the development of hip flexion contractures and the patients should be so instructed. The use of crutches without a prosthesis also encourages bad habits such as propping the short above-knee stump into the "V" of the crutch for support. If this habit is allowed to persist, flexion contractures may be promoted, (Fig. 11.3).

The use of immediate postoperative fitted prosthesis has decreased the number of joint contractures, particularly in the short below-knee amputee. In the usual rigid plaster dressing, the knee joint is maintained in only a few degrees of flexion and this minimizes any type of contracture at the knee. If a rigid plaster dressing is not used in the below-knee amputee, then it is important that the patient is put into a regular physical therapy program to extend his knee completely several times a day to avoid flexion contractures.

Fifteen degrees of flexion contracture at the knee is the maximum that is permissible for a reasonable prosthetic fitting. If the patient develops a knee flexion contracture of more than 15°, the patient should undergo daily physical therapy in the form of ultrasound to the posterior joint capsule and the hamstring tendons, followed by massage and passive joint stretching—with considerable discomfort to be endured by the patient. These contractures are better avoided than treated.

The patient with a Chopart or Lisfranc amputation is usually a good candidate for an equinus ankle joint contracture because of the overpull of the gastrocnemius. It is difficult at these amputation levels to prevent such a contracture; however, if during the surgery all the extensor tendons are reattached at the ends of the remaining bone, they will to some degree, counterbalance the strong pull of the gastrocnemius. If the patient develops a fixed equinus deformity of the ankle then it might be necessary to lengthen the Achilles tendon or perhaps even perform an ankle fusion to maintain a plantigrade attitude of the foot stump on the floor.

Do Not..
..HANG STUMP OVER BED
..SIT IN WHEELCHAIR WITH STUMP FLEXED
..PLACE PILLOW UNDER HIP OR KNEE
..PLACE PILLOW UNDER BACK CURVING SPINE
..LIE WITH KNEES FLEXED
..REST AK STUMP ON CRUTCH HANDLE
..PLACE PILLOW BETWEEN THIGHS
..ABDUCT AK STUMP

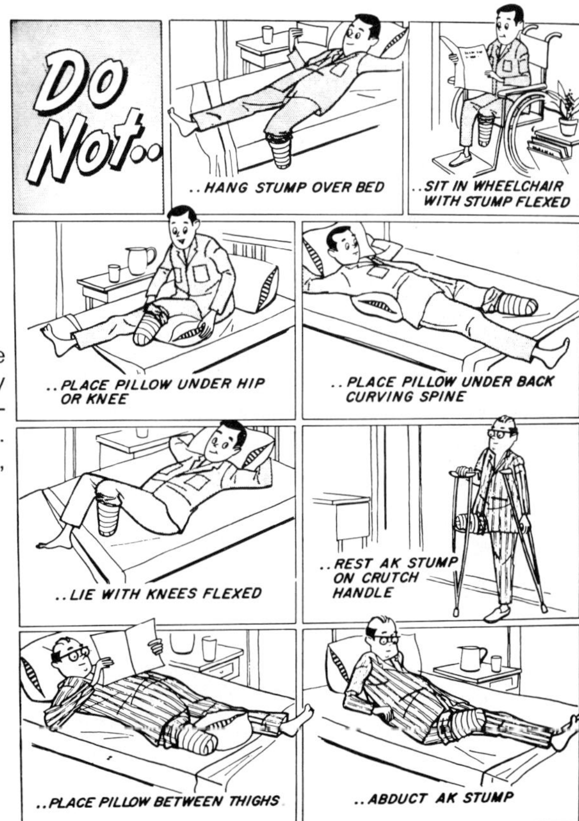

Fig. 11.3. Positions to be avoided by lower extremity amputees during the immediate postoperative period. (Courtesy of Bennett Wilson, Jr.)

BONE SPUR FORMATION

It is not common to feel the bony spur underneath the skin by palpating the stump, but it might be seen quite often on an X-ray film. These bony spurs, if small, are not presenting any problems, such as pain, so they are not an obstacle in the fitting of a definitive prosthesis. It is rare to see a resection being necessary for a spur in a healed amputation stump. Thompson (24) believes that most bone spurs are caused by retained tags of periosteum and so the operating surgeon is warned to resect the periosteum carefully by a sharp scalpel section, severing the bone at the same level, and thus avoiding the retention of periosteal tags on the amputation stump. He also advises not to strip the periosteum proximally from the bone ends since, in some instances, this may lead to the formation of a bone sequestrum, which subsequently may result in a draining sinus in a healed amputation stump (Fig. 11.4). If drainage persists from an amputation stump it is advisable to obtain an X-ray view of the stump in order to ascertain whether there is a ring sequestrum present. Drainage usually persists until the bone sequestrum is removed.

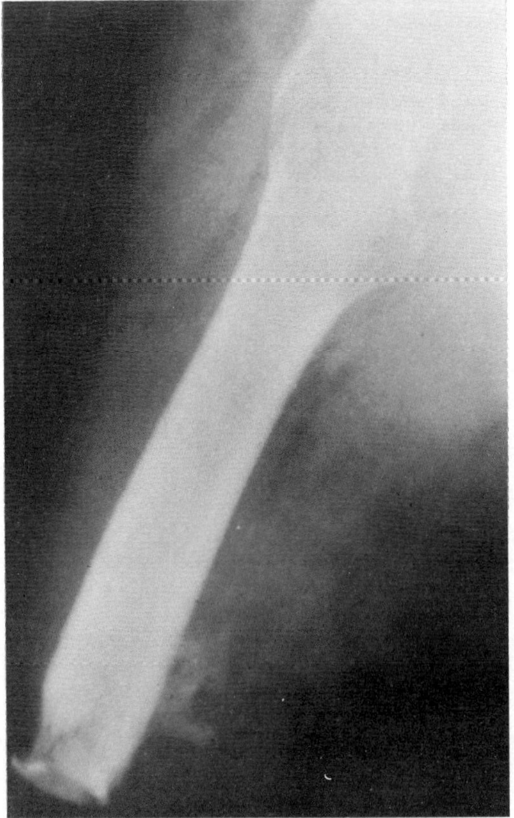

Fig. 11.4. Sequestrum at the distal end of femur which needed excision. (Courtesy of Dr. Thompson.)

STUMP EDEMA

In amputation stumps that are not treated with rigid plaster dressing, stump edema is a common problem in the preprosthetic period. In spite of using an elastic compression dressing, stump edema will develop and further, if the compression dressing is poorly applied, the edema may not be symmetrical (Fig. 11.5). The patients, nursing staff, and the physical therapists are advised to maintain a compression wrap on the stump, replaced every 6 hours until a definitive prosthetic fitting. The patient also is advised not to take off the compression for more than 15–20 min at any given time. However, performance of poor wrapping by the patient or the untrained nurse on the ward often leads to poor results. If the patient wraps the above-knee stump and does not include the end, a dumbbell-shape stump may result. Sometimes the above-knee amputee may only partially bandage the stump rather than bandaging fully into the groin and the adductor roll may develop, which may hinder the fitting of a definitive prosthesis. The above-knee stump should be wrapped completely into the groin area, maintaining the placement by a spica bandage above the waist. Newer methods include

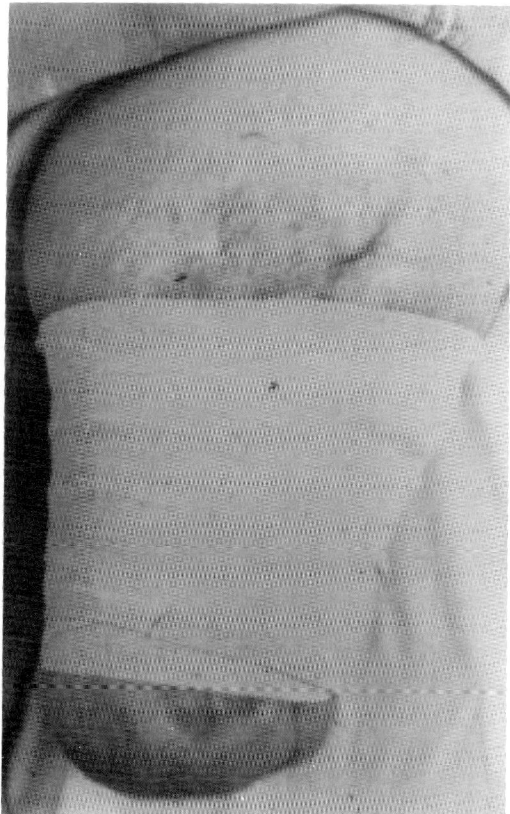

Fig. 11.5. Detrimental stump wrapping.

elastic stockinette drawn on the stump or using air inflated air boots, (Fig. 11.6–8), using 20–40 mm Hg pressure.

PHANTOM LIMB AND PHANTOM PAIN

Phantom limb sensation is a normal phenomena after amputation of a limb. The patient experiences sensations which seem to come from the missing limb which may be accompanied by a tingling sensation. At first the phantom sensation can be so deceptive that the patient may attempt to scratch his chin with the absent hand or to walk on his missing leg. With the passage of time, phantom sensation tends to diminish in a manner which has been described as "telescoping into the stump," but occasionally it may persist for years or decades. The last sensations to disappear are those which seem to originate from the thumb or index finger or from the great toe which may be perceived by the patient as directly attached to the stump.

The limb is an integral part of the body continuously bombarding the sensory cortex with tactile, proprioceptive and occasionally painful stimuli which are remembered largely subconsciously as part of the body image. After amputation of the limb, these remembered perceptions produce phantom sensation, which may even include the feeling of a ring, wristwatch or bracelet worn on the phantom hand or wrist. Deformity of a limb present before amputation usually continues to be perceived in the phantom, and pain which has persisted in the limb a long time prior to amputation

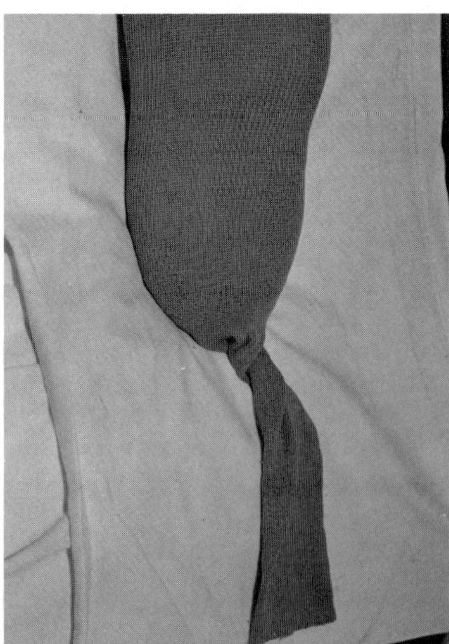

Fig. 11.6. Early postoperative below-knee stump with elastic compression to reduce edema.

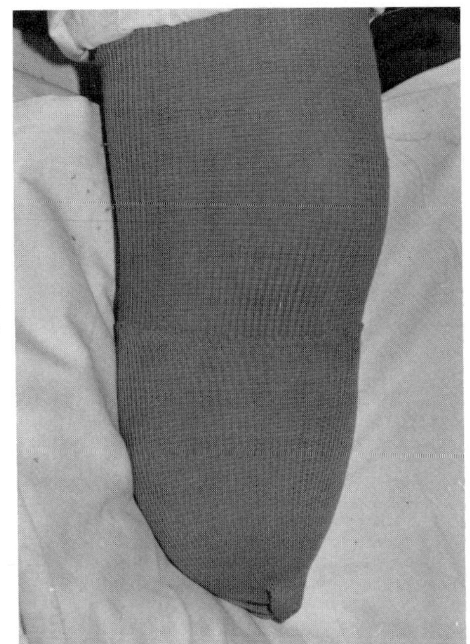

Fig. 11.7. Second layer of elastic stockinette drawn over the stump to further increase compression.

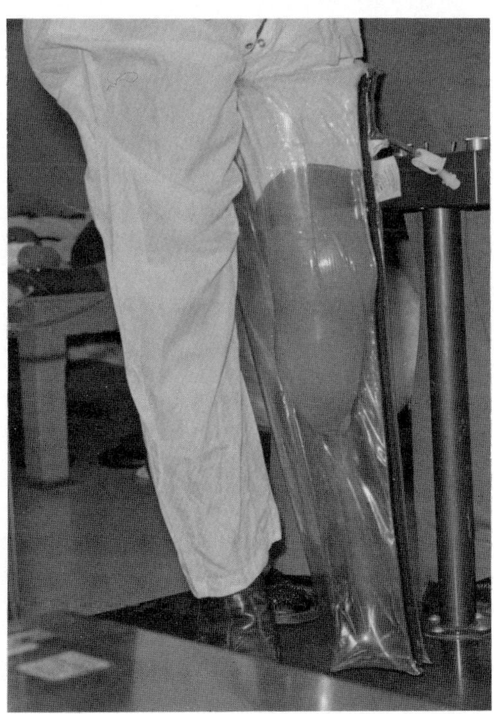

Fig. 11.8. Plastic air-inflated boot that can be put on the stump to further eliminate edema.

increases the likelihood of phantom pain. Anesthetic limbs leave no phantom after amputation and gradual loss of an extremity, as in leprosy, usually is not associated with phantom pain. Children with congenital absence of a limb or who have a limb amputated before the age of 6 do not have phantom sensation.

Phantom pain, in contrast to phantom sensation, does not occur normally after amputation, but one out of every two or three patients complains of it at some time. It is severe in 5%–10% of patients who undergo amputation. Phantom pain is variously described as cramping, crushing, burning, or shooting and may be intermittent or continuous, frequently waxing and waning in cycles of several minutes duration. It is localized in the phantom, not the stump, and is often perceived as a painful twisting discomfort, as for example, a clenching of the fist with the fingernails digging into the palm. Phantom pain may be precipitated or intensified by any contact, not necessarily painful, with the stump or with the trigger area on the trunk, contralateral limb or head. A neuroma may occasionally be present in the stump, but 80% of patients with phantom pain have no detectable abnormality of the stump. Phantom pain may also be triggered by urination, defecation, sexual intercourse, and cigarette smoking.

Historical Aspects of Phantom Limb

Aaronson (1) informs us that the literature on this subject extends back at least 400 years when Ambroïse Paré, in 1579, described the phantom complaints accompanied by severe depression. According to Aaronson, Guenoit was the first person to describe phantom phenomena as hallucinatory and to describe telescoping, that is, the shortening of the phantom until the most distal part approximates to the end of the stump.

Weir Mitchell (14) reporting on 86 amputees following the American Civil War, recorded an incidence of phantom phenomena as high as 90% and found that telescoping could continue for as long as 24 years. Toward the end of the 19th century, treatment of phantom pain was attempted with injections of cocaine, and the passage of electric current into the stump. In spite of some claims of success, most therapists continue to believe that the phantom is derived from central sources. In the 20th century, more interest was shown in the psychological aspects of phantom phenomena and in 1923, Schilder (22) theorized that a phantom was partly an imaginary sensation with a narcissistic explanation, namely the love of one's own body and denial of self-incompleteness.

In the decade between 1930–1940, concern with treatment was paramount. Mescaline, for example, was used for treatment and it was claimed that the phantom shrank and then lost feelings of continuity. Subsequently, there were many reports of good results following alcohol injections into the stump, sympathectomy, presumably to improve the blood supply and neurosurgical procedures ranging from peripheral nerve section, posterior root resection, cordotomy, thalamotomy, cortectomy of the sensory cortical field to frontal lobectomy. None has been consistently successful. Bonica (3) writing in 1953, stated that total spinal anesthesia will not remove phantom pain although the stump is totally devoid of sensation. Bonica reported that pain in the phantom limb often was increased during spinal anesthesia and he suggested that the pain could not, therefore, be due to afferent peripheral flow. This is in accordance with the previous failures to relieve phantom pain by interrupting the sensory pathways at various levels.

Theories on Phantom Pain

Gate Theory. There was another surge of neurological interest following the publication of the "gate" theory of pain by Melzack and Wall (13) in 1965. This theory proposed that the dorsal horns of the spinal cord act like a gate, capable of modulating somatic input before perception and response occurs. It was suggested that the filtering of input by this neuromechanism is determined by the relative activity of large-diameter fibers (A_β) and small diameter fibers (A_δ and C), the whole being under influence of descending impulses from the brain. This led to a new concept of stimulating the nervous system to produce inhibition of pain-transmitting mechanisms. Melzack (12), working with amputees, wrote in 1971 that the loss of sensory input after amputation would decrease tonic inhibition in the reticular system and increase a selfsustaining neuroactivity, which would explain prolonged pain. He suggested that after a local anesthetic block had been carried out, the prosthesis could be fitted. It would stimulate the patient to move and hold objects, these activities producing pattern inputs from the muscles, in particular, which would disrupt the rhythmically firing neuron pools and abolish pain. The concept of stimulation rather than of severing the nerve supply was attractive, and it was claimed that electrical stimulation of the large fibers was assumed to close the gate and would alleviate pain for prolonged periods. Recently, a further development is being investigated. Electrodes are placed on the surface of the dorsal columns of the spinal cord in patients suffering from intractable pain (20). Given a small transmitter control box, the patient is able to stimulate himself. Sufficient time has not elapsed to evaluate this procedure, but one wonders, considering the affective component of pain, if there is reciprocal inhibition to be considered in the psychological meaning of the term.

Psychological Theories. In 1957, Murphy (15) called attention to the extent of psychological disturbance and stressed the mourning for the lost part and the development of grief reaction. Parkes (17) has written extensively in this same vein, stressing that grief is a universal reaction to loss, and he views the phantom limb as part of a mourning syndrome. "Just as the widow finds it hard to believe that her husband is dead, and often has a strong sense of his presence, so the amputee has difficulty in accepting the loss of his limb and he continues to feel that it is present." Parkes and Napier (19) liken the immediate reaction of numbness, disbelief and severe distress, later to be followed by insomnia, anorexia, depression of cognitive functions and associated irritability and bitterness, with the bereavement symptomatology. They stress, however, that the situation is different in that the amputee had a direct connection to the missing limb through the nerves to the central connections and part of this connection remains intact.

Central Origin Theory. Many theories of central process responsible for phantom pain and phantom limb have been proposed. Briefly, the central bias concept suggests that the brain-stem reticular formation tonically inhibits or biases transmission of the somatic projection system at all synaptic levels (8). When a large proportion of sensory fibers is destroyed by amputation of a limb, the input to the reticular formation is reduced and its inhibitory influence decreased. Serotonin (5-HT) is thought to be the most important neurotransmitter in central modulation of pain. Evidence from animal studies suggest that 5-HT modulates pain centrally under normal conditions and deficient 5-HT decreases sensitivity to painful stimuli (9, 23). Lysergic acid diethylamide (LSD-25) and other lysergic derivitives antagonize or potentiate, depending on the dose, 5-HT in animals and is similar to that in humans (5). LSD-25 increases brain concentration of 5-HT by reducing its turnover altering its uptake and retension (6, 21). Fanciullacci *et al.* (8), studying a small group of amputees used subhallucinogenic doses of LSD-25, found that these small doses were effective in ameliorating phantom limb pain suggesting a central site of action and facilitatory effect of 5-HT. The plasma levels of LSD-25 reached a maximum of 10 ng/ml immediately after intravenous administration and was 5 ng/ml at 1 hour after injection, concentrations which would not produce an antiserotonin effect peripherally.

Incidence and Clinical Presentations of Phantom Limb and Phantom Pain

Carlen *et al.* (4), studying 73 Israli male soldiers injured in the Yom Kippur War in October 1973, came up with rather interesting details about amputees. All subjects interviewed immediately after the amputation experienced some phantom limb sensation. Sensations were felt immediately after injury in 33% of all amputees. Another 32% felt phantom sensation within 24 hr of amputation. The remaining 35% felt phantom sensations within a few weeks of injury. The reason for delay in reporting the onset of sensation was because they were unconscious or had amnesia or were critically injured. Descriptions of phantom limb sensation varied. Mentioning in order of frequency they are jabs, strong currents, pins and needles, burning, knife-like pressure, and cramps. Movements of phantom limbs were a frequent phenomena. Forty-five per cent of the amputees replied affirmatively when asked about phantom limb movements. Telescoping, wherein the phantom foot or hand is felt to be closer to the stump end than one would anatomically expect, was noted in 45% of the amputees on interview. Often the hand or foot was felt to be in the stump itself, even when the amputation was above the knee or elbow. This phenomenon usually took a few weeks to develop and the day after, the position of the distal part of the phantom remained unchanged. Abnormal stump sensation, associated with urination, defecation and ejaculation also was noted. Some of those visceral body functions that are under considerable autonomic nervous control tended to cause a burning sensation at the end of lower limb stump and, in a few patients, in the phantom. Forty-five per cent noted that urination caused a burning sensation in the stump end. Thirty per cent felt this sensation with defecation as well. Six per cent experienced burning with ejaculation, defecation, or urination. This sensation usually came with the onset of urination or with the straining associated with defecation. There are also aggravating or relieving factors. Almost all amputees were more aware of the phantom when they thought about it or when they were quietly resting, particularly at night, just before falling asleep. Soon after amputation some noted aggravation of phantom limb phenomena when touching or hitting the stump, but most found that hitting, stroking, tapping, or squeezing a part of the stump tended to relieve bothersome phantom phenomena. Common relief was obtained in lower limb amputees by patting the posterior thigh over the sciatic nerve. Early on, some amputees noted that causing muscles in the stump to contract aggravated the phantom phenomena. However, most noted that after a week or two, active stump exercise reduced the phantom sensations. Physically and mentally active amputees had fewer problems with phantom sensations. Sensory examination of the stump may show abnormalities. All patients showed areas of abnormal sensitivity in the stump whether or not they are complaining of pain at the time of amputation. This universal phenomena had been previously described by Noordenbos (16). Close to the skin flap scar, there was a 2–4 sq. cm. area of hyperpathia.

Management of Phantom Limb Sensations and Phantom Limb Pain

Nearly every amputee experiences phantom limb sensations soon after an amputation. The natural phantom sensations usually disappear over a period of months to years. Nothing needs to be done except reassurances to the patient that it is a natural process and that it is likely to resolve over time.

The mystery of phantom limb pain is compounded by the unpredictability of usual therapeutic measures. While it is difficult to develop a strict treatment protocol for all patients with phantom limb pain, an outline of general approach to their management will be presented (2). A thorough history taking should be undertaken which needs to include questions about the patient's family background, level of education, history of injuries, if any, cooperation of the employer, lawsuits pending or in progress, description of the pain, attitude towards physician, current medications, attitude of family toward patient and his/her problem, feelings of hopelessness, etc. While a carefully taken history often may be more rewarding than the physical examination, the latter must not be neglected. The limb stump, particularly the scar, is inspected for tender or poorly healed areas, including evidence of trauma from a poorly fitting prosthesis. Subcutaneous masses may indicate the presence of neuromata, bone fragments, stitch abcess, or actual infection. Most patients with stump problems should have an orthopaedic evaluation prior to attempting specific therapy for pain relief. However, patients with tender areas in well-healed scars that aggravate or precipitate phantom limbs and pain sometimes obtain excellent and long lasting relief from simple infiltration of local anesthetic into the tender area. These injections often need to be repeated at a weekly or longer intervals and may be more effective when steroids are combined with a local anesthetic, especially when nerve entrapment or neuroma formation is suspected. The combination of triamcinolone (Aristocort) 20–40 mg and lidocaine (Xylocaine) 50 mg often is used for this purpose. Those areas on the stump which trigger phantom pain and which respond to local anesthetic, but which consistently recur, are sometimes amenable to revision of the surgical stump or to excision of neurotoma. Examination of the stump may reveal signs of altered sympathetic activity, such as excessive sweating, vasoconstriction, decreased temperature or hypersensitivity to light touch. Skin temperature differentials may be obvious to touch but the direct measurement by skin thermistor is preferable. Thermography may be useful but the abscence of an opposite limb stump for comparison, in many patients, makes interpretation difficult.

A history of aggravation of phantom pain by autonomic functions, such as micturition and defecation, suggest that afferent impulses in the sympathetic nervous system may be involved in the phantom limb pain (10). In these patients, sympathetic nerve blocks may produce relief of symptoms which could be made permanent by doing a sympathectomy. The results, however, are not consistent. Decreasing afferent nerve traffic from the amputee stump is not the only way to relieve phantom pain. Many patients discover for themselves that application of heat or cold, simple rubbing or tapping or applying their prosthetic limbs for pressure on their stumps bring relief. In a similar fashion, transcutaneous electrical nerve stimulation may prove helpful. Usually one electrode of the transcutaneous nerve stimulator is positioned over the trigger area or an area where pressure or tapping reduces pain while the indifferent electrode is placed 10—20 cm proximally, usually over a major nerve to the extremity. Rate and intensity of stimulation are adjusted to the most effective and comfortable levels, stimulation then being used for 10–20 min, one to four times daily, or as needed for pain relief. A stimulator is loaned to the patient for 3 to 4 weeks of home trial, after which he may purchase one if desired.

Psychologic factors are involved with phantom pain as suggested by the response to distraction, conditioning, hypnosis, and other forms of psychotherapy. Parkes (18) found that people who are rigid and compulsively self-reliant are more prone to develop chronic phantom pain. He felt that this type of personality reacts to an amputation by suppressing true emotions and maintains self-esteem by denial. This type of patient might benefit from counseling prior to amputation so that the patient may become able to express his true grief. Families also should be taught to reinforce the patient's ego in such situations. Some degree of mental depression is common in these patients who often are unable to work or even sleep because of chronic unrelenting or frequently recurring episodes of intense pain. Sympathetic understanding by the physician and reassurance that different techniques may succeed where others have failed are essential. The physician, regardless of the field of his specialty training, can provide some psychological support and therapy. It was found that amitriptyline (Elavil) 50 mg at bedtime and later increased to 100–150 mg at bedtime is a useful antidepressant drug to provide restful sleep without undue sedation during the day. Mehta (11) and others have reported electroconvulsive therapy to be beneficial to some of these patients. Elliott *et al.* (7) report that carbamazepine (Tegretal) is a good drug in the management of patients who are having disabling phantom symptoms after amputation. They found that a dosage of from 400–600 mg/day to be effective in alleviating both the lancinating type of phantom pain and the hallucinatory type of phantom experience. They also suggest a 6 weeks trial of this drug before ablative neurosurgical procedures are considered.

Postprosthetic Complications

SKIN COMPLICATIONS

Skin problems constitute the major percentage of complications even after the patient begins using a definitive prosthesis. In the early days of use of a prosthesis, a previously healed scar may show evidence of breakdown or blister formation (Fig. 11.9). This may be due to stretching of the scar from use of a prosthesis or undue pressure or friction from the prosthetic socket. The skin breakdown or the scar breakdown may be managed by not using the prosthesis for a few days and wrapping the stump to avoid edema and maintain good circulation. If the scar area heals and the patient is then able to wear the prosthesis satisfactorily, nothing further needs to be done. Sometimes, return to the use of the prosthesis may result in a second breakdown and this may suggest poor prosthetic fit or the need for a surgical revision of the scar. Partial thickness skin grafts over the stump may be

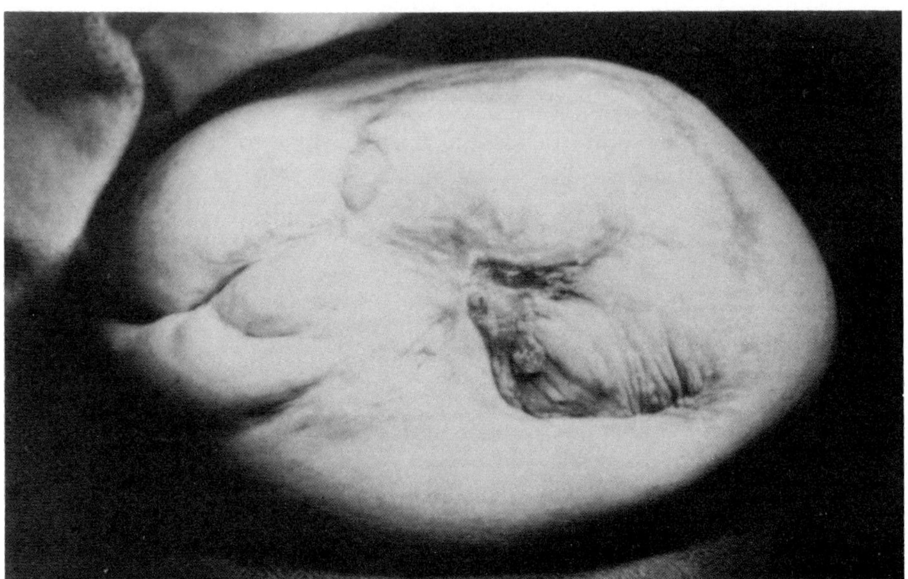

Fig. 11.9. Scar breakdown after prosthetic usage in an above-knee stump.

satisfactory for prosthetic usage if they are small and if they are not at the major weight bearing area. However, if the skin-grafted section is adherent to a bone in a weight-bearing area, and cannot be loosened by massage, the skin graft area may ulcerate and require a stump revision, application of a full thickness graft to the area, or perhaps use of a prosthesis that minimizes weight bearing in the skin grafted area. In some cases, in the below-knee amputee, use of a corset may relieve some of the weight bearing from the upper end of the tibia. Some amputees may even need an ischial weight-bearing seat so as to relieve more weight bearing from the upper end of tibia. If a draining sinus develops during the wearing of a prosthesis and refuses to heal after several days of nonuse of the prosthesis, it may indicate the presence of a foreign body within the stump. This foreign body may be an avascular bone fragment produced perhaps by overzealous periosteal stripping at the time of surgery. Healing of the area will follow only after the foreign body is removed.

In the early days of definitive prosthetic use, the stump should be repeatedly inspected by the patient, the therapist, or the physician, as the case may be, so as to detect any evidence of blister formation or skin abrasion. Any undue prominences in the prosthetic socket often may encourage development of skin blisters or, in some instances, skin ulceration. If local skin lesions are found, the socket should be inspected thoroughly to decide whether it needs "relief." Sometimes blisters may occur in an area of usual weight bearing, in which case it may be concluded that the local skin is not sufficiently tolerant of the socket pressure. In such a case, the prosthesis usually should not be worn until the blister or ulcerated area is healed. When the area is healed, the prosthesis is again worn, usually for shorter periods, or until skin tolerance to prolonged weight bearing is adequate.

In some amputees in whom open end below- or above-knee sockets have been utilized, or in situations in which the socket becomes ill-fitting because the stump has shrunk and the patient has lost weight, the proximal tightness of the socket that develops may produce terminal stump edema. If the edema persists, stasis eczema may develop which leads eventually to a chronic state known as verrucose hyperplasia. These skin changes may develop from open end sockets or be instances of poor fit at the proximal end of the socket, what the prosthetist often referrs to as "choking." This problem can be solved by providing a new well-fitted socket with the use of total contact and this usually clears up the most stubborn case of verrucose hyperplasia (Fig. 11.10).

In the above-knee socket, snug fit is a requirement which predisposes to the development of a sebaceous skin cyst. It is well known that the above-

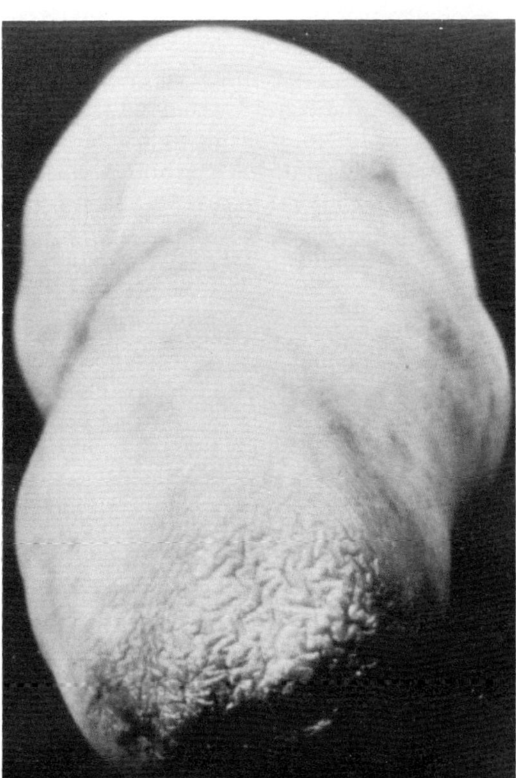

Fig. 11.10. Verrucose hyperplasia in a below-knee stump.

knee amputee, while performing normal gait, develops considerable amount of torque that needs to be absorbed at the interface between the stump and the socket. This torque effect is usually concentrated at the brim of the socket where sebaceous glands are abundant, grinding dead skin flakes into the sebaceous gland openings, and plugging them so as to encourage sebaceous cyst formation. When these cysts become infected, drainage usually ensues. The infected sebaceous cyst usually requires adequate drainage and perhaps enucleation of the cyst wall. For this reason the amputee should be educated well with the necessity of adequate hygiene of the stump. Dead skin flakes and debris should not be allowed to collect in any area of intimate socket contact. Local skin bacteria counts may be decreased by using a medicated soap, such as Phisohex. When sebaceous cysts become painful, with a resultant inability to use the prosthesis, surgical excision may be indicated before infection develops.

In some instances, patients might develop local skin friction resulting in small cornified skin areas similar to "corns" that appear on the foot. It might be necessary to resect the cornified areas, or at least pare them down so that local pressure no longer causes discomfort. In some patients when the recurrent cyst or corn formation becomes a major problem, inserting a rotator in the prosthesis may reduce the recurrence by reducing the torque at the stump socket interface.

Peripheral neuropathy may be an extra finding in amputees with diabetes mellitus, which may result in loss of skin sensation over the stump and may lead to skin breakdown. Without the normal protective skin sensation, skin blistering and ulceration may become far advanced before the amputee is aware of its presence. These patients should inspect their amputation stumps daily to minimize skin complications.

REDUNDANT SOFT TISSUE

Some surgeons, from a misplaced sense of sympathy for the amputee, may leave behind a considerable amount of soft tissue as a cushion over the end of the bone. This extra soft tissue may develop edema which may persist and progress to eczema and then ulceration. If the redundant soft tissue is a small amount it may slowly shrink and no intervention may be needed. However, if the redundant soft tissue is large, it is wise to surgically resect the redundant soft tissue.

Sometimes, development of a bursa occurs when pulling of muscle tissue over the bone end is accomplished (myoplasty) and this may be treated with injection of hydrocortisone acetate. Occasionally it might necessitate revision of the stump to resect the redundant muscle tissue.

NEUROMA OF STUMP

Every effort should be made to transect the major nerves at least several inches above the stump and, further, that the nerves be excised with a sharp knife rather than cut with scissors. It has not been found satisfactory to ligate the nerve or inject it with a noxious substance, such as alcohol or phenol. A neuroma is produced by excessive growth of the axons in an attempt to reach into the distal nerve segment. These axons of the cut end of the nerve growing into the soft tissue at the end of the stump are turned back on themselves, thus producing a small ball of nerve tissue which is labeled a neuroma. Most of these neuromas are placed in normal soft tissue, 1″–2″ proximal to the stump end, and should not cause too much trouble for the patient nor require any particular treatment. Sometimes painful subcutaneous neuroma often may be accommodated within the socket by sufficient "socket relief." Thompson (24) mentions that only a few neuromas, those that have become attached to the scar on the stump end, or that may have been buried in the bone, may require surgical excision.

BONY OVERGROWTH

A special problem called bony overgrowth may develop during prosthesis usage in children. This condition, in which femur, tibial or humeral bone ends may grow and in some instances actually may protrude through the skin, may require surgical revision. This bone growth is believed to be due to appositional bone accretion and is not apparently related to a epiphyseal bone growth. It is therefore advisable and satisfactory simply to adequately to resect the protruding bone and reclose the amputation stump. Parents may be advised, however, that the problem may recur and require another, or several more, minor surgical operative procedures before the child becomes mature.

REFERENCES

1. Aaronson, L. M. The Psychological Adjustment of the Orthopedic Patient. Ph.D. Thesis, University of Liverpool, 1968.
2. Blankenbaker, W. L. The Care of Patients with Phantom Limb Pain in a Pain Clinic. *Anesth. Analg., 56:* 842–846, 1977.
3. Bonica, J. J. *The Management of Pain*, 1st ed., p. 994. Lea & Febiger, Philadelphia, 1953.
4. Carlen, P. L., Wall, P. D., Nadvorha, H., and Steinbach, T. Phantom limbs and related phenomena in Recent Traumatic Amputations. *Neurology, 28:* 211–247, 1978.
5. Costa, E. Effects of Hallucinogenic and Tranquillizing Dryer on Serolinin-Evoked Uterine Contractions. *Proc. Soc. Exp. Biol. Med., 91:* 39–41, 1956.
6. Diaz, J. E., and Huttunen, M. O. Persistent Increase in Brain Serotinin turnover After Chronic Administration of LSD in the rat. *Science, 174:* 62–64, 1971.
7. Elliott F., Little, A., and Milbrandt, W. Carbamazepine for Phantom-Limb Phenomena. *N. Engl. J. Med.*, 678, 1976.
8. Fanciullacci, E., *et al.* Phantom Limb Pain: Subhallucinogenic Treatment with Lysergic Acid Diethylamide.
9. Harvey, J. A., and Lints, C. E. Lesions in the Medial Forebrain Bundle: Delayed Effects on Sensitivity to Electric Shock. *Science 48:* 250–252, 1965.
10. Maloney, P. R., Jr. Phantom Sensation with Urinary flow. *JAMA, 218:* 1052, 1971.
11. Mehta, M. *Intractable Pain. Major Problems in Anesthesia Series*, vol. 2, W. W. Muslin, W. B. Saunders, Co., 1973.

12. Melzack, R. Phanton Limb Pain: Implications for Treatment of Pathologic Pain. *Anesthesiology, 35:* 409, 1971.
13. Melzack, R., and Wall, C. D. Pain Mechanism: A New Theory. *Science, 150:* 971, 1965.
14. Mitchell, S. W. Injuries of Nerves and their Consequences, Lippincott, Philadelphia, 1874.
15. Murphy, W. F. Some Clinical Aspects of the Body Ego. *Psychoanal. Rev., 44:* 462, 1957.
16. Noordenbos, W. *Pain*, p. 182. Elsevier-North Holland, Amsterdam, 1959.
17. Parkes, C. M. Bereavement. Studies of Grief in Adult Life, p. 184. Tavistock, London, 1972.
18. Parkes, C. M. Factors Determining the Persistence of Phantom Pain in the Amputee. *J. Psychosom. Res., 17:* 97, 1973.
19. Parkes, C. M., and Napier, M. M. Psychiatric Sequelae of Amputation. *Br. J. Hosp. Med., 4:* 610, 1970.
20. Riding, J. E., and Lipton. Relief of Pain. In *Recent Advances in Surgery. No. 8*, chap. 1, Churchill, Livingston, London, 1973.
21. Sankar, D. V. S., Sankar, D. B., Phipps, E., and Gold, E. Effects of Administration of Lysergic Acid Diethylamine on Serotinin Levels in the Body. *Nature, 191:* 499–500, 1961.
22. Schilder, P. *The Image and Appearance of the Human Body*, pp. 63–70 and 297, Wiley, New York, 1953.
23. Tenen, S. S. The effects of *p*-chlorophenylalamine, a Serotinin Depletor, on Avoidance, Acquisition: Pain Sensitivity and Related Behavior in the Rat. *Psychopharmacologia, 10:* 204–219, 1967.
24. Thompson, R. G. Complications of Lower Extremity Amputation. *Orthop. Clin. North Am., 3:* 323–338, 1972.

12

Child and Juvenile Amputee

D. A. GIBSON, M.D., F.R.C.S.(C)

There is a sense in which serving a juvenile amputee is just fitting a smaller limb to a smaller person. Saying that exhausts the similarities between the management of juvenile and adult amputees, leaving many areas of profound difference.

The congenital amputee starts life that way. Dealing with him is also dealing with his parents. The stump is unlikely to resemble a standard surgical stump at a site of election. Prosthetic parts of the appropriate size may not be avalable on the market. Training a child in the use of a limb is geared to his age and developmental stage. Supervision and management patterns are modified by the child's growth. As the patient reaches the late teens, all factors fade and merge into an adult situation.

The views expressed in this chapter were developed by the author while consulting in the Amputee Clinic at the Ontario Crippled Children's Centre in Toronto, and references to our clinic experience refer to this facility.

Incidence of Congenital Amputations

IN POPULATION AT LARGE

The incidence of congenital amputation is hard to be sure of because there are variations in terminology and of reporting practices.

In Ontario in a 3-year period there were 395,517 live births. Ninety-three were reported to have a "reduction deformity of the upper limb," 46 with a "reduction deformity of the lower limb," 8 more with reduction deformities of a limb unspecified. The total is 147 cases, or less than 0.37 cases/1000 live births (4).

Some years ago the World Health Organization (WHO) surveyed some 24 centers around the world and the incidence of reduction deformities varied from 1.78/1000 to 0.1/1000, averaging 0.21/1000 (5).

WITHIN OUR CLINIC POPULATION

Terminology is a real problem when discussing the congenitally limb deficient child. If we use terms valid for the surgical amputee, we encounter a number of situations which really do not quite correspond. Many attempts have been made to develop a perfect classification of congenital limb deficiencies, none entirely satisfactory (9). Franz and O'Rahilly (7) in 1961 published the most useful classification currently available. It makes sense but, even with it, there are patients for whom an accurate classification is difficult. Sometimes it is not clear what anatomical bone is represented by a residual odd-shaped bone element and sometimes it is clear, as a child grows and ossification proceeds within a cartilage model, that the original classification is not accurate. In these circumstances, a description of the defective limb must be included in the record, in addition to the classification. Fortunately, these problems are more academic than clinical as we fit the limb in accordance with the gross appearance and function.

In the Franz-O'Rahilly classification (7), an absent limb is an amelia and a partial limb is a hemimelia. Hemimelias are further described in two ways, each with a pair of adjectives. One pair is "intercalary" indicating a segment lost with distal limb present, or "terminal", indicating that the whole limb or ray distal to a certain point is missing. The other pair is "paraxial" indicating a ray defect (*e.g.* radial ray) or "transverse" meaning the whole limb is absent beyond that point.

The use of the two descriptive terms, together with the name of the missing bone, identifies the deformity effectively for communication and classification purposes. This may sound complicated but really it is not, and a few attempts at classification of specific limb deficiencies, with reference to the article, will make it clear and easy to remember.

In our clinic we use these terms for classification and for precision, but for everyday speech and when dealing with common deficiencies we tend to revert to the simple descriptive language "congenital below-elbow amputation" and so on. We reserve the more complex terms for situations where a simple short term is inadequate.

In our clinic, out of a patient load of about 560 children, 72% have congenital limb deficiencies. Of this group, in turn, 60% have upper limb defects, 30% have lower limb defects, and the rest have some combination of the two.

Figure 12.1 indicates the distribution of levels of amputation in the upper limb, and Figure 12.2 indicates the levels in the lower limb. There is some overlap as a few children appear in both upper and lower limb figures.

Etiology of Congenital Amputations

Unfortunately, no system of classification helps with the etiology. A few congenital amputations are clearly the result of congenital constriction

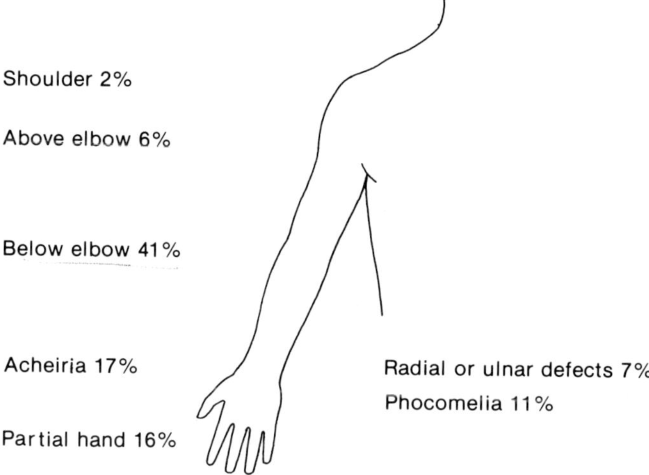

Fig. 12.1. Levels of amputation in 310 congenital upper limb amputations in 282 patients.

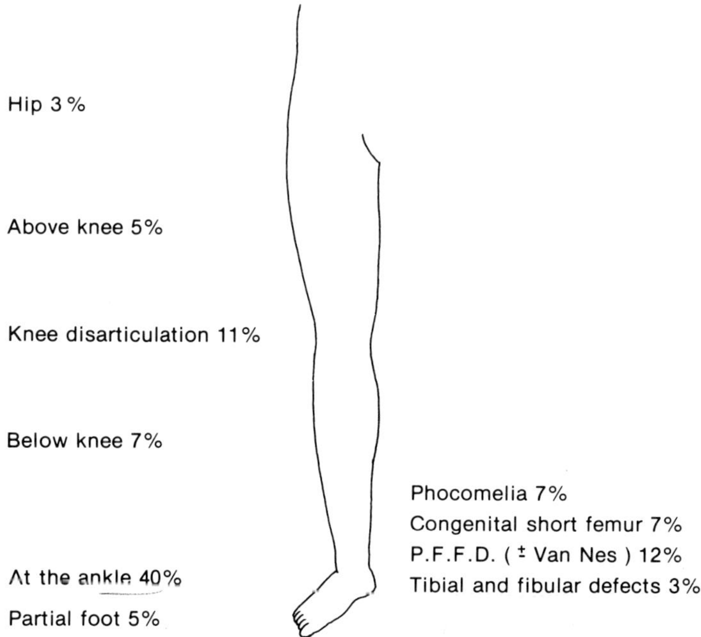

Fig. 12.2. Levels of amputation in 177 congenital lower limb amputations in 152 patients.

bands which had progressed antenatally to complete amputation. Babies have been born with the amputated limb floating free and expelled at the time of parturition. This is the exception.

Some deformities are familial. A mother with a radial hemimelia brought her daughter with a radial hemimelia. A father who brought his son had a tibial hemimelia, and so did the child.

The majority, however, must represent an injury to, or a failure of, the limb at an early stage. The thalidomide tragedy which produced characteristic limb deficiencies when the mother used thalidomide in the first 6 weeks of pregnancy, provided evidence that intrauturine poisoning of this kind does occur. It is probable that many of the defects we see have a similar causation, but from an agent which we have not the wit to identify. In taking the history of a limb-deficient child, therefore, we should look for a family history of a limb defect, and for a history of any untoward circumstance, drug, illness or accident during the early part of the pregnancy.

Surgical Considerations in Management of Congenitally Limb-Deficient Child

There is a basic principle here that no form of reamputation or removal of the unusual appendages should ever be done until all parties concerned in the decision have got full peace of mind that it is right. Sometimes, this involves waiting a long time, but it is better so than to remove some part of a child's body and have lingering doubts and resentments harbored by the parent.

Upper limb amelias (Fig. 12.3), above-elbow amputations (Fig. 12.4), and below-elbow amputations (Fig. 12.5) are not helped by any form of surgery. Lengthening a short below-elbow stump with grafted skin cover has been attempted but substitutes a stump with uncomfortable scars and an insensitive tip for the natural comfortable stump. With modern sockets and

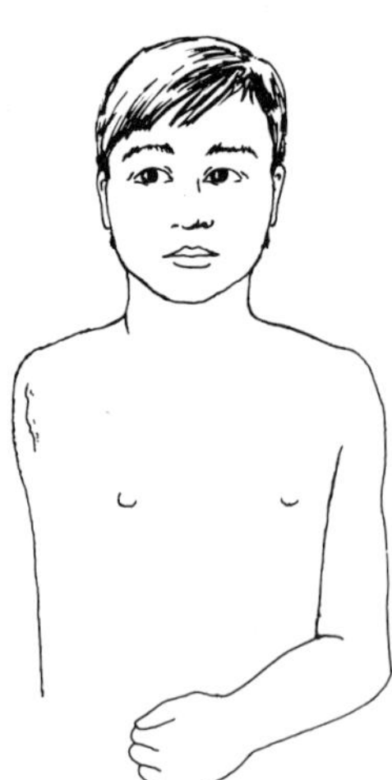

Fig. 12.3. Right upper limb amelia. This corresponds to a shoulder disarticulation. Sometimes, even the pectoral girdle element may be absent, and the deficiency resembles a forequarter amputation.

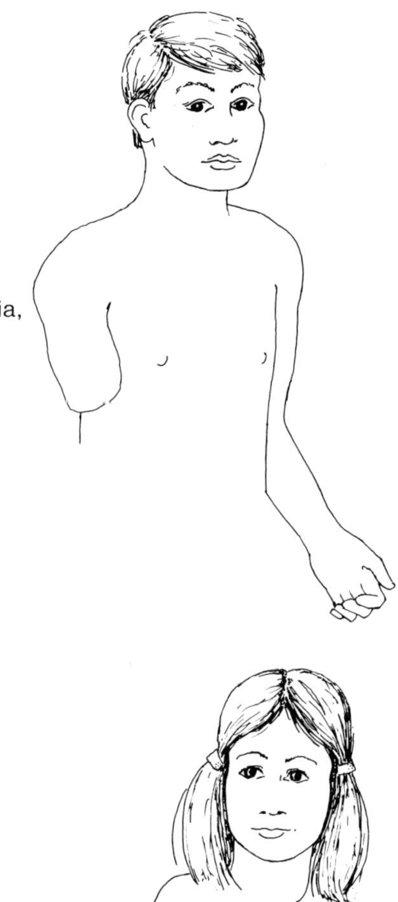

Fig. 12.4. Right terminal transverse hemimelia, above-elbow.

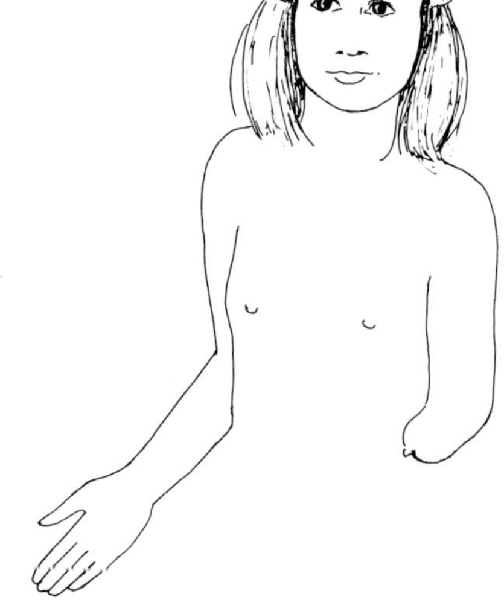

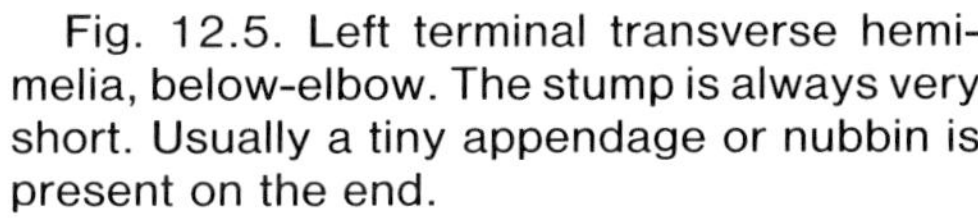

Fig. 12.5. Left terminal transverse hemimelia, below-elbow. The stump is always very short. Usually a tiny appendage or nubbin is present on the end.

techniques, even the short stumps can be well fitted without surgery. A fairly common stump is the acheiria (Fig. 12.6), or short forearm with a soft tissue wrist element which is mobile. Fingers are represented only by nubbins on a pedicle containing neither tendon nor bone. Our policy with

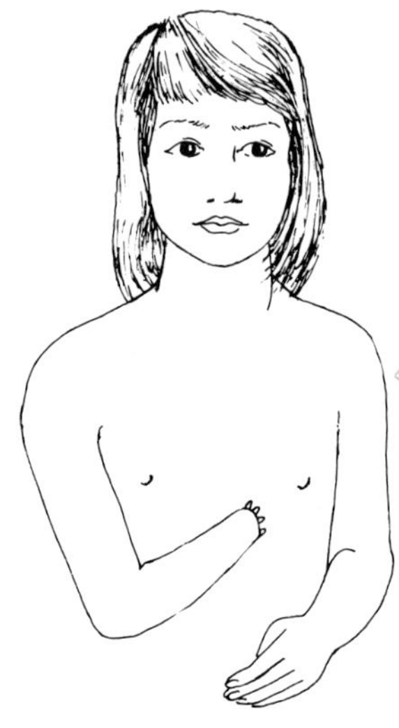

Fig. 12.6. Right terminal transverse hemimelia, wrist level, or acheiria. There is voluntary movement of small wrist soft tissue elements but the excursion is small.

these nubbins has been to leave them alone, unless they actually cause trouble by becoming irritated inside a socket or by some activity of the child.

The place of surgery for the partial hand is more important and more difficult. Children with a terminal paraxial radial hemimelia lack a thumb and the question arises whether a radially located digit can be rotated and stabilized in a thumb-like location. This gives opposition and improves grasp. Whether it is going to be functional or not depends to a large extent on the quality of control present in the finger to be moved. Sometimes, in other partial hand deficits, function can be improved by stabilizing weak digits, deepening clefts and potentially, in the future transplantation of toes or fingers, using microvascular techniques to obtain good sensory function and vascular supply. None of these should be done in infancy. All of them should be done only by an experienced hand surgeon and, before anything is done, a careful documentation of existing function together with the predicatable functional loss as well as the anticipated functional gain should be recorded and discussed with the family.

Phocomelic upper limbs (Fig. 12.7), should be left alone as finger function available in these small deformed hands may be useful to control electric switches even if it is too weak to provide a sturdy grasp.

In the lower limb, because the need for lower limb function is at once more absolute and also vastly simpler than with the upper limb, the place of surgery is more easily defined, although still often controversial. Congenital amputations at any level quite often require revision and, when they do, the indication is obvious difficulty with the present fitting and some anticipated improvement in function or comfort with the new postsurgical fitting. The difficulty comes with the deformed deficient limbs such as those in sacral agenesis, the proximal femoral focal deficiencies, the fibular and tibial hemimelias, congenital pseudoarthroses of the tibia, short limbs, and foot deformities.

Lumbosacral agenesis is so rare that few surgeons have a series. It may be managed by leaving the child alone surgically and providing a wheelchair for outdoor use. It may be managed by amputating both lower limbs at the hip level and fitting a prosthetic bucket with limbs (15). We have not done this. It also may be managed by disarticulating the knees which are usually fixed in profound flexion, using the autogenous tibial bone to provide some stability between the thoracic spine and pelvis. This has the advantage of controlling the concertina effect seen in these children which allows the chest to crumple down on the pelvis, and yet leaves the thighs for prosthetic fitting. Function, however, is disappointing and laborious because, in this condition, hip movement and power are always impaired. Even with these limitations, however, it is probably the best way to serve these children. Careful evaluation of the child's urological and rectal function should precede any decision making as these are also affected.

Proximal femoral focal deficiency, (Fig. 12.8) is a complex defect varying from one extreme where only a tiny nondescript particle of bone represents the whole femur to the other where the femur is apparently complete and merging into the "congenital short femur." These variations are well described in Aitken's classification (1).

The problems in dealing with a given child are surgically complex and only a few basic observations can be offered here.

1. The important issue in terms of eventual function is hip stability. If there is no femoral head, the hip function will always be poor and the child will always limp with a Trendelenburg lurch. If the femoral

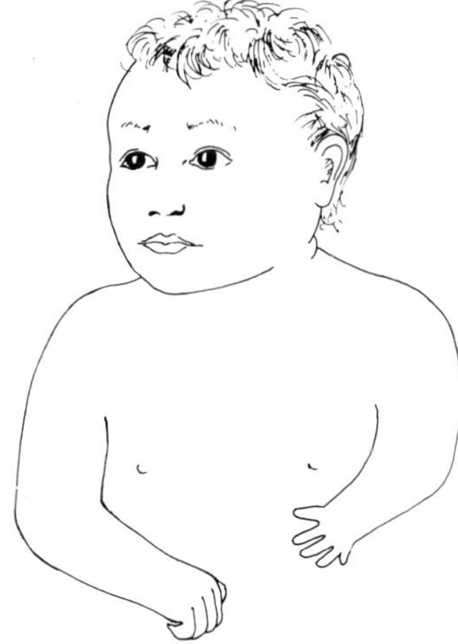

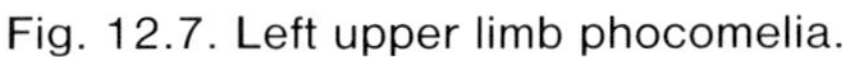

Fig. 12.7. Left upper limb phocomelia.

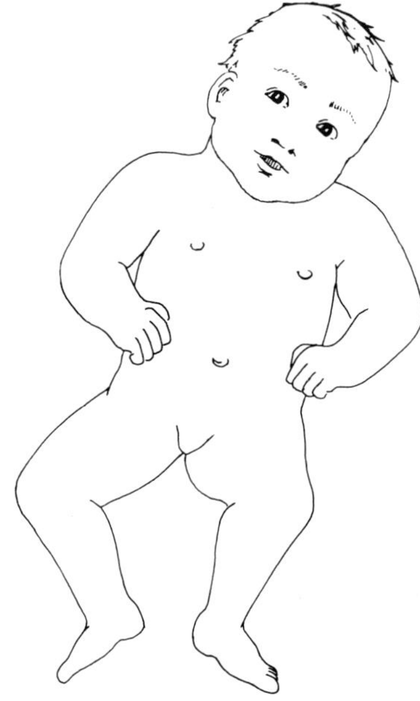

Fig. 12.8. Left proximal femoral focal deficiency (PFFD).

head is there, surgery for the upper femur should wait until all the cartilaginous elements have become bony and then the upper end of the femur should be reconstructed to stabilize the relationship of the limb to the pelvis. This will give a much improved gait, although probably with some continuing hip abductor weakness. If the upper end of the femur is present and solid, hip function will be good.

2. In severe deformity, the hip and knee are fixed in flexion. This militates against satisfactory fitting and the desired ischial bearing, as an apparent pistoning effect is created, even though the stump is not going up and down in the socket. Early fusion of the knee has been advocated for this and should be done with great care to avoid damaging the lower femoral and upper tibial epiphyses (10). The hip flexion deformity improves as the infant grows (11).
3. It is sometimes possible to rotate the tibia to use the ankle joint and its muscle control to activate the prosthetic knee (20). The decision here depends on how short the limb is, determining where the rotated ankle would be in relation to the opposite knee, and the mobility and quality of control over the ankle. Where rotation surgery is planned, it should be deferred until the early teens as muscle pull, which after the operation is in a spiral direction, will cause derotation in a younger child (12).

When the ankle on the short side is low then the choice exists between doing leg lengthening procedures, time consuming and full of hazard as they are, or of amputating to facilitate prosthetic fitting. This is not an urgent decision as the situation can be handled until everybody's desires and thoughts and plans are clear by fitting a prosthesis over the plantar-flexed ankle.

Patients with fibular hemimelia or absent fibula (Fig. 12.9) may have a fairly good foot on a rather short leg. They can walk with or without a prosthesis. The problems they encounter, however, are:

1. Shortness,
2. Valgus deformity and displacement at the ankle,
3. Valgus deformity of the knee.

The shortness is managed prosthetically. Excision of the fibrous mass representing the fibula lateral to the ankle may reduce the tendency for the foot to be pulled into valgus and make it possible to stabilize the ankle within a prosthetic socket. This prosthesis uses an equinus position of the ankle to compensate for shortness of the leg. This may be all that the child needs, but often a progressively uglier fit, or pressure areas over the toes or medial malleolus, will make it obvious that the child would function better

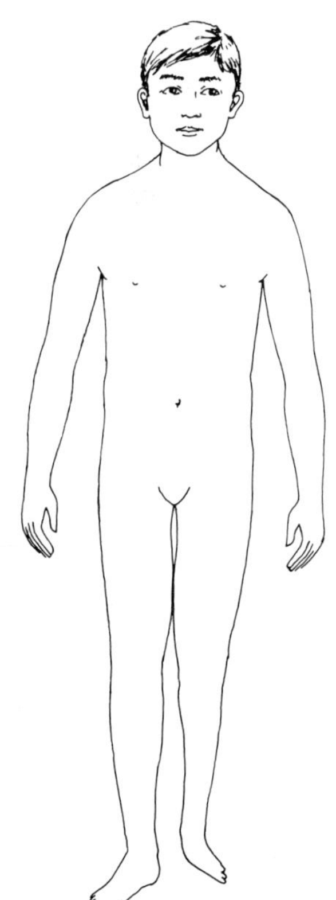

Fig. 12.9. Left fibular hemimelia. Here the distal ray is lost and the lateral toes are missing, but sometimes the foot is whole.

after a Syme's amputation. The valgus deformity at the knee can, in mild degree, be accommodated by medial displacement of the foot on the prosthesis, but where this is becoming increasingly awkward and ugly, a tibial osteotomy is justified.

Patients with a tibial hemimelia or absent tibia (Fig. 12.10), have no real stability around the knee. The upper end of the fibula can be implanted between the femoral condyles, and the distal end into the tarsus (2, 3) but we believe the resulting limb, necessarily braced, is less satisfactory than a knee disarticulation fit with a good prosthesis.

Congenital pseudoarthrosis of the tibia may, on occasion, be prevented by the identification of a prepseudoarthrosis showing up as a cortical thickening with obliteration of the medullary cavity and, sometimes, the formation of a cyst at the level which will become the pseudoarthrosis. If this is recognized, a protective removable walking cast made of suitable plastic can be supplied and actual fracture may not occur.

Once a fracture has occurred, the controversy is on. There are many schools of thought and a series large enough and well enough controlled to give a dogmatic answer has not yet been published. A number of observations can be made, however:

1. Early attempts to obtain union are seldom successful.
2. It is possible to persevere with repeated surgical attempts to obtain union to the point where a large part of the child's early life is spent in an institution. This is to treat the lesion rather than the child.

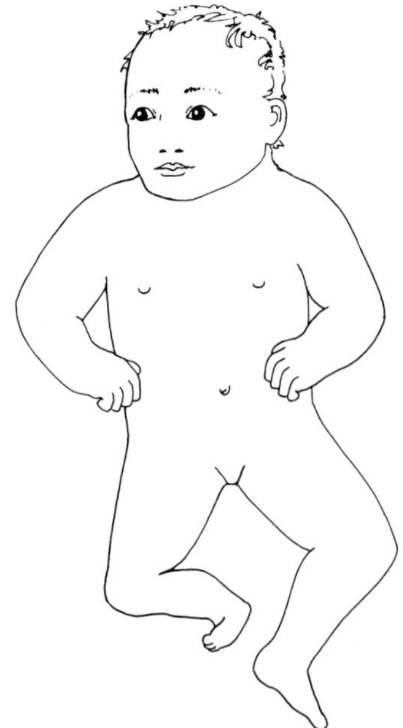

Fig. 12.10. Right tibial hemimelia. The fibula is present but does not articulate with femur or foot, so the limb assumes a bizarre position.

3. Even when union is achieved after numerous operations the end result may well be such a scarred, disfigured and short leg that the only way to obtain reasonable cosmesis (for a woman especially) and function is to do a Syme's amputation below the surgical triumph. The only achievement of the surgery, therefore, was to give an unnecessarily long below-knee stump covered with scars.
4. Late attempts to secure union, in adolescence, are much more likely to be successful than early ones.

It seems reasonable, therefore, to treat an established pseudoarthrosis in a below-knee removable plastic walking cast, taking weight on the patella tendon and tibial flares for some years.

Then one very careful attempt should be made to secure union, either by a massive bypass graft or massive onlay graft with rigid fixation. If this is not successful, a below-knee amputation should be done to provide function without further loss of time, and without more hospitalization, morbidity and uncertainty. The function will be excellent, especially as the stump, although more scarred than some, will still be a good one. In the future, living bone grafts kept alive by microvascular anastomoses may radically improve what can be done for these patients.

The management of a short limb, otherwise normal, depends on the etiology and the extent of the shortness. In general, congenitally short limbs do not do well when subjected to surgical lengthening so, if the extent of the shortness is more than can well be managed by contralateral appropriately timed epiphyseodesis, the option of managing it by a Syme's amputation and a prosthesis is certainly a valid one.

Foot deformities, if modest, can be hidden in a shoe, sometimes with special modifications or a silastic fill-in. Where the deformity is too unshapely to permit normal footwear, everybody will be delighted if a surgical procedure permits the child to be shod with an off-the-shelf product. Theoretically, it is immoral to operate on a living foot to make it fit a manufactured shoe, but where doing this simplifies the child's life, restores his self-image as "a normal" and relieves his parents of enormous costs for custom footwear recurring for the rest of a life it is justified.

Surgical Considerations in Management of Acquired Amputations in Childhood

INCIDENCE OF ACQUIRED AMPUTATIONS IN CHILDHOOD

Acquired amputations in childhood account for more than 150 children attending our clinic. One-third of these are children with upper limb amputations, two-thirds with lower limb amputations. Malignant disease accounts for 4 in the upper limb and 28 in the lower limb. The rest are due to accidents—motor and farm vehicle accidents, burns, train accidents, vascular catastrophies and so on.

AMPUTATIONS FOR MALIGNANT DISEASE IN CHILDHOOD

Malignant tumors calling for amputation are quite rare producing only about 8% of our clinic load. Theoretically, there are many tumors of soft tissue and of soft tissue within the bone, and actual bony tumors, which could justify amputation surgery. At a practical level, however, osteogenic sarcoma is the tumor for which most amputations are done.

For a long time, amputation was the only way to treat this disease and it was recognized that even in centers with good results the mortality was high in spite of amputation (6, 13). Pre- and postsurgical radiation had little impact on the survival rates. We continued to amputate because death from secondaries was easier than death from a painful fungating primary with bleeding. Then two changes occurred. The first was that in Toronto we began to see an occasional survivor and the second was that methotrexate and adriamycin with citrovorum rescue became widely used with an increased survival (16, 17). This is believed to be dependent on the surgical removal of the main mass of the tumor.

Our practice now when we believe our patient has an osteogenic sarcoma is to obtain a consultation with an oncologist, confirm the diagnosis unequivocally with a biopsy and paraffin section, and proceed to amputation within a few days. These patients are usually teenagers and the psychological trauma they suffer is enormous. Use of an instant fit is helpful for this group of patients, although in general with children it does not seem necessary.

The level of amputation is one where all the bone affected is ablated. The one exception to this may be in the femur where a small lesion at the lower end has on a number of occasions been managed by an amputation at the level of the lesser trochanter. This gives a stump which is much easier to fit and on which the patient walks better than with a hip disarticulation. On one occasion the tumor recurred in the stump of femur which was then removed with no further local recurrence.

These children are difficult candidates for rehabilitation. Their morale is depleted by the magnitude of the surgery and the uncertainty of the prognosis. Their vitality and vigor is sapped by the very chemotherapy which may save their lives. Their parents may well be so overwhelmed with grief and anger that they find it very difficult to support these children as they may need to be supported. If they do well, our rehabilitation efforts will be appreciated. But if they die, these efforts will be criticized. If staff pushed these patients to make the effort required to become good users, we will be censored for making the patients' last days hard by bullying them when there was no point. If staff have not worked hard with them, we will be considered to have given up without trying, indeed, not to have bothered because the prognosis was poor. Clearly, great sensitivity and judgement is needed in managing the rehabilitation of these children (and appreciation is a bonus for the therapist, not an objective).

AMPUTATIONS AFTER TRAUMA

Even in today's exciting climate of limb replantation and with the improved techniques of microscope-assisted vascular and neural surgery now available, children will still lose limbs from accidents, most of them preventable.

The surgical considerations special to childhood amputation surgery for trauma are of importance. Many of these factors apply also to any amputation surgery in childhood:

Graft skin. Graft skin on a stump often can become satisfactory in a child when it would not be expected to do well in an adult. Thus, for example, knee function may be saved by an amputation through the tibia even if good skin is only available for part of the stump. Graft skin will thicken and tolerate being in a socket better in children than in adults (19).

Preservation of growth potential. In a lower limb, every effort should be made to save the lower femoral epiphysis even if this means taking bone out of the shaft of the femur. Loss of the epiphysis where most of the length of femur is grown will result in an above-knee stump which becomes progressively shorter in relation to the patient's size as he grows.

Foot. A midfoot amputation, while generally frowned on in an adult limb-fitting center, can give many years of service to a child, leaving tissues useful in providing an excellent, definitive stump should revision be required later.

Burn. Where the accident has involved a high-voltage electrical burn, tissues within the limb may be more damaged than the skin. Thus, it is sometimes possible to save a short below-elbow or below-knee stump and get good skin cover, but end up with a rigid joint precluding both satisfactory fit and adequate function. If, in these patients, elbows and knees are saved, it is well to warn the family a revision may be needed and imperative to institute early movement in the joint on a very disciplined basis (8).

Revision. It is normal for above-elbow and below-knee amputations done in childhood to require revision. This is because the spur of new subperiosteal bone which usually forms at the end of an amputated bone is thrust downwards and eventually through the thin skin over the tip of the stump by the rapidly growing upper humeral epiphysis and upper tibial epiphysis. Much of the growth of the upper limb occurs at the upper end of the humerus and much of the growth of the lower limb takes place at the upper end of the tibia. These are very active growth areas without which the stump would not continue to be adequate into adult life. These epiphyses are saved, therefore, knowing revision will be needed.

Efforts have been made to eliminate the problem of the terminal spur by special care in the repair of the periosteum, by covering the bony stump with muscle, by cushioning the end of it with a silastic cap, and so on. So far, no solution to this problem has been found and we continue to revise these stumps as necessary, often several times during the growth period.

Knee Disarticulation. In children this is a good amputation. It preserves the valuable lower femoral epiphysis. The long anterior flap in a child has a good blood supply. A four-bar linkage can be used to give a good prosthetic knee joint mechanism. The end-bearing quality is saved. In many children as they grow, the femoral condyles do not grow as fast on the amputated side as on the normal side so that the unattractive bulbous shape of the stump is no longer conspicuous.

Tibiofibular Synostosis. In performing a below-knee amputation in adult life, the surgeon may choose to fix the lower end of the fibula to the tip of the tibia to give a solid lower end to the stump. In a child, this is a mistake as the proximal fibula grows faster than the proximal tibia and gradually forces the whole stump into varus. For the same reason, the fibula should be amputated well above the level of the tibial amputation.

Syme's Amputation. In adults, this amputation gives a bulbous stump which is hard to fit cosmetically. In children, the distal end of the tibia and fibula do not grow normally in width after a Syme's and, by adult life, will provide a very durable end-bearing stump, usable by itself in an emergency, and easy to fit cosmetically.

When the operation is done in infancy, the parents should be warned that a revision may be needed later. This is because periosteal separation of the heel pad from the os calcis takes with it the calcaneal apophysis, to which the tendoachilles is still attached. This will not adhere to the shaved cartilage surface of the lower tibial epiphysis and is pulled up behind the lower end of the tibia as the child grows. There, it forms a bony mass which may or may not complicate fitting. Sometimes it actually facilitates suspension, and other times it is just awkward and requires revision.

AMPUTATION FOR INSENSITIVE LIMB

Children with insensitive limbs due to spina bifida or other neurological deficit may develop trophic ulcers on their feet, even septic arthritis and osteomyelitis. They also may develop deformities from which a simple solution would appear to be an amputation and a prosthesis. Unless the amputation can be taken back to an area which will give a stump with feeling, it is not a good solution to such problems because the patient really needs sensation in the stump to warn of excessive pressure, impending skin breakdown, and the limits of use which the stump can tolerate.

REDUCTION OF GIGANTISM

Children may develop localized gigantism associated with anomalies of vasculature or with neurofibromatosis. Partial amputations in the lower limb will provide a satisfactory solution to problems of footwear and function.

AMPUTATIONS FOR VASCULAR DISEASE

Embolic phenomena associated with meningococcemia can produce localized areas of gangrene requiring amputation, as can frostbite and embolic phenomena associated with cardiac disease.

Psychological Aspects of Management for Child Amputees

PARENTAL INVOLVEMENT

A new amputee baby, whether by birth or surgery, creates a terribly upsetting experience for the parents. Anger, guilt, denial, a continuing sense of disappointment and resentment, are all natural for them. Most of these parents are very young adults who had never really recognized the possibility that parenthood might involve them in tragedy of this order. The stress of this situation may well break a family, leaving the child, who will need more support than most, with only one parent.

It is of great importance, therefore, that time be spent with the parents during which they must be convinced that:

1. It is not specifically anybody's fault. Otherwise, the mother will always feel guilty and father may readily blame her. (Sometimes there clearly is blameworthiness involved in the creation of an accident situation, and counselling here is important.)
2. The handicap is one which can be overcome.
3. Their child has the prospect of participating happily in most normal activities of life.
4. They must work, and work faithfully, with the prosthetic facility during the patient's childhood and bring him or her up to do the same in adult life.

In continuing contact with these parents it is important for the clinician to realize that although the parents and their child receive much help at a prosthetic clinic, they continue to bear heavy burdens emotionally, financially, for transportation, for time lost from work, and in relation to inconvenience occasioned by having to arrange for repairs to the limb and for supervision of its proper use and care at home. They may well be looking for more help with their problem than our society gives them. And, paradoxically, the place where they can voice their felt needs is the one place where people are already doing all and more than they can to help. Many parents of "normal" children have periods of frustration and a sense of being subjected to unreasonable demands, and these normal feelings in the case of an amputee child tend to get concentrated on the disability and on the prosthesis. It is not useful for the amputee clinic team to resent such behavior on the parent's part. It is more useful for them to be patient, explanatory and supportive. In this way, they can continue to meet the needs of the child. The time spent to win the parents' support and cooperation is of great importance to the child because so often it is parental attitudes which determine "patient acceptance" of the prosthesis.

The parents have real needs in relation to the prosthesis also. Traditionally, for an upper limb, a hook has been recognized as providing superior function to an artificial hand. Fortunately, we are moving into an era when we can expect to have available prosthetic hands with good function in a range of sizes suitable for children of all ages. This will really help many parents to accept a prosthesis for a child. It is much easier for an individual to accept the odd look of a hook for himself than it is for him to sit back and watch his child with a hook in place of a hand. This parental agony has been firmly overruled in the past, but will be more sympathetically considered in the future.

As the child grows and leaves the home setting, his or her psychological needs begin to compete with those of the parents. Most children of kindergarten age are tolerant of differences encountered in other children. The amputee child will be accepted fairly easily by his peers but the teachers may need support around the nature and function and care of the prosthesis.

In public school, children are of an age where they can be exceedingly cruel to their peers and it is a big effort to cushion the entry of an amputee child into a new class. Thus the teacher or parent or therapist, depending on who is able and comfortable with a class and the task, should give a "show and tell" session with the prosthesis. Display the stump, remove the prosthesis, demonstrate its function, be matter of fact about the disability, emphasize the usefulness and ingenuity of the device, explore all the "unknown" in the situation, let other children handle the device, and the amputee becomes no longer the object of fear, misunderstanding, scorn and cruelty, but the hero of the moment, the center of attention.

By high school age, children are capable of more thoughtfulness and conscious support for the handicapped, and a small party of friends is a more appropriate setting for the display and explanation of a prosthesis. Each friend then becomes unwittingly a person who can justify the prosthesis and its use to the rest of the class.

Adolescence is well recognized as a difficult interval between childhood status and the independence of adult life. For the amputee, it is also a time when the realization that the amputation and the prosthesis are for ever begins to sink in. This new insight may create its own additional stresses. Quite casual comments, not even necessarily directed to the amputee, can color his/her reaction to his/her future and to his/her prosthesis. Such comments may induce behavior others do not understand. There are no simple solutions to these problems. Understanding, patience, and good will from the amputee clinic staff must help, as will peer group interaction, appropriate sporting activities and, where wanted, prevocational assessment and counselling.

It is of importance to note that a high percentage of traumatic amputees in childhood, such as the children who get into trouble jumping freight trains, climbing transformer poles, and so on, are ones who were in difficulty and had been recognized to have a behavior problem or had been in some way socially disadvantaged before their accident. Clearly, these children will be difficult to rehabilitate in a full psychosocial as well as a physical sense after their amputations. They may well represent one category of amputee for whom the amputation situation might have been preventable (8).

Special Considerations for Fitting Congenital and Juvenile Amputees

TIMING

The time for fitting a lower limb prosthesis is soon enough to permit the infant to learn to walk. The stage of motor development, that is when the infant is beginning to pull up on furniture, is probably a better guide than a particular age in months, although for many patients this means about 10 months of age. The best time for the upper limb is not so obvious. Indeed, a congenitally one-armed person becomes so skilled in the use of the normal arm that the physical need for the prosthesis is open to challenge. Nevertheless, if the patient can use a prosthesis as a helping hand, function will be improved and so will body image for the patient and cosmesis for the public.

Once it is decided that this patient with an upper limb amputation should use a prosthesis eventually, there is little doubt that early fitting improves acceptance, improves the naturalness with which the patient wears the limb, and improves the skill with which he or she operates it. The accepted practice now is to fit as sitting balance is developing ("fit with sit"), so allowing 1) the sense of balance to develop with two arms instead of one, 2) the child to learn to crawl with upper limbs of comparable length and; 3) the child to learn from an early age that help is available for the normal hand.

TERMINAL DEVICE

In the upper limb fitting for an infant, we use a passive hand. The handlike shape improves acceptability. The next stage is a spring-loaded hook or hand in which parents can place a toy or cookie.

Later, when activation is introduced, we tend to use a hook or Child Amputee Prosthetics Program (CAPP) device for its functional potential, but allow parents to participate in the choice of a terminal device. We recognize increasingly (and it is we who are changing rather than the parents) a need on the parent's part to see a handlike terminal device on the child.

Some children are fitted not only with a hand, but also with a hook to use for special activities. Some are fitted with a hand, but with a special detachable terminal device, to permit specific functions such as holding a hockey stick or throwing a tennis ball. Others are fitted with a purely cosmetic device that will tolerate water for swimming. There is really no limit to the need for imagination and ingenuity here if we are to achieve our goal of permitting the amputee child to participate fully in life.

In the lower limb, the issue of the terminal device is much simpler. We have found solid ankle cushion heel (SACH) feet functional and durable. The sizes need changing to fit into the shoe which is the pair to the one on the opposite side. Both girls and boys may need two prosthetic feet for different heel heights. Almost routinely, and in spite of explanations and exhortations, children turn up in clinic with a changed heel height, different from the height for which the SACH foot was set. The cushioning effect of the heel is modified by changes in the rigidity of the heel counter of the shoe.

ACTIVATION

The age at which a child can learn to operate a cable-activated hook or hand varies widely. We do not have a good gauge for this and possibly one reason is that the amount of use to which a child will put an activated terminal hook is a factor not only of his own motor development but also of his mother's or his attendant's enthusiasm and skill in working with him. Thus, we will give an infant a cable-operated hook at about 12–14 months and, wit a bright child and a mother who is at home and enthusiastic, the child learns to use it quickly. Another child apparently at the same stage of motor development may be fitted, but with little use apparent 3 months later because the child has spent all day in the care of an indifferent baby sitter. Again, early fitting with an activated (cablc operated) terminal device permits the child to find out naturally how to operate the limb effectively from his or her own earliest practical age.

SERVICING

An adult or an older child will complain if an upper limb is not functioning well. A younger child will either reject it, just objecting to putting it on or carrying it around passively until the next clinic visit. It is, therefore, necessary to train parents to identify malfunction and educate them about the importance of servicing should poor function develop between scheduled checkups.

GROWTH FACTOR

One would expect sockets supplied in infancy to become too tight and small very quickly because of rapid growth. Fortunately, this is not so, for the infant has a chubbiness about his stump which gives way over a period of time to a firm, thinner subcutaneous layer, so that the stump does not grow as fast as its owner. With appropriate relief from time to time, a socket will last about 2 years and sometimes even longer.

More conspicuous is the need to lengthen lower limb prostheses regularly and change the foot size, and to lengthen the forearm and change the hook or hand size of an upper limb prosthesis.

In the upper limb, the need to adjust the harness size and the control straps also calls for relatively frequent checks.

FOLLOW-UP INTERVAL

The need to keep the limb in good repair, the extraordinarily hard use to which children put their limbs, the need to accommodate growth, and to encourage increases in function as the child develops, all point to frequent clinic visits as desirable. The convenience of the family, reduction in time lost from school and from parents' work and in travel and the need to keep the load on clinic staff to a minimum all point to longer intervals. The compromise will be influenced by how far away the patient lives, and the attitude and responsibleness of the parent and what facilities or skills they may have for minor repairs near home. Usually with younger children we suggest every 3 months and for older children every 6 months, but the figure is arbitrary.

ACHEIRIA

A patient with a below-elbow amputation clearly benefits from a prosthesis. A patient with part of a hand clearly does not, although a cosmetic device for social purposes may at times be appreciated and used in adolescence and later. But what of the child with a classical acheiria? The forearm bones are present, but short. Usually there is some firm tissue in the area which should be carpal bones which is under voluntary control although it wiggles through only a very short range. Fingers are represented only by functionless nubbins. The stump is covered with sturdy palmar skin and is highly sensitive.

We have tried to improve the function of these stumps by providing an opposition post against which the carpal elements can grasp; even a voluntary opening self-locking spatula, providing for the patient the ability to grasp objects of widely varying size (14). All these devices, however, obstruct the use of the stump as a sensory organ and, for this reason, are often rejected by the patient. This is true, even where the child has become highly skilled in its use and worn the device for months. We now offer only a simple spatula and let the child try it out and use it if he finds it helpful.

TRAINING

Training an infant or a young child in the use of a prosthesis clearly differs from training an older child or adult. Explanations, persuasion and direction are major techniques for the older child. With little ones, however, it is a matter of putting the limb on the child and then demonstrating to the child and mother or father how it works. When the child opens the terminal device or grasps with it, there is pleasure and encouragement. With an upper limb, cookies and toys are legitimate bribes. When the parent and child combination have grasped the concept, they go home and the parent becomes the trainer and succeeds in this task just as she does in training a child in any other task.

With little children, prostheses are kept simple. With older ones, they are as complex as they would be for an adult. Somewhere in between is the child who, it is believed, could operate a more complex upper limb prosthesis with appropriate training and parental support. Here it is necessary to educate the parent in detail, not only about the care and operation of the prostheses but also about concepts such as planning a whole action ahead of time, setting elbow and wrist units appropriately before the hand is advanced, and so on. They will be able to impart these concepts over a period of time. Frequent contact is necessary to sustain their enthusiasm and vision for what may be achieved.

Training for the lower limb amputee involves frequent attendance for two purposes. Firstly, the tolerance of a new stump to the socket needs tight supervision and, secondly, the alignment can only be finalized during the period when the limb is being used. Parents are encouraged to stay nearby with the child and participate in the whole process. Admissions are reserved for children from distant places or with special problems.

Again, in the matter of stump sock and socket care, the parents are trained in the first instance and the child later as he grows. It is not unlike teaching a child to wash or to clean his teeth.

SELECTION OF PROSTHETIC COMPONENTS

For the children, the selection is determined not only by the level of amputation but also by the motor developmental level of the wearer and the desires of the parents, and the availability of components of the right size.

Thus, in the upper limb, a terminal device could be an infant hand, a passive-opening, elastic-band-closing hook into which a parent could put things, or an activated hook or CAPP device, an activated hand, a purely cosmetic hand, an electric hand (switch or myoelectrically controlled) or a custom-built device for a specific purpose.

The wrist unit could be rigid, friction controlled or electrically activated. The elbow could be rigid, friction controlled, under conventional cable-locking and unlocking control, manually locked, or electrically powered. The shoulder will be friction controlled. Harnessing can consist of a simple chest strap, or shoulder loops connected by a ring at the back, or by special frames in plastic or aluminum, designed to fit a child's particular needs.

In the lower limb, the terminal device is a SACH foot, but the knee prescription varies considerably. Sometimes no knee unit is fitted and the child walks with a straight leg. In older children, free swinging, single-axis knee units are used, with an extension assist elastic strap. Later again, the knee unit will be changed to available pneumatic or hydraulic designs with swing phase control.

More choice exists when it comes to suspension. For a below-knee amputee, the patella tendon bearing socket with a suprapatellar strap is satisfactory, but a patella tendon bearing supracondylar socket with high side flanges and a medial wedge, obviates the need for the suprapatellar strap. Where there is great instability of the knee, a thigh corset with lateral knee hinges, old-fashioned as it may be, is useful on rare occasions. For a delicate stump which needs time to toughen up, an ischial-bearing thigh corset with a slip socket (which pistons gently on a light spring) is useful on a temporary basis, leaving the stump with its normal knee control function, but reducing its weight-bearing requirements (18).

Again, at a higher level of amputation, suspension is the area where choice exists. For a good stump, a suction socket eliminates the need for straps. Not all stumps can tolerate a suction socket, however, and for these a Silesian band is appropriate. It is rare to require a belt with a hip hinge.

MULTIPLE AMPUTEE

Training for children with multiple amputations clearly takes more time, during which the need for other assistive devices may be identified and met. This sort of complex training is time consuming because a small child's attention span is short. It makes great demands on the personality, patience and persistence of the therapist. Conversely, the rewards for the patient in improved ability to live independently are extensive and exciting.

INTERMITTENT UPGRADING OF SKILLS

A child amputee, particularly with an upper limb prosthesis, can be expected to enlarge his repertoire of skills as he grows and his neuromuscular abilities develop generally. To do this he will, from time-to-time need training sessions, suited to his current age and stage.

IMMEDIATE POSTOPERATIVE FIT

The teenager undergoing planned amputation for osteogenic sarcoma is a good candidate for this approach, but in general for children it does not accelerate final fitting or contribute to better end function. Some exuberant children are hard to control on an instant fit leg and threaten the amputation flaps.

ELECTRICALLY POWERED SWITCH-OPERATED PROSTHESES

These are useful for the upper limb amputee with only a tiny phocomelic hand, or a very short stump, even a bit of clavicle. The prosthesis is harnessed to the trunk and the active member moves freely to operate the conveniently located switch.

This system is useful for preschoolers and the switch system can be extended to control more activities as the child grows.

Place of Myoelectric Fittings in Childhood

At the amputee clinic at the Ontario Crippled Children's Centre, we have been privileged to collaborate with the Bio-Engineering Institute of the University of New Brunswick, where there has been a special interest in developing myoelectric control systems. We also have been privileged to have on our staff a highly skilled prosthetist who has made myoelectric fittings his major concern. This combination of circumstances has made it possible for us to prescribe a very large number of myoelectric fittings and see them functioning successfully and the wearers functioning happily.

Our custom has been to review our teenage patients as they come through clinic, looking at the use to which they put their prostheses, their patterns of life and their desires, and then to recommend to some of them that they change from a conventionally controlled prosthesis to a myoelectrically powered prosthesis. Out of a number of such fittings, few have reverted to the conventional prostheses.

Most of these patients from our clinic have been adolescent girls with a below-elbow amputation for whom the major attraction of the myoelectric forearm and hand has been the elimination of all harnessing.

The advantages of such myoelectric fittings are:

1. Elimination of harnessing
2. Increased gripping power
3. Improved appearance and freedom in clothing fashions
4. Improved function in awkward positions that make operating a cable control difficult
5. Less fatigue.

The disadvantages are:

1. High cost
2. Service facilities are few and more servicing is required
3. Increased number of socket adjustments are needed with growth
4. Malfunction of batteries in extremely cold weather
5. Slight motor noise
6. Batteries run down
7. Motor and batteries are heavy.

It is clear to us that such fittings are highly satisfactory to the users. We recognize that great care in the selection of control sites and in the crafting of the socket are necessary for these fittings and are more critical for them if success is to be achieved than in conventional limbs. We do not have any way of proving that we have prescribed too many or too few.

It has not been our custom to fit preschool children with myoelectric prostheses, for the reasons which used to be advanced many years ago for not fitting little children with upper limb prostheses at all. These reasons are cost, and the questionable ability of the child to learn to use and care for the device. We have now made conventional limbs sufficiently versatile and sturdy that we do fit small children with them and find that they are excellent users by adolescence and throughout adult life—and that they are the more skilled for having started early. It seems probable that as our skills in making dependable and satisfactory myoelectric prostheses improve, we will find that early fitting will result in improved function and use of these limbs, also, later in life.

To do this, however, calls for not only new skills in miniaturization of components but new ingenuities in training small children to regulate anything through a myoelectric interface.

It is clear to us working with these children, that the whole area of prosthetic fitting and management for these young amputees, be their condition congenital or acquired, is filled with potential for progress. We find this stimulating and exciting.

REFERENCES

1. Aitken, G. T. Proximal Femoral Focal Deficiency. In *Limb Development and Deformity: Problems of Evaluation and Rehabilitation*, Edited by C. A. Swinyard. Charles C Thomas, Springfield, Ill., 1969.
2. Brown, F. W. Construction of a Knee Joint in Congenital Total Absence of the Tibia (Paraxial Hemimelia Tibia). *J. Bone Jt. Surg., 47A:* 695–704, 1965.
3. Brown, F. W., and Pohner, W. H. Construction of a Knee Joint in Meromelia Tibia (Congenital Absence of the Tibia) A Fifteen-Year Follow-up Study. *J. Bone Jt. Surg., 54A:* 1333, 1972.
4. Congenital Anomalies reported by Physicians, Live births and Stillbirths. Ontario 1969–1971, Govt. of Ontario, Ottawa, 1973. Special Report No. 50.
5. Congenital Malformations. Bull. WHO, Vol. 34 Suppl., 1966.
6. Coventry, M. D., and Dahlin, D. C. Osteogenic Sarcoma, *J. Bone Jt. Surg., 39A:* 741, 1957.
7. Frantz, C. H., and O'Rahilly, R. Congenital Limb Deficiencies. *J. Bone Jt. Surg., 43A:* 1202–1224, 1961.
8. Galway, H. R., Hubbard, S., and Mowbray, M. Traumatic Amputations in Children. Personal communication, 1979.
9. Kay, H. W. A proposed international terminology for the classification of congenital limb deficiencies. *Orthotics Prosthet., 28:* 33–48, 1974.
10. King, R. E. Some Concepts of Proximal Femoral Focal Deficiency. *J. Bone Jt. Surg., 49A:* 1470, 1967.
11. King, R. E., and Marks, T. W. Follow-up Findings on the Skeletal Lever in the Surgical Management of Proximal Femoral Focal Deficiency; *Interclin. Inf. Bull., 11:* 1–4, 1971.
12. Kostuik, J. P., Gillespie, R. G., Hall, J. E., and Hubbard, S. van Nes Rotational Osteotomy for Treatment of Proximal Femoral Focal Deficiency and Congenital Short Femur. *J. Bone Jt. Surg., 57A:* 1039–1046, 1975.
13. Marcove, R. C., Miké, V., Hajek, J. V., Levin, A. G., and Hutter, R. V. P. Osteogenic Sarcoma Under the Age of Twenty-one. *J. Bone Jt. Surg., 52A:* 411–423, 1970.

14. MURRAY, J. F., SHORE, B., AND TREFLER, E. Prostheses for Children with Unilateral Congenital Absence of the Hand. *J. Bone Jt. Surg., 54A:* 1658–1664, 1972.
15. RUSSELL, H. E., AND AITKEN, G. T. Congenital Absence of the Sacrum and Lumbar Vertebrae with Prosthetic Management. *J. Bone Jt. Surg., 45A:* 501–508, 1963.
16. SONLEY, M. J., BOBECHKO, W. P., AND SIMPSON, J. S. Adjuvant Therapy with Adriamycin and Methotrexate in Osteogenic Sarcoma. *Ann. R. Coll. Physicians Surg. Can.*, 60, 1979.
17. SUTOW, W. W., SULLIVAN, M. P., FERNBACH, D. J., CANGER, A., AND GEORGE, S. L. Adjuvant Chemotherapy in Primary Treatment of Osteogenic Sarcoma. *Cancer, 36:* 1598–1602, 1975.
18. THOMSON, H. G., AND BOCHMAN, D. The Skin-Grafted Below-knee Stump: Can knee Function Be Salvaged? *Can. J. Surg., 13:* 37–40, 1970.
19. THOMSON, H. G., MARTIN, S. R., AND MURRAY, J. F. Grafted Juvenile Amputation Stumps—Are they durable? *Plast. Reconstr. Surg. 65:* 195–198, 1980.
20. VAN NES, Rotation-plasty for Congenital Defects of the Femur. Making Use of the Ankle of the Shortened Limb to Control the Knee Joint of a Prosthesis. *J. Bone Jt. Surg., 32B:* 12, 1950.

13

Reintegration and Adjustment as Seen By the Amputee

HUGH C. CHADDERTON, C.M., C.A.E.

It should be made abundantly clear, at the outset of this chapter, that the successful rehabilitation of an amputee, while often resulting in an outlay of some magnitude in terms of money, in reality costs nothing. To the contrary, the successful transition of an amputee from a somewhat costly patient to a productive member of the labor force represents a rich reward for society. Furman (4) gives a number of illustrations. Some are obvious, and deal with cases where, by reason of successful rehabilitation, an amputee became employable. Some of the other illustrations, however, show considerably more insight. For example, the investment in providing for prostheses for an aged person, and training such persons in the use of artificial arms and legs, is not only contributing to the well-being of the aged amputee, but there is the additional benefit when it frees a son or daughter, who might otherwise be required for duties as an attendant, to join or rejoin the labor force.

The statistical data quoted in this (4) told of some 7118 amputees who were fitted with prostheses and retrained in 1956. Only 2568 of them were working before rehabilitation and their total annual earnings were $5,080,800. After rehabilitation the number had increased to 6133 with earnings of $14,277,700. Impressive figures even for that preinflationary period.

As we intend to show in this chapter, the reintegration of an amputee is an area which involves many disciplines, governments at all levels and both medical and educational institutions. It is submitted, notwithstanding, that the major contribution in rehabilitation can, and must, come from the amputees themselves. Without their desire to succeed, applied with a generous measure of ingenuity, improvisation and sheer determination, very little can be accomplished.

The world of the amputee, although defined by the common denominator of amputation, is nonetheless a wide and varied constituency. Longevity has its rewards—and its own particular set of problems, including a high number of amputations from cardiovascular diseases, and from diabetes and cancer. It is believed that some 80% of amputations are now caused by disease.

Accidents from power machinery, recreational vehicles and the tools and playthings of a highly mechanized society are, as expected, bringing a higher toll in the number of amputees who fall victim to the jet age—and all that it implies. Farm machinery and automobile accidents are, as well, among the chief cripplers.

It is interesting to reflect that amputation due to accident can leave a different mark on the psyche of the amputee, depending upon the circumstances under which the accident occurred. This often raises questions of guilt and blame, directed inwardly in some instances to the amputee himself or herself, *i.e.* "Was this a self-inflicted casualty?" Blame is sometimes laid by the amputee on the doorstep of others if the circumstances of the accident would appear to support this. These illustrations are given to support the contention that amputees, even within the category of those arising from accidents, can be very much of a mixed bag.

There is, as well, the often tragic circumstance of the congenital amputee. In such instances it is necessary to face the initial decision: that is, should an amputation be done, or should an attempt be made to fit a prosthesis incorporating the vestigial limb? Congenital amputees bring to the fore another set of problems of a psychological nature. Is there a hereditary factor on one side of the family? Did the mother bring on the birth defect by some specific act, such as ingestion of a harmful drug? It is not unknown for parents to take on to their shoulders a load of self-guilt which leaves them wondering whether the birth of a child with a deformity is a form of punishment.

Those who suffer amputation by reason of war-incurred disability are, in one sense, more fortunate. Under ordinary circumstances, they can point to the amputation with justifiable pride; the result of an honorable wound incurred in combat in the defence of one's country. Here, too, there is an area for so-called "hang-ups" if the amputee, or his friends and relatives, begin to question too deeply into the motives and factors which brought the battle casualty into a theater of war, where exposure to the enemy resulted in grievous dismemberment.

Setting aside all attempts at psychology, a simple fact becomes very clear indeed. There is absolutely nothing to be gained (and the risk of increased disability can result) if the amputee attempts to dwell upon the reasons for having become an amputee. Those involved in amputee care—and the amputee—must strive never to look back. The goal should be occupational and social rehabilitation. Nothing else matters.

From the time of surgery until return to a normal life in the community, the majority of amputees are beset by many doubts and fears (8). The problems involve relationships with the medical staff, the physical therapist, the prosthetist; and with family (including those with whom there are the closest ties) and with friends. A major concern also is the amputees' place in the work force and the reaction of employers and fellow employees.

Possibly one of the greatest misunderstandings arises because those around the amputee—in hospital, in the home and at work—are hesitant about how to make the approach. They know not whether to extend sympathy, and are fearful that if they do, they may be rebuffed. Contrariwise, if they treat the new amputee in a cavalier manner, making light of the disability, it may lead to the accusation that they neither care nor understand. Most amputees do have the need for assurance and constructive advice but because amputation is very much of a visible disability, there is usually a hesitancy on the part of others to consider amputees as normal, healthy individuals who want, and need, to take their place in society.

It was the finding of Kerr and Brunnstrom (7) that excess sympathy—and too-readily offered physical aid by family, friends and work acquaintances to relieve the amputee of physical tasks (or in some instances complete avoidance of mentioning the amputation)—could lead to a conclusion on the part of the amputees that they are in the category of permanent cripples.

The only certain solution is within the competence of the amputees themselves. They must learn to recognize these attitudes on the part of others, and to realize that they are based on misunderstanding and a lack of knowledge concerning the disability of amputation. If, however, the amputees will make their own evaluation of their abilities and potential, and make constructive plans for the future, they will be well beyond the stage where the thinking of others can influence their attitudes.

It is too much to expect that the amputee will be considered as a fully able-bodied person. The "wooden leg" or "empty sleeve" syndrome will prevent this, and even with the advent of prostheses which stress cosmesis, it will, indeed, be an extremely clever person who can hide forever the fact that he or she has an amputation. Once the psychological and physical factors of amputation are accepted, the amputee is no longer in danger of being affected or hindered by others; and can then get on with the job of returning to as nearly a normal life as possible.

Vocational Rehabilitation for Amputees

The question of education and training for an amputee, to provide skills which can be translated into earning capacity, should be approached on the basis of two principles. These are:

1. The fullest possible use must be made of the facilities available to the able-bodied.
2. The amputee must be prepared to make any adjustment necessary so that full advantage can be taken of such facilities.

The opportunities for vocational training will, of course, vary from one geographical location to another and will depend, in some measure, upon government- and privately-sponsored institutions. Some generalizations can, however, be made which will be valuable in assessing the amputee's problems.

For example, it is often a mistake for the amputee to assume that the officials charged with the responsibility for administration of academic and vocational training institutions are fully enlightened in regard to the rights of the disabled in respect of eligibility. There are countless cases on record where administrators have gone to very considerable lengths to devise plausible, if totally invalid, reasons to deprive amputees of entitlement to participate as members of a student body. Where this happens amputees, and those responsible for their well being, must insist that access be available. If necessary, any denial of such rights should be brought to the attention of the body politic and should be pursued, even to the threat of exposure in the media. In most countries, human rights legislation exists which guarantees access on an "equal opportunity" basis for the disabled. If necessary, an application should be made to the appropriate jurisdiction such as the Human Rights Commission, Ombudsman, etc. Harsh measures, yes, but sometimes the only answer to inhuman rejection of the rights of the disabled.

The Canadian Human Rights Act (1977) provides that " ... every individual should have an equal opportunity with other individuals to make for himself or herself the life that he or she is able and wishes to have ... without being hindered or prevented from doing so ... by discriminatory employment practices based on physical handicap." This Act applies to all Federal Government agencies and to business and industry under Federal jurisdiction. Similar laws have been enacted by each of the 10 Canadian provinces.

The definition of "physical handicap" in the Canadian legislation (Federal) is quoted below:

> " ... 'physical handicap' means a physical disability, infirmity, malformation or disfigurement that is caused by bodily injury, birth defect or illness and, without limiting the generality of the foregoing, includes epilepsy, any degree of paralysis, amputation, lack of physical coordination, blindness or visual impediment, deafness or hearing impediment, muteness or speech impediment, and physical reliance on a seeing eye dog or on a wheelchair or other remedial appliance or device."

Where access is available, the onus is often on the amputee to make the special effort required to ensure that full benefit can be derived from the education and training available. Some frequent examples:

1. Special arrangements in respect of transportation to and from the facility, and in some instances within the institution, so that the

trainee can be at the proper place at the proper time in accordance with the syllabus and timetable of the course of study involved.
2. Adaptive equipment to enable an amputee to take part. This may require special ingenuity of the educator, the prosthetist and the amputee.

The situation of Phyllis G. comes to mind.

> She was a bilateral above-elbow upper extremity amputee. She had learned to write with her feet but when she entered the University stream, the volume of written work called for some improvision. The problem was overcome by the provision of a tape recorder with a mask, so that she could dictate her notes without disturbing the other students. The Prosthetic Department made her a special fitting for an above-elbow prosthesis which allowed her to carry and manipulate the tape recorder.

In certain circumstances amputees should consider an on-the-job training program, particularly where they may have neither the capabilities nor the inclination to tackle academic or vocational training in an institutional atmosphere. For such persons, it is sometimes possible to work out special arrangements with an employer, under which training can be given on a quasiapprenticeship basis. Quite often, inasmuch as the employer will not benefit immediately from the production of the amputee during the training period, an arrangement must be entered into where no salary is paid, and/or where the employer receives some financial subsidization from government or private sources in respect of the training being provided. Experience would indicate that, even in the most extreme cases, persons disabled from multiple amputation can engage in training or retraining so long as they are prepared to make the effort.

A case in point is Bernadette L.

> She is a bilateral above-knee amputee, having lost both legs in a tragic farm accident when she was 3 years of age. At 16, she realized that there would be unusual difficulties in job placement. She visited an employment counsellor, learned that she could carry out clerical and executive duties, and set about to obtain the necessary education and training. On graduation she entered employment as an "intake" counsellor in a Social Welfare Agency. She relied entirely on normal resources for her training although she did require special assistance in connection with transportation and accommodation.

"Yes you can" is probably the most important lesson to be learned by an amputee in connection with employment potential. A secondary requirement is to seek out sources which may be of assistance. There are few, if any, training facilities specificially designed for amputee needs. Moreover, "mainstreaming" is a popular and current trend which means, simply, that the amputee should make use of the same educational facilities as other persons. Any limitations of the disability should be compensated for by attitude, improvisation and ingenuity.

Where necessary, special arrangements concerning transportation and accommodation may be required, particularly in the case of multiple amputation. The amputee must not be reluctant to put forward strong arguments for the right to training and education, despite any handicap. Educational authorities in most jurisdictions are not permitted, by law, to discriminate against the disabled in the matter of provision for education. In the event that amputees encounter difficulty in this area, they should have no qualms about seeking support from both public and voluntary agencies.

Medical social workers and persons in other disciplines who have a responsibility for amputee care and management should be prepared to support the amputee's cause in assuring that access is not denied to such facilities because of the disability.

Social Activities

A lesson to be learned early in the life of an amputee is that the public cannot always be expected to understand that the amputee has the same desires in respect of enjoyment of life as other persons. In carving out a social life which has meaning and quality, the amputees must learn to accept any indication of rejection by their peers with good grace. Very often, the general population tends to regard an amputee with an air of mystique. They have trouble in understanding how a person can cope with the loss of one or more of the major extremities. The attitude is, in many instances, one of ill-conceived curiosity. Amputees should be counselled to speak freely and frankly about their amputation. They should approach their social life with acceptance of the fact that amputation does make them somewhat different. They should be prepared to explain, however, that anatomical loss of a limb or limbs, while representing some limitation in regard to mobility or function, can, with the utilization of the remaining faculties, allow the amputee to enjoy an interesting and rewarding experience in social life.

Mr. Herbert Marshall, the well known British actor, was an amputee who appeared in more than 200 motion pictures. He was urbane, scholarly and a pleasant companion. Most people never knew that he wore a below-knee prosthesis. Social activities present no barrier whatsoever for the amputee who is well adjusted and who accepts the uniqueness of amputation.

Recreational Activities

Recreational activities are a different matter. In this area, amputees must learn to "cut the coat according to the cloth." They must come to a personal decision, first and foremost, that amputation will impose some physical limitation. Once they have had an opportunity of measuring this, they can develop for themselves a recreational life-style which makes allowances for the effects of the disability. There are very few recreational pursuits which are denied to even the most seriously handicapped amputee.

Karl H. is a bilateral above-knee amputee with extremely short stumps and a partial loss of function in one arm.

> He took up golf after his accident, balancing in a form of "tripod" with his two artificial limbs and his injured arm, and swinging at the golf ball with his remaining arm. He has a 16 handicap, which is better than 75% of the members of most golf clubs in North America.

Lloyd E. is a bilateral below-elbow amputee.

> He swings righthanded. He has had his golf clubs adapted with a bayonet attachment which fits into the left prosthesis in place of the normal hook. A "sleeve" takes the place of the hook of the right arm and fits over the bottom half of the grip on the golf club shaft. He, too, has a 16 handicap.

Amputees who can walk, can participate in cross-country skiing; and, with practice, they will find that the gliding action of the skis allows them to cover a great deal more territory than they can negotiate by mere walking. Usually they will have no trouble keeping up with nonamputated companions. Cross-country skiing is an excellent sport for those with upper extremity amputations too, and there are adaptors for artificial arms which clamp on to ski poles.

Below-knee amputees who are downhill ski enthusiasts usually have a prosthetist design an artificial limb which tilts forward to allow for the normal knee bend required in this activity.

Single above-knee amputees usually use the "track three" method, leaving off their prosthesis and skiing on the good leg with outrigger miniature skis attached to ski poles.

Swimming is a rewarding form of recreation for all amputees—even those with triple amputation. Lower extremity amputees will often use waterproof prostheses, designed specifically for aqua sports. Any good prosthetist can manufacture such prosthesis from one of several designs available. The so-called "swimming leg" is particularly useful for those who intend to swim in natural surroundings, such as a beach, where it is necessary to walk into the water. (Incidentally, many leg amputees use a waterproof limb for showers, changing to their "street" leg for everyday use.)

There are other sports for which adaptive equipment is available for the amputee. Fishing, rowing, golf, bowling, sailing and horseback riding are some of the recreations in which amputees can excel. A word of caution here. The objective, for most amputees, should be to enjoy the sport, realizing the handicap which may be placed upon them, and which may understandably affect their ability to compete with able-bodied persons.

It is of interest, in this respect, to understand the derivation of the word handicap. In ancient times in England, when a race steward desired to impose a handicap on a particular horse to even the odds in a race, he would require the rider to place his hand inside his cap, thus having to control his steed with only one hand on the reins; hence, the term hand-in-cap, conveniently shortened to handicap.

The statement is made by Adams *et al.* (1) that it is an obvious but frequently overlooked fact that the physically handicapped are otherwise normal individuals who have some degree of physical deficit. Hence, their need for an interest in play, recreation and social activities is usually very similar to that of able-bodied persons. They point out, as well, that recreational activities for the physically disabled are quite often involved with treatment procedures to provide an effective and vigorous program to assist patients in regaining use of their injured bodies.

In studying the needs of the amputee population it is necessary to break them into two groups, or possibly three. The unilateral below-knee or below-elbow amputee can usually attain satisfactory proficiency in most sports. The only exclusion would possibly be team sports requiring considerable physical activity, *e.g.* American football. The degree of difficulty will be increased for the unilateral above-knee amputee who would obviously experience more restrictions than the below-knee amputee, but who can, nevertheless, with instruction and adjustment—and possibly with adaptive equipment—manage to enjoy many sports. The multiple amputee will encounter more severe difficulties but, again, with proper training and equipment the adjustment can be made to permit the development of a satisfying involvement in sports.

Adaptive equipment is readily available for the following sports.

Golf. The leg amputee (single) should consider installation of a rotator in the prosthesis. The single arm amputee can have a "sleeve adaptor" made with a bayonet attachment to lock into the prosthesis. The sleeve has an opening to insert the thin part of the shaft of the club; then the shaft is pulled down causing the sleeve to tighten over the grip.

Hunting. Lower limb amputees usually experience no difficulty. For arm amputees a specially-designed hook is available for holding and firing pistol, shotgun or rifle.

Target and Trap Shooting. For upper-limb amputees a special stand can be constructed with tripod legs with a shaft, bent at right angles, to which a chain is attached. The chain can be clipped onto the rifle or shotgun. There are several adaptors for prosthetic hooks which will allow an arm amputee to shoot a pistol, using his prosthesis.

Baseball. There is a hook, commercially available, for the below-elbow amputee designed to hold a baseball glove.

Bowling. Attachments for holding a bowling ball may be purchased commercially.

Fishing. A harness and special fishing pole for upper-limb amputees is available commercially. This will hold the rod so that a single upper-limb amputees can use their other hand to reel in fish. A bilateral upper extremity amputee (with one amputation below-elbow) can use this equipment, with an adaptor for the below-elbow prosthesis to operate the reel mechanism.

Gardening. The upper-limb amputee can adapt many tools to be used with prostheses. The "farmer's hook" is a versatile terminal device which is available.

Swimming. The prosthetists are now able to fabricate waterproof limbs. No special equipment is required for the below-knee (BK) amputee. For the above-knee (AK) amputee, there is available, commercially, a special waterproof limb which has a nylon bolt through the knee. This bolt can be removed and the prosthesis can be packed into a suitcase. These prostheses for lower-extremity amputees are particularly useful for wading.

Skiing. Adaptors are available for ski poles for the arm amputee. The BK amputee usually skis with both legs and can have the prosthesis adapted to normal skiing stance. The AK amputee usually skis using the "track three" method with special crutches to which is attached to short skis called outriggers. They are available from prosthetic supply firms.

Consumer Participation in Amputee Care

Probably the most important factor in the life of an amputee is the prosthesis. Bill C. was a middle-management executive who lost his lower limbs below the knee on military service in World War II.

> He returned to his prewar employment and with hard work, grit and determination, reached a position of some responsibility after 20 years. During this time, he wore less-than-adequate prostheses, mostly through his own negligence. He was reluctant to take time to ensure a proper fit; and when confronted by indifferent prosthetists, he failed to insist on his right to decent and comfortable limbs. This was holding back his progress in his employment; and, in that he was devoting most of his energies to remaining mobile in his job, he found it difficult to enjoy any family life or recreation. Fortunately improvements in prosthetics caught up with him and when, at last, he was properly fitted, he was able to tackle his employment with renewed vigor, with resulting promotions which had been long overdue. Also, he was able to make important changes in his lifestyle with the result that he commenced to enjoy golf, cross-country skiing and curling—all being pursuits in which he could engage with his family.

This case history has a moral for all amputees. In most instances, the fitting techniques and available hardware exist which should result in an adequate prosthesis. Very often, however, this requires patience, understanding and knowledge on the part of the amputee, together with the willingness to cooperate with the clinic team.

The first point of contact by the amputee will be with the doctor—usually an orthopaedic surgeon or specialist in physical medicine. Amputees must be prepared to sketch out what they expect of their prostheses. In some cases, financial considerations will be involved but, even if amputees must dig a little deeper into their own pockets, it will pay dividends to ensure that there are sufficient funds to finance the prosthetic requirements. The medical social worker can play an important role at this juncture if outside financing is required.

During the clinic experience, the amputees will have an opportunity to avail themselves of the services of the physiotherapist. This will be a very important facet of the prosthetic procedure, particularly if it is necessary to retrain certain muscles.

Also, general physical fitness is important, in that the wearing of a prosthesis consumes more energy and can place additional stress upon the remaining limb, and the spine—specifically the lumbar area for lower extremity amputees and the cervical area for those with an amputation of an upper extremity.

In the final analysis, it is the prosthetist who will carry the major share of the burden of ensuring that the amputee is properly fitted. A close and harmonious relationship between the prosthetist and the amputee is essential. This will be enhanced if the amputee makes an effort to understand the prosthetist's problems and limitations, at the same time showing such perseverance as might be necessary to work in a cooperative manner toward a comfortable and functional prosthesis.

Much is written about the responsibility of consumers to shop around, to get to know the product, and to be in a position to ensure that they are getting their money's worth. It is recommended that, in the matter of an artificial limb, the amputee (who is the consumer) will be well advised to learn as much as possible about the prosthetic craft, and the techniques and hardware available. They should use this knowledge to discuss their problems with all members of the clinical team. It is a cardinal error, however, to insist on a type of fitting or limb which may be contraindicated by the type of amputation, medical condition or other factors. In short, the amputees' knowledge always should be used in conjunction with the recommendations of the professionals involved. The amputees should have sufficient information, though, to recognize if they are getting the runaround and to make a decision as to whether the prosthesis, from various points of view—including comfort and function, is the best that is available under the circumstances.

Philosophy

The amputation of a limb or limbs is translated into the anatomical loss of a major portion of the body—with subsequent loss of function, only part of which (under even the most favorable circumstances) can be restored by prosthesis. Depending on the individual, amputation can bring with it a host

of other problems, one of which is loss of "body image." There may be psychological hang-ups and the amputee might show an inclination to wonder about acceptance by family, friends, employer and members of the public.

The amputee should forego any such thoughts. If a "loser's psychology" is allowed to develop the amputee is simply inviting additional difficulties which will make rehabilitation more difficult. Possibly the most important single achievement is for amputees to put themselves in the "winners' circle." The simple fact of being able to overcome a major disability will require a great deal of courage and, having overcome the disability, that courage can be put to excellent use for the remainder of the amputees' lives. Amputees are different, but that very difference makes them something special. They can build on the inner resources which will make them better persons. There is no disadvantage in having a limb amputated. Quite the contrary. It is a badge of honor which sets the amputee apart. It can represent an added dimension in life which will bring out qualities which otherwise might have lain dormant.

In the area of philosophy, amputees must adopt a very special feeling for their prosthesis. The author has known thousands of amputees, and has had the benefit of the experience, related to him by the first major group of amputees in history; namely, the survivors of World War I.

Prior to that war, persons with major wounds seldom survived. The evolution of amputation as a successful technique in the treatment of gangrene and other complications from gunshot wounds in World War I resulted in the first large group of amputees in history.

Many of those men wore crude appliances. Given the fact that the vast majority of them returned to the unskilled labor force from which they had been recruited, they had, of necessity, to rely on their artificial limbs in order to earn a livelihood. The one significant lesson learned by them—and very quickly—was to develop a sense of pride and ownership in regard to their prostheses. Their secret was to "learn to love" the artificial leg or arm; to think of it as part of themselves. The amputee who, consciously or subconsciously, rejects the prosthesis is in for a great deal of trouble.

Psychological Adjustment

Friedmann (3) suggests that psychology is often neglected or glossed over in most works dealing with the rehabilitation of the amputee. He finds this unfortunate and suggests that treating the psychological problems faced by the amputee might have more significance than the quality of the surgery or the nature of the prosthetic device.

It seems obvious that, to achieve successful reintegration, the clinical team, and the amputee, must develop a strong psychological base. It is reasoned that amputation, viewed in the subjective sense, is often considered as mutilation. If ignored, the psychological shock can hinder readjustment.

There is, as well, a strong involvement of society with the amputee in that amputation is an obvious disability which is often misunderstood by a public whose attitude towards the amputee is one of traditional isolation and segregation.

Friedmann (3) concludes that education of the nondisabled is sorely needed to allow satisfactory growth of social and recreational, as well as vocational, interaction between the able-bodied population and the amputees. Until this becomes a reality, amputees must learn to survive. They can do this by recognizing the potential psychological problems, and learning to adjust to them. This will require a strong effort of will but the amputee should not be reluctant to ask for assistance from the clinical team and, in some instances, from other amputees who have successfully overcome the psychological pitfalls of amputation.

The new amputees have to be well prepared mentally as well as physically. One area where psychological problems may arise is frustration. The amputees with high hopes who are adapting well to their prostheses may find that they just cannot quite do many of the things they felt they should be able to manage. Obviously, cases such as double lower limb amputees use one hand most of the time to maintain balance. As a result there are sporting, social and manual activities they will find they cannot manage at first. This becomes a challenge to the amputees' ingenuity.

Consumer Feedback

The results of a survey of 19 organizations belonging to the World Veterans Federation, in 14 countries (2), indicated that the major complaints of amputees included: poor fitting; poor dissemination of knowledge to doctors and amputees regarding new prostheses; lack of opportunity for input from amputees at the research level; and inadequate measures to deal with phantom and stump pain. The survey indicated improvements suggested by amputees, as follows: decrease in weight of prostheses; reduction in maintenance for swing and stance phase control units; development of recreational prostheses; and more frequent checks through use of X-ray and film techniques, particularly during the break-in period of a new appliance.

Generally, it seems possible to observe that the feelings of an amputee, as a patient, or of the amputee as a consumer in respect of prostheses, have not been seen as a major consideration by the various disciplines involved in amputee care. Possibly, there are good reasons for this attitude, if it does exist. Certainly the situation must be avoided wherein the patient or consumer is attempting to dictate to the professionals who have been trained in the field of amputee management. On the other hand, it would be prudent to ensure that those responsible for delivering amputee care are not depriving themselves of a valuable source of feedback concerning the efficacy of treatment methods, or of prosthetic fitting techniques or hardware. Another concern is that, if the patient/amputee is not encouraged to participate in the process of treatment and restoration of function, vital information which might otherwise contribute to recovery and rehabilitation may be denied the doctor, the physical therapist or prosthetist.

Sequelae of Amputation

The survey of the 19 veterans organizations (2) reported that persons who had worn prostheses for 25 years or more showed increasing concern in regard to the development of consequential disabilities arising from amputation. These include: premature arthritic changes in spine and remaining limb; circulatory problems; and gastrointestinal problems due to long-standing discomfort, and to ingestion of drugs to control pain.

Medical histories on long-time amputees will undeniably show a very distinct pattern of the sequelae of amputation, which manifests itself in new medical conditions which are secondary to the primary condition of loss of limb. Compensation agencies responsible for the administration of legislation which provides additional compensation for such disabilities which develop, in whole or in part as a consequence of amputation, will be aware that such sequelae are very real. A long-time study of these problems by The War Amputations of Canada indicates that, while the development of such sequelae is inevitable, it can be retarded, and possibly the effect can be lessened, if the amputee, and those responsible for his care, will take necessary precautions to ensure that he/she has a properly-fitting prosthesis which is prescribed in accordance with the indications of the amputee and other factors such as his/her physical make-up and his/her employment. Also, it goes without saying, that if the amputee can initiate and maintain a program of physical exercise, designed to develop the nonamputated parts of the body and the interrelated muscles, ligaments and tendons, the incapacity of such sequelae can be minimized.

It has long been suspected that major amputation can lead to arteriosclerotic heart disease. Further confirmation of this is reported by Hrubec and Ryder (5). This study concluded that there was a significant relationship between amputation of a lower limb at or above the knee and the onset of arteriosclerotic heart disease, and that there was an even greater relationship between bilateral lower limb amputation and arteriosclerotic heart disease. The "modifiable risk factors" included: 1) obesity; 2) sedentary life style; and 3) psychosocial tension (5).

All of these factors are an obvious sequelae of amputation. The study states that sedentary life-style appears important in relation to cardiovascular disease of amputees. There was an increase in coronary deaths among groups of less active males as compared with active cohorts.

In summary, this study indicates that veterans with proximal traumatic amputations subsequently had excessive mortality due to cardiovascular disease. From the data presently available, the most likely factors of importance include increased sedentary life-style among amputees, and increased emotional stress caused by amputation.

The Hrubec-Ryder report (5) does not make a finding in specific terms, to the effect that lower limb amputation leads to obesity, which is considered as one of the causes of increased risk. It should be accepted, as a matter of course, that by reason of enforced sedentary life-style, a lower limb amputee would have a tendency towards overweight; thus, the obesity factor would apply in assessing the additional risk regarding the development of arteriosclerotic heart disease and its possible consequence of loss of life expectancy.

REFERENCES

1. ADAMS, R. C., DANIEL, ALFRED N., AND RULLMAN, L. *Games, Sports and Exercises for the Physically Handicapped*, Lea & Febiger, Philadelphia, 1972.
2. CHADDERTON, H. C. Prosthesis, Pain And The Sequelae Of Amputation As Seen By The Amputee. *J. Int. Soc. Prosthet. Orthot., Vol. 2,* 1978.
3. FRIEDMANN, L. W. *Rehabilitation of Amputees, Rehabilitation in Medicine.* Elizabeth Licht, New Haven, Conn., 1968.
4. FURMAN, B. *Progress in Prosthetics*, United States Department of Health, Education and Welfare, Washington, D.C., 1962.
5. HRUBEC, Z., AND RYDER, R. A. *Report to the Veterans Administration, Department of Medicine and Surgery, on Service Connected Traumatic Limb Amputations and Subsequent Mortality from Cardiovascular Disease and Other Causes of Death*, United States Veterans Administration, Washington, D.C., 1978.
6. KENDALL, H. O., KENDALL, F. P., AND BOYNTON, D. A. *Posture and Pain*, R. E. Krieger, Huntington, N.Y., 1970.
7. KERR, D., AND BRUNNSTROM, H. *Training of The Lower Extremity Amputee*, Charles C Thomas, Springfield, Ill., 1956.
8. MELZACK, R. *The Puzzle of Pain*, Penguin Books, Baltimore, 1973.
9. WILSON, A. B. JR. *Limb Prosthetics*, 5th ed. R. E. Krieger, Huntington, N.Y., 1976.

14

Current Trends in Amputation and Prosthetics

S. N. BANERJEE, B.Sc., M.B.B.S., F.R.C.P.(C)

The impetus for the current developments in amputation surgery and prosthetics came primarily during and after the Second World War and subsequent Korean and Vietnam wars. During the postwar period the civilized world was confronted with thousands of young amputees and health professionals throughout the world realized their lack of knowledge and technical expertise to deal with this problem adequately. Also, the increasing trend towards socialized medicine during this period, made increasing demands from the inadequate existing facilities responsible for the long-term care of amputees.

In early 1945 the Surgeon General of the United States requested the National Academy of Sciences to provide guidance to his office regarding the care of thousands of young veterans returning from war. In the same year the National Academy of Sciences established a research development program in cooperation with universities and industrial laboratories (49). Although initial emphasis was on design and development of various components, it was apparent that basic knowledge regarding mechanics and kinesiology was lacking. The Biomechanics Laboratory at the University of California at Berkeley and Los Angeles were established to answer some basic fundamental questions regarding amputees and prosthetics. In 1947 the Department of Veterans Administration in the United States became actively involved in this early effort of research and development by providing funds for research efforts. As these programs grew in scope, the National Academy of Sciences established the Committee on Prosthetics Research and Development which provided guidance and coordinating role through symposia, publication and continuing education courses.

Similar efforts were being made in Canada through the Department of Veterans Affairs and in the early 1960s by establishing research groups in Montreal, Winnipeg, Toronto and New Brunswick. In England, the Limb Fitting Centre at Roehampton was responsible for providing prosthesis to war veterans of the First World War and, with the introduction of the National Health Scheme in 1948, became actively involved in research and development. Subsequently, several centers were established in the United Kingdom including the Dundee Limb Fitting Centre. During this period similar research and development efforts were being carried out in West Germany, Italy, Denmark, Sweden, Russia, Yugoslavia and Poland.

In order to coordinate and disseminate information throughout the world in areas of research development and education, the International Society for Rehabilitation of the Disabled created the Committee on Prosthetics, Braces and Technical Aids in 1951, with Headquarters in Copenhagen. This group with able leadership by Dr. Knud Jansen sponsored several symposia and the first such symposia on prosthetics was held in Copenhagen in 1957. The proceedings of the meeting were published by the Research Board of the National Academy of Sciences in the United States (51). This International Committee established the International Society of Prosthetics and Orthotics (ISPO) in 1970, working in close cooperation with the Rehabilitation International (49). Through its publication and Annual Meeting and sponsored courses, the International Society helped to bring together health professionals from all corners of the globe in sharing their knowledge and expertise regarding the disabled.

Amputation Surgery

The ability of an amputee to function at his highest possible level is dependent to a large extent on the surgeon's skill and knowledge regarding amputation and prosthesis. If the patient undergoes an unnecessary high level of amputation and the residual limb is poorly shaped and painful, even the best prosthetist in the world will not be able to help the patient to achieve a maximum possible functional level. This is more important when dealing with an elderly dysvascular patient.

Immediate Postsurgical Fitting

In 1959 Mazet *et al.* (cited in Ref. 30) studied 1356 leg amputations in patients over 55 years of age and found 90% had above-knee amputation and only 10% were fitted with prosthesis. In 1961 Berlemont *et al.* (3) drew attention to the benefits of immediate postsurgical fitting and Weiss soon emphasized the need for maintenance of neuromuscular pattern in the residual limb. These two basic principles combined with measurement of distal arterial pressure and skin blood flow have brought about revolutionary changes in the rehabilitation potential of all elderly dysvascular amputees who form the largest number among all amputees today.

Burgess *et al.* (6) applied the principles of immediate postsurgical fitting and maintenance of neuromuscular pattern in elderly dysvascular patients with meticulous care of surgical technique and judiciously delayed weight bearing. He proposed that the timing of weight bearing and ambulation be dependent upon the general medical state of the patient and vascularity of the residual limb. When immediate weight bearing was contraindicated, the residual limb was kept immobilized in a plaster cast and a decision regarding weight bearing was made after the first cast change. The main purpose of the application of rigid dressing was to promote wound healing by reducing edema and isolating the surgical wound from external environment. Following this technique, Burgess *et al.* (7) reported results on 177 patients undergoing amputation for vascular insufficiency. A total of 193 amputations of the lower extremities were done and the initial levels were above-knee in 28, below-knee in 157, Syme in 2, and knee disarticulation in 3 patients. The final levels were above-knee in 40, knee disarticulation in 3, below-knee in 145, and Syme in 2 patients. In spite of this overwhelming evidence, the technique has not achieved universal popularity and deleterious effects of the technique has been reported.(9)

Other Forms of Immediate Postoperative Fitting

The immediate postoperative fitting as suggested by Berlemont *et al.* (3), Weiss (48a), and Burgess *et al.* (6) requires application of a plaster cast in the operating room and subsequent attachment of pylon. However, expertise required to carry out such a program may not be available in all hospitals and, also, frequent wound inspection is not possible through a plaster cast. Because of these difficulties, alternative methods have been introduced to achieve the same goals of prompt wound healing and early ambulation.

AIR SPLINT

Little (25) introduced the use of pneumatic weight-bearing prosthesis as an alternative to application of rigid plaster cast in the operating room. The pneumatic prosthesis consisted of an inflatable plastic bag mounted inside an aluminum frame pylon connected to a SACH foot. Eight patients with obliterative vascular disease were fitted with the inflatable plastic bag in the operating room and the bag inflated to 25 mm Hg and maintained for 48 hr. After 48 hr, the dressings were changed and the patients were allowed partial weight bearing with the specially designed pneumatic prosthesis. All patients achieved primary healing. Kerstein (21) and Sher (41) reported similar results with the use of pneumatic long leg splint alone.

In spite of the ease of application and the favorable results, this method so far has not enjoyed the same popularity as the plaster cast application. In our limited experience, leakage, perspiration problems during the summer and limited weight-bearing capability are major drawbacks of this method.

SEMIRIGID DRESSING

Ghiulamila (12) offered an excellent alternative to plaster cast application in the operating room. He used Unna's paste as a compressive bandage to promote healing and to prevent edema in 11 patients with below-knee amputation. After skin closure, a layer of gauze and Telfa is applied. A strip of clean adhesive plastic is applied over the dressing in order to isolate the surgical wound from Unna's paste bandage which is wrapped over the adhesive plastic. After 24 hr, a temporary prosthesis can be applied for weight bearing and progressive ambulation. After 2 weeks the sutures are removed and Unna's paste bandage is reapplied. Four to five weeks after surgery, Unna's paste bandage is discarded and a temporary prosthesis is remolded. The patient is fitted with a permanent prosthesis 2 months after surgery. All patients achieved primary healing and there were no untoward complications recorded. Warren (48) described favorable experience in six patients but used plaster cast over Unna's paste bandage when weight bearing was desired.

CONTROLLED ENVIRONMENT TREATMENT

Redhead and Snowdon (36) at the Biomechanical Research and Development Unit at Roehampton have developed a unique approach to wound healing of extremities called Controlled Environment Treatment (CET). In this approach, the bare residual limb after surgery is placed in a transparent plastic bag which is connected *via* a flexible hose to a console containing an air compressor with controls regulating temperature, humidity, timing and sterility of air sample. This treatment is continued for 24 hr/day until healing is achieved. Since their initial presentation at the First World Congress of ISPO in 1974, several centers in the United Kingdom and the United States of America have favorable results with the technique. Burgess and Pedegana (5) reported their initial experience with CET treatment along with four other centers in the United States. All participating centers had favorable experience with CET treatment. Several advantages of the CET treatment were reported by the participating centers which includes adequate edema control, with uniform pressure, minimal discomfort experienced by the patients, and easy visual inspection and palpation of the wound without disturbing the sterile environment. The major disadvantages were delayed weight bearing, restricted mobility and lack of contouring of the residual limb. The authors recommended further multicenter control trials of the treatment method.

Selection of Amputation Level

The selection of the appropriate level of amputation is guided by various factors which include the patient's ability and potential to use a prosthesis, availability of suitable prosthesis for the selected level and potential for achieving satisfactory stump healing. The surgeon will have to take various factors into consideration but his immediate concern is to achieve satisfactory healing without subjecting the patient to serial amputations. The healing of the stump is of the utmost concern to the surgeon when dealing with an ischemic lower extremity. In the past, decision regarding the specific level was made on the basis of clinical findings regarding the circulatory state of the extremity and arteriography. However, arteriography and presence or absence of peripheral arterial pulse do not provide adequate information about blood flow and healing potential of the involved extremity.

Murdoch (29) asserted that arteriography presents the vascularity at a disadvantage and Burgess *et al.* (7) supported this view. After reviewing 177 patients who had undergone amputation for peripheral vascular disease, Burgess found no correlation between the demonstrated level of obstruction on arteriography and stump healing. Similarly, the presence or absence of popliteal pulse did not have any correlation with healing of below-knee stump.

DISTAL ARTERIAL PRESSURE

Strandness *et al.* (43) emphasized the importance of measurement of distal arterial blood pressure in peripheral vascular disease and Neilsen (31) stressed the reliability of indirect systolic blood pressure measurement using strain gauge technique, and the results were comparable to pressures measured by intraarterial recording. In recent years transcutaneous Doppler ultrasound has been used in measuring arterial pressure along the major arteries in the extremities. This method has gained popularity because of the ease of operation and availability of the instrument in most hospital intensive care units. Wagner (47) reported that healing can be predicted with 90% accuracy when the ischemic index was over 0.35 in patients with arteriosclerosis and over 0.45 in diabetics. He defined ischemic index as a ratio of blood pressure at the selected level of surgery measured by the Doppler method and by arm systolic pressure. Barnes *et al.* (1) reported correlation between systolic blood pressure exceeding 70 mm Hg and healing of below-knee amputation. However, in a later series Barnes and colleagues (2) cautioned that segmental blood pressure measured by Doppler ultrasound is a fallible guide for wound healing at below-knee or foot level. In this series of 122 lower limb amputations, 24% of foot amputations failed to heal with ankle systolic pressure above 60 mm Hg—which has been suggested in the past as the requirement for healing. Similarly, in the below-knee group there was no significant difference in mean systolic pressure between the healed and nonhealed group. Digit photoplethysmography to determine pulsatile flow was found to be more sensitive in predicting healing in foot amputation. Lee (24) found blood flow measurement by electromagnetic flow meter, more accurate in predicting healing of amputation stump than Doppler pressure, especially in patients with severely calcified noncompressible vessels where excessively high Doppler pressure may be encountered in spite of severely reduced blood flow. He found calf flows in excess of 35 ml/min were indicative of probable healing at below-knee level and calf flows in excess of 60 ml/min predicted healing of more distal amputation of foot and toes.

SKIN BLOOD FLOW

Wound healing following amputation is dependent on an adequate blood flow to the skin at the site of amputation. Skin blood flow can be measured by using different forms of ^{133}Xe radioisotope clearance as described initially by Bohr (4) and later by Sejrsen (39). Moore (26) measured skin blood flow using ^{133}Xe clearance in 30 patients undergoing below-knee amputation. He found that three patients having blood flow below 0.6 ml/100 g of tissue/min failed to heal at below-knee level. Holloway and Burgess (18) studied skin blood flow in 26 patients undergoing below-knee amputation by measuring blood flow in both anterior and posterior skin preoperatively and 4 and 8 weeks after amputation. They could not identify a critical flow level below which wound healing would not occur. However, they believed that flows of 1.0 ml/100 g/min or below should be viewed as borderline where healing may not occur or may be very slow. The other interesting finding was that skin flow increased in all patients postoperatively and reached a level equal to that for the normal control group by 8 weeks. They concluded that, in many instances, a nonhealing below-knee stump may heal following local revision after an appropriate delay of 4–8 weeks following the initial surgery. Moore *et al.* (27) in a current series of 45 lower extremity amputations reported a minimum flow of 2.4 ml/100 g/min is required for satisfactory wound healing at below-knee as well as other levels of amputations. Kostiuk and co-workers (22) using an epicutaneous method of ^{133}Xe flow measurement reported a critical value of 1.5 ml/min/100 g of tissue.

It appears that critical value for skin blood flow for stump healing is dependent on various factors, *i.e.* method used, frequency and time of measurement, operative technique, etc.

Besides arterial pressure and skin blood flow measurement, other methods have been described in predicting wound healing following amputation. Holstein and co-workers (19, 20) correlated wound healing with distal skin perfusion pressure. They determined skin perfusion pressure (SPP) as that external counter pressure sufficient to stop washout of radioactive isotope (^{131}I or ^{125}I antipyrine mixed with histamine) injected intradermally. They concluded that SPP measurement is a reliable method in predicting wound healing and pressures below 30 mm Hg are associated with poor healing in both below-knee and above-knee levels.

Infrared thermography provides information regarding temperature distribution in the affected limb. Spence and co-workers (42) reviewed thermograms of 104 patients undergoing amputations and concluded that thermogram is a reliable indicator of the level of amputation. By using a set of criteria (*i.e.*, bilateral temperature assymmetry, analysis of longitudinal thermal gradient and the presence or absence of local hyperthermia) they were able to select a thermographic amputation level with a success rate of 80% at above-knee, through-knee and below-knee level. In the case of partial foot amputation, thermography was less reliable. Out of 22 partial foot amputations, 11 patients achieved primary healing, but thermogram predicted successful amputation only in 5 cases. The authors felt that this inadequency of thermography was related to inflammatory reaction often present in ischemic feet.

In the last 10 years, considerable advancement has been made in applying noninvasive methods for hemodynamic evaluation of an ischemic limb. The healing potential of an amputation stump at a selected level of amputation can be predicted with a fair degree of preciseness when the surgeon's clinical judgement is augmented by information regarding distal arterial pressure, skin perfusion pressure and skin blood flow. The ultimate aim still remains the achievement of healing at the lowest possible level without subjecting the patient to multiple unnecessary surgical procedures.

PERMANENTLY ATTACHED PROSTHESIS

The amputee's ability to walk with a lower extremity prosthesis is dependent on the comfort of socket fit. The difficulties encountered by the prosthetist in providing a comfortable socket fit can be reduced significantly if the pylon can be attached to a permanently implanted obturator. Hall and Mallow (15) and their co-workers at Southwest Research Institute in Texas, have done considerable animal work by implanting an intramedullary rod attached to percutaneous load-bearing skeletal extension (PLSE) in Spanish goats. Several Proplast- and velour-coated prostheses have lasted up to 12 months without any adverse effect. In the initial phases of the experiments, they used bone cement as an anchoring material for stabilizing the intramedullary rod. But recently (16) sintered titanium fiber-coated intramedullary rods have been used with reasonable success. Similar animal experiments have been carried out by Fernie and co-workers (10) in Toronto using pigs as models. The major difficulties still remain with adequate bonding of the intramedullary prosthesis to bone and creation of a permanent seal between skin and protruding obturator.

LIMB PROSTHETICS

The introduction of four basic socket types for Syme, below-knee, above-knee and hip disarticulation amputation in the mid-1950s brought about a major change in lower extremity prosthetic fitting. Since then, major developments in lower extremity prosthetics have been in application of newer plastic material for socket fabrication and design of newer components, especially various types of knee units. In upper extremity prosthetics, the most notable developments have been in the area of powered prostheses.

LOWER EXTREMITY SOCKETS

Since its introduction in 1955, the quadrilateral socket still remains the most universally used socket for above-knee amputation. The socket was designed on the basis of sound biomechanical principles, and casting and alignment technique of the socket is well standardized so that similar fitting procedure is followed by all well trained prosthetists.

TOTAL SURFACE-BEARING SELF-SUSPENDING ABOVE-KNEE SOCKETS

Redhead (35) at the Biomechanical Research and Development Unit at Roehampton, England, has designed a new type of above-knee socket with total surface support rather than primary weight bearing on ischial tuberosity. The basic principle in fabrication of the socket requires that the stump be stretched distally, making the stump longer and thinner. This is achieved by fitting with a "compliant socket" made from a sleeve of elasticized material, and the distorted shape is then fixed by applying a plaster of Paris bandage. Extensive testing has been carried out regarding weight-bearing characteristics of the socket by placing pressure transducers at strategic locations on the stump socket interface. This socket has been available for routine use in England since 1974. It appears that this type of socket may be indicated in patients who are unable to tolerate significant weight bearing at the brim and ischial tuberosity.

BELOW-KNEE SOCKETS

The fitting of below-knee amputees with patellar tendon bearing (PTB) socket has become universal since its introduction by Radcliffe and coworkers in 1958. In spite of its universal use, some patients experience difficulty in using a PTB socket. Various attempts have been made to improve suspension system and comfort of socket fit, although the basic design of the socket has remained unchanged. The PTS (Pierquin 1964, cited in Ref. 13) and Kondylen Betrung Münster (KBM) (Kuhn 1966, cited in Ref. 13) sockets are two examples of modified PTB sockets for better suspension. Both sockets are self-suspending over the femoral condyles and provide additional mediolateral stability. Although both sockets can be used by many below-knee amputees, patients with short stumps, with or without mediolateral instability of the knee, are ideal candidates for PTS or KBM sockets. Other methods of improving suspension are elastic rubber sleeve suspension and PTB suction socket. Elastic rubber sleeve suspension can be added to any PTB socket or its variant and reduces pistoning of the stump into the socket. It also creates negative pressure inside the socket during swing phase providing suction effect. This method was developed at the University of Michigan Medical Center in Ann Arbor by Chino and coworkers (8). The authors had extensive experience with this system using a PTB socket with silicone gel liner.

The PTB suction socket was designed by Grevsten and Marsh (13, 14) at

Upsala University in Sweden. The prosthesis was initially designed for below-knee amputees who experience recurrent skin irritation and ulceration. The criteria for using suction socket are stumps longer than 125 mm and the presence of a reasonable amount of soft tissue.

ULTRALIGHT BELOW-KNEE PROSTHESIS

A below-knee prosthesis with PTB socket supracondylar cuff suspension made of laminated plastic weighs much less than the amputated limb, but many elderly amputees find them heavy and difficult to maneuver. Wilson (50) at the Moss Rehabilitation Hospital (1976) has developed a light weight below-knee prosthesis made of a polypropylene sheet. The prosthesis consists of an inner socket of PTS type, an outer shank and molded foot, and a sole and heel section (Fig. 14.1). The prosthesis weighs 60% less than standard below-knee prosthesis. The initial acceptance by patients has been quite favorable.

SYME SOCKETS

Canadian Syme prosthesis is universally used for fitting of Syme amputation. Efforts have been made to reduce breakage and also provide better ankle and foot action. Winnipeg Syme prosthesis was developed in Winnipeg, Canada, with cut-outs on medial and lateral walls and a specially

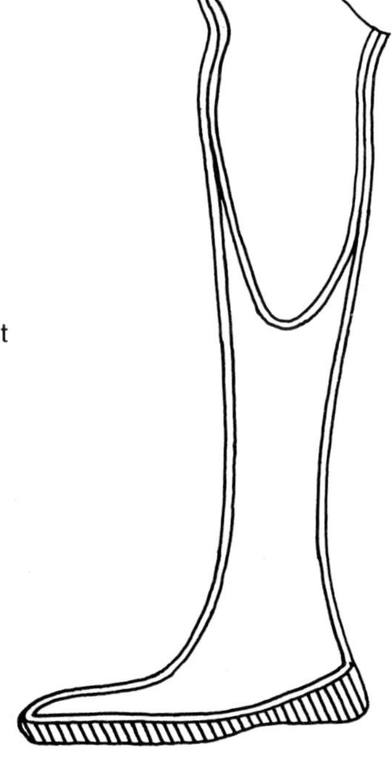

Fig. 14.1. Moss Rehabilitation Hospital ultralight below-knee prosthesis.

designed foot to provide more flexibility. The amputee dons the prothesis from the top. The stump should have well trimmed malleoli and the amputee should be able to tolerate end bearing. Ricci and Gabourie (37) have designed a polypropylene Syme prosthesis which weighs one-third to one-half of the standard Canadian Syme prosthesis. The prosthesis consists of a polypropylene socket with front fenestration attached to a custom-made foot with heel and sole cushion, rubber toe cap and foam-filled keel (Figs. 14.2 and 14.3). If the residual limb is bulbous, a pelite pad is added over the medial aspect. The prosthesis is durable, light, and patients prefer the smooth ankle action.

COMPONENTS

Since the early days of prosthetic fitting, efforts have been made to design various artificial joints so that they simulate normal anatomical joint action as much as possible. In the past, most above-knee amputees have been fitted with prostheses consisting of single axis knee joint with built in friction system to control swing phase. However, the anatomical knee is polycentric with varying friction depending on cadence.

Knee Joints

In order to provide increased stability in stance phase and increased knee flexion during swing phase, various polycentric knee units have been used

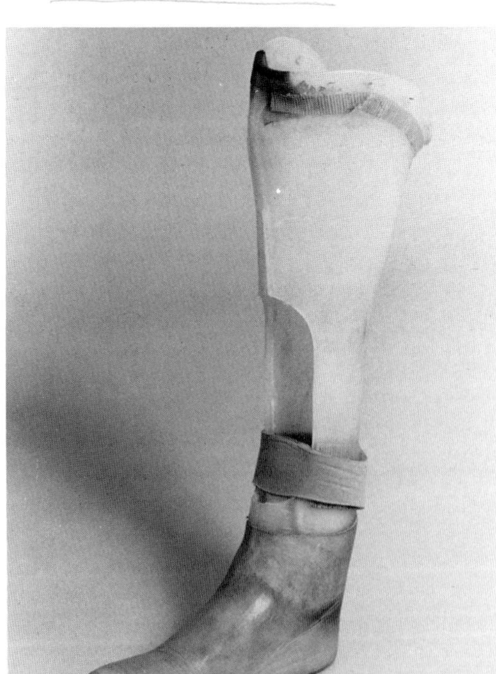

Fig. 14.2. Lightweight polypropylene Syme prosthesis designed by Ricci and Gabourie (37).

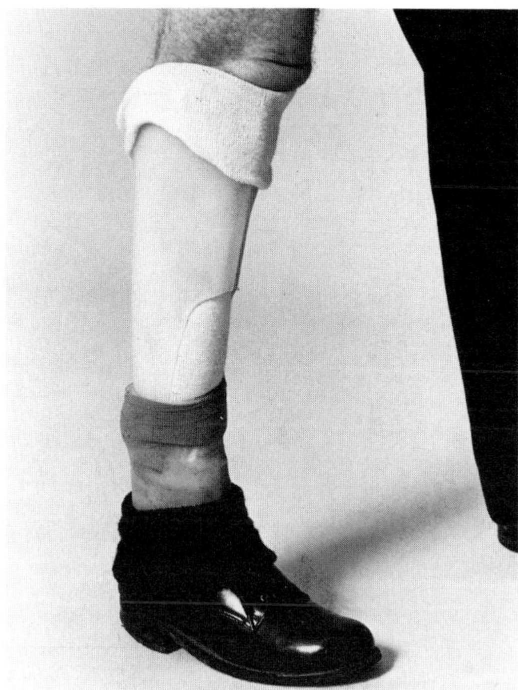

Fig. 14.3. Lightweight polypropylene Syme prosthesis, design by Ricci and Gabourie (37), in use.

in the past. Radcliffe (34) has pointed out that prosthetic knee stability is dependent on interaction of several variables which include muscle moment around the hip joint generated by the amputee, knee moment created by friction system in the artificial knee, length and load of the prosthesis, the vertical height of the instantaneous center of knee rotation of knee unit, and the distance of center of rotation from hip/heel line. The UCBL four-bar linkage knee (Fig. 14.4) was designed taking into consideration these variables so that the instantaneous center of knee rotation stays high during the first 10° of knee flexion, providing the amputee with knee stability when the stability is disturbed accidentally. By keeping the knee center high, it has been possible to have the center of rotation of the knee in front of the hip/heel line at the end of stance phase, which allows the amputee to have better control and stability of the knee. A pneumatic swing control system can be added to the unit to provide better control of swing phase. Based on similar principles, a six-bar linkage knee has been designed by the Biomechanics Laboratory of the University of California at Berkeley, suitable for knee disarticulation amputees (Fig. 14.5).

Swing Phase Control

The major objectives of a swing phase control system is to simulate action of the quadriceps and hamstring muscles in order to provide smooth flexion and extension during swing phase. It also should automatically change the

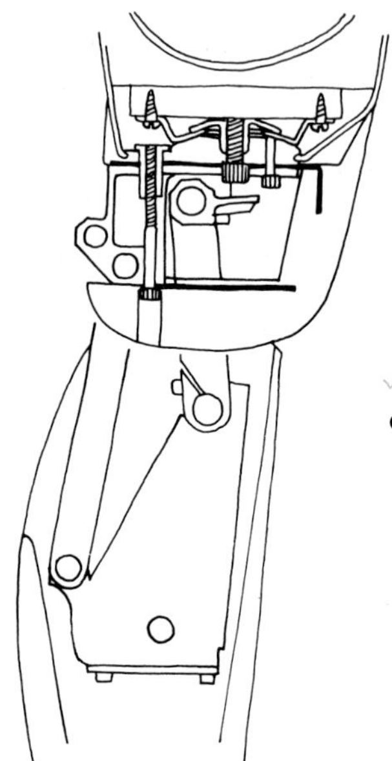

Fig. 14.4. University of California Biomechanics Laboratory (UCBL) four-bar linkage knee unit.

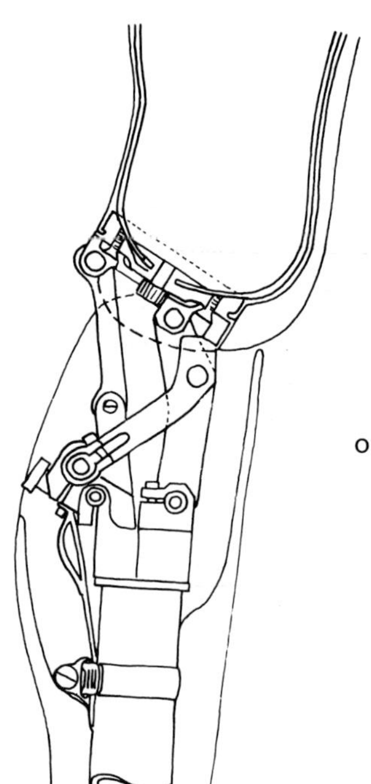

Fig. 14.5. University of California Biomechanics Laboratory (UCBL) six-bar linkage knee unit.

resistance pattern with varying cadence. A hydraulic cylinder with multiple holes in the wall of the cylinder can offer the above functions by reducing the available flow by movement of the piston.

The SNS Mauch hydraulic swing phase control system (Fig. 14.6) manufactured by Mauch Laboratories of Dayton, Ohio, has undergone fairly extensive clinical trials and is suitable for young athletic type above-knee amputees. In this unit, stance and swing control mechanism can operate simultaneously or independently, depending on the amputee's need. For example, an amputee is able to go down the stairs step-over-step and the stance control system will provide resistance to knee flexion. However, during bicycling, the amputee can disengage the stance control system in order to achieve free knee flexion. The unit is equipped with a selector switch which allows the amputee to lock the knee when desired.

Ankle and Foot

The SACH foot is universally used for lower extremity amputees, but, because of very limited movement in the mediolateral plane, the amputee finds it difficult to walk on rough terrain. The Greissinger multiaxial foot, manufactured by Otto Bock Company, allows dorsal and plantar flexion, as well as movements simulating eversion and inversion (Fig. 14.7).

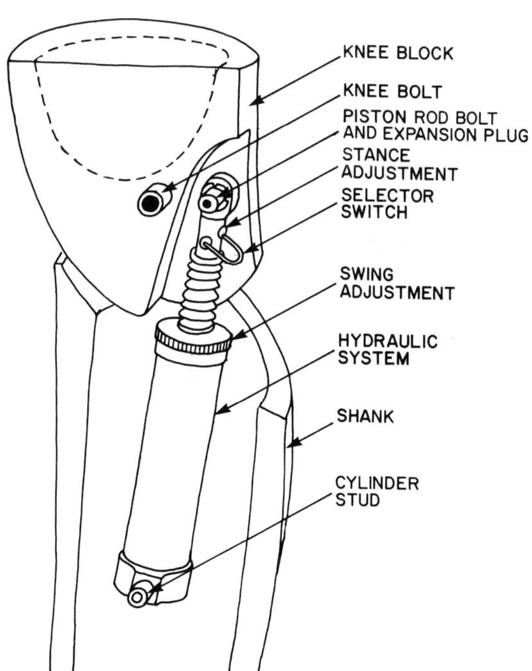

Fig. 14.6. SNS Mauch hydraulic stance and swing phase control.

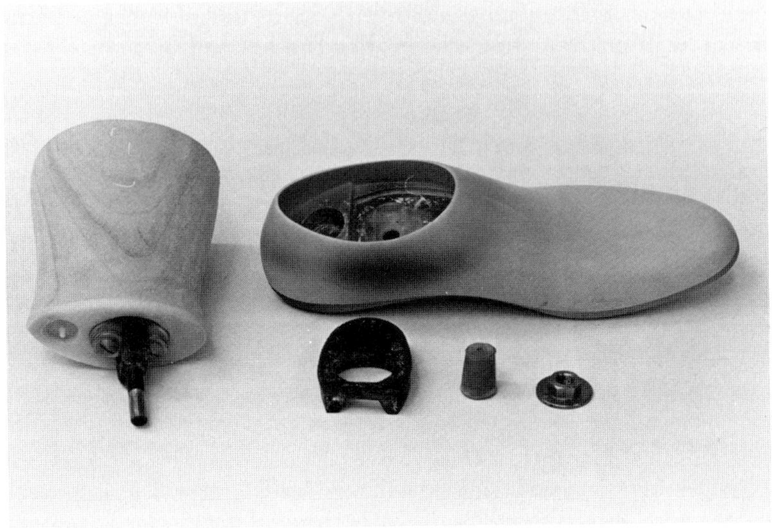

Fig. 14.7. Greissinger multiaxial foot.

MODULAR PROSTHESIS

With the advent of early postoperative fitting, the need for modular system as the initial prosthesis has increased, especially at the above-knee level. The modular system has been used in the United States since the 1950s, although, Foort (11) and associates in Winnipeg, Canada, were the first to carry out extensive clinical trials. Since then, several systems have been available in the market—*i.e.*, Hosmer, U. S. Manufacturing, Blatchford, and Otto Bock. The Blatchford and Otto Bock systems have the added advantage of alignment device incorporated in the prosthesis. Although the above-knee modular system is used more frequently than the below-knee system, it appears that, with further improvement in the systems regarding fit and durability, more amputees will be fitted with modular prosthesis in the future. The University of California Biomechanics Laboratory in Berkeley, has designed a new below-knee modular prosthesis (17) (Fig. 14.8). The prosthesis consists of a plastic shell on which the socket is mounted. An aluminum adapter connects the socket to the pylon and the UCBL metal keel SACH foot. A spherical coupler between the plastic shell and pylon allows ±5° of alignment change. The unit is covered with a polyethylene foam cover. The system is currently undergoing clinical trial.

UPPER EXTREMITY PROSTHETICS

The developments in upper extremity prosthetics have been rather slow, possibly due to a relatively small number of patients, also, most unilateral upper extremity amputees are able to function independently without the aid of a prosthesis.

EXTERNALLY POWERED PROSTHESIS

The most significant development in upper extremity prosthetics in the last 20 years has been in the area of externally powered prosthesis, possibly triggered by the thalidomide tragedy. Through the years, various types of power source and control systems have been used, but battery-powered myoelectrically controlled prosthesis, or a similar system, functions quite satisfactorily. However, for short below-elbow amputations or amputations at a higher level, the University of New Brunswick (UNB) three-state myoelectric control may be more suitable because of the reduced number of control sites. In a recent clinical evaluation (32), nine patients with very short below-elbow stumps, were fitted with a self-suspending Munster socket and an Otto Bock hand with three-state UNB myoelectric control. The patients were found to be unsuitable for the standard Otto Bock control system, because of the unavailability of two interference-free control sites in residual forearm. The patients' acceptance was 100% and the major disadvantage cited by patients was the lack of feedback regarding pinch force.

Externally Powered Hook

Amputees using conventional prosthesis can achieve a higher functional level and dexterity with a hook, rather than a mechanical hand. Therefore,

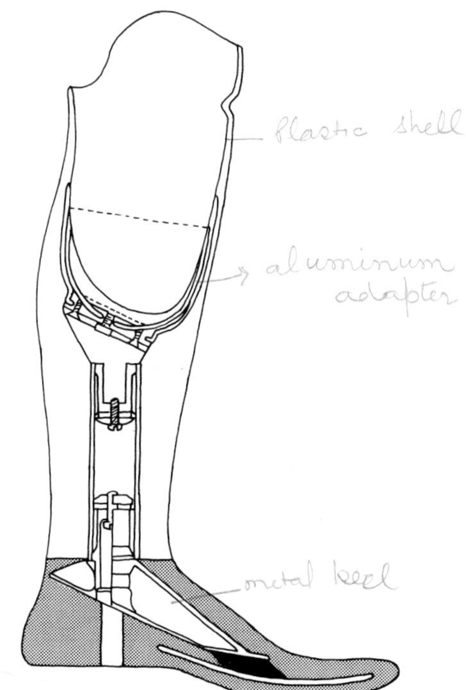

Fig. 14.8. University of California Biomechanics Laboratory (UCBL) modular below-knee prosthesis.

it is expected that an externally powered hook will be more functional than a hand. However, at present a reliably powered hook is not available for day-to-day use in a clinic setting. The Michigan external power system for Hossmer-Dorrance 10X and 10P hooks is available (Fig. 5.47 Chapter 5) but extensive clinical trials with this system have not been done.

Northwestern University, Prosthetics Research Laboratory has designed an interchangeable powered hook (44) and hand and there have been several modifications of the initial design of 1976. The so-called synergetic hook is capable of generating pinch force of 25 lb and has a closing time of 350 msec from full open position. The system has undergone limited clinic trials and patient response has been favorable (45).

Upper Extremity Prosthesis with Sensory Feedback

Normal hand function is dependent on both motor and sensory control. An artificial hand replaces parts of motor function, but the amputee loses tactile and proprioceptive feedback in order to control grasp or pinch force. Efforts have been made to provide sensory feedback to the amputee regarding pinch force by implanting a strain gauge in the index finger of an Otto Bock electrically powered hand (40). The output from the strain gauge which is proportional to pinch force, activates the stimulus generator. The stimulus generator delivers an electrical pulse to the stump lasting 10 msec. A slow pulse (1/sec) indicates weak pinch and a faster pulse (10/sec) strong grasp.

A more sophisticated system to provide supplemental sensory feedback regarding grasp force and hand opening, has been developed at the University of California in Los Angeles (33). The system used a Veterans Administration/Northwestern University (VA/NU) myoelectric hand fitted with a strain gauge to measure grasp force and a potentiometer to measure hand opening. The feedback is provided through two stimulating concentric silver electrodes placed around the residual forearm.

It is apparent that supplementary sensory feedback will be helpful to an upper extremity amputee in order to achieve better control of the operation of the terminal device. At present, no system is available for routine use in clinics. More experimental work is needed in this area.

Conclusions

During the post-World War II period considerable advancement occurred in amputation surgery and limb prosthetics. However, there are still many areas in limb prosthetics that deserve further work. The Rehabilitation Services Administration in the United States of America sponsored a series of workshops entitled "The Current Status of Prosthetics and Orthotics and Trends of Future Research and Development" and the last workshop was held in Miami, Florida in April 1977. The recommendations of the panel on upper and lower extremity prosthetics identified several areas on which future work is needed. In upper extremity prosthetics (23), the need for better packaging (improved material for cosmetic gloves, self-suspension, self-containment and general aesthetics) and commerical availability of better components for high bilateral amputees were recommended. In lower extremity prosthetics (28), the need for better knee and ankle joints and lighter durable modular components, was identified. The concluding remarks of the co-chairmen of the workshops, "It is obvious that much has been achieved over the past few years, but it is equally as obvious that we still have a long way to go" are still valid today.

This brief summary may reflect the author's bias towards applicability of new technology in day-to-day patient care. Many areas of basic research, as well as many innovative techniques and components, have not been discussed, because of the constraints of space. However, continuing work in both basic research and application of new technology to patient care are essential for improvement in the quality of care of all amputees.

REFERENCES

1. Barnes, R. W., Shanik, G. D., and Slaymaker, E. E. An Index of Healing in Below-Knee Amputation; Leg Blood Pressure by Doppler Ultrasound. *Surgery, 79:* 13–18, 1976.
2. Barnes, R. W., Thornhill, B., Nix, L., Rittgers, S. E., and Turley, G. Prediction of Amputation Wound Healing. Roles of Doppler Ultrasound and Digit Photoplethysmorgraphy. *Arch. Surg., 116:* 80–83, 1981.
3. Berlemont, M., Weber, R., and Willot, J. P. Ten Years of Experience with the Immediate Application of Prosthetic Devices to amputees of the Lower Extremities on the Operating Table. *Prosthet. Int., 3:* 8–18, 1969.
4. Bohr, H. Measurement of the Blood Flow in the Skin with Radioactive Xenon. *Scand. J. Clin. Lab. Invest.,* Suppl. 99, *19:* 60, 1967.
5. Burgess, E. M., and Pedegana, L. R. Controlled Environment Treatment for Limb Surgery and Trauma. (A Preliminary Report) *Bull. Prosthet. Res., 10-28:* 16–57, 1977.
6. Burgess, E. M., Romano, R. L., and Zettle, J. H. Amputation Management Utilizing Immediate Postsurgical Prosthetic Fitting. *Prosthet. Int., 3:* 28–37, 1969.
7. Burgess, E. M., Romano, R. L., Zettl, J. H., and Schrock, R. D. Amputations of the Leg for Peripheral Vascular Insufficiency. *J. Bone Jt. Surg. 53A:* 874–890, 1971.
8. Chino, N., Pearson, J. R., Cockrell, J. L., Mikishko, H. A., and Koepke, G. H. Negative Pressure During Swing Phase in Below-Knee Prostheses with Rubber Sleeve Suspension. *Arch. Phys. Med. Rehabil., 56:* 22–26, 1975.
9. Cohen, S. I., Goldman, L. D., Salzman, E. W., and Glotzer, D. J. The Deleterious Effect of Immediate Postoperative Prosthesis in Below-Knee Amputation for Ischemic Disease. *Surgery, 76:* 992–1001, 1974.
10. Fernie, G. R., Kostiuk, J. P., Lobb, R. J., Pillar, R. M., Wong, E., and Binnington, A. G. *J. Biomed. Mater. Res., 2:* 883–891, 1977.
11. Foort, J. Modular Prosthetics—A Philosophical View. *Prosthet. Orthot. Int., 3:* 140–143, 1979.
12. Ghiulamila, R. I. Semirigid Dressing for Postoperative Fitting of Below-Knee Prosthesis. *Arch. Phys. Med. Rehabil., 53:* 186–192, 1972.
13. Grevsten, S. Ideas on the Suspension of the Below-Knee Prosthesis. *Prosthet. Orthot. Int., 2:* 3–7, 1978.
14. Grevsten, S., and Marsh, L. Suction Type Prosthesis for Below-Knee Amputees. A Preliminary Report. *Artif. Limbs, 15:* 78–80, 1971.

15. Hall, C. W., and Mallow, W. H. Permanently Attached Artificial Limbs. *Bull. Prosthet. Res. 10-31:* 136–145, 1979.
16. Hall, C. W., and Rostoker, W. Permanently Attached Artificial Limbs. *Bull. Prosthet. Res. 10-34:* 98–100, 1980.
17. Hoagland, F. T., Jergesen, E., Radcliffe, C. W., Lamoreaux, L. W., Cunningham, D. M., and Stout, G. Modular below-knee Prosthesis. *Bull. Prosthet. Res., 10-34:* 87, 1980.
18. Holloway, Jr., G. A., and Burgess, E. M. Cutaneous Blood Flow and its Relation to Healing of Below-Knee Amputation. *Surg. Gynecol. Obstet. 146:* 750–756, 1978.
19. Holstein, P., Dovey, H., and Lassen, N. A. Wound Healing in Above-Knee Amputations in Relation to Skin Perfusion Pressure. *Acta. Orthop. Scand., 50:* 59–66, 1979.
20. Holstein, P., Sager, P., and Lassen, N. A. Wound Healing in Below-Knee Amputations in Relation to Skin Perfusion Pressure. *Acta. Orthop. Scand., 50:* 49–58, 1979.
21. Kerstein, M. D. Utilization of an Air Splint after Below-Knee Amputation. *Am. J. Phys. Med., 53:* 119–126, 1974.
22. Kostiuk, J. P., Wood, D., and Hornby, R. The Measurement of Skin Blood Flow in Peripheral Vascular Disease by Epicutaneous Application of ^{133}Xeon. *J. Bone Jt. Surg., 58:* 833, 1976.
23. LeBlanc, A. Upper Limb Prosthetics—Current Status and Future Needs. *Orthot. Prosthet., 31:* 6–9, 1977.
24. Lee, B. Y., Trainor, F. S., Kavner, D., McCann, W. J., and Madden, J. L. Noninvasive Hemodynamic Evaluation in Selection of Amputation Level. *Surg. Gynecol. Obstet. 149:* 241–244, 1979.
25. Little, J. M. A Pneumatic Weight Bearing Temporary Prosthesis for Below-Knee Amputees. *Lancet, 1:* 271–273, 1971.
26. Moore, W. S. Determination of Amputation Level. Measurement of Skin Blood Flow with Xenon 133. *Arch. Surg., 107:* 798–802, 1973.
27. Moore, W. S., Henry, R. E., Malone, J. M., Daley, M. J., Patton, D., and Childers, S. J. Prospective Use of Xenon 133 Clearance for Amputation Level Selection. *Arch. Surg., 116:* 86–88, 1981.
28. Muilenburg, A. The Current Status and Future Needs in Lower Limb Prosthetics. *Orthot. Prosthet., 31:* 10–13, 1977.
29. Murdoch, G. Levels of Amputation and Limiting Factors. *Ann. R. Coll. Surg. Engl., 40:* 204–216, 1967.
30. Murdoch, G. Research and Development within Surgical Amputee Management. *Acta Orthop. Scand., 46:* 526–547, 1975.
31. Nielsen, P. E. Digital Blood Pressure in Patients with Peripheral Arterial Disease. *Scand. J. Clin. Lab. Invest., 36:* 731–737, 1976.
32. Paciga, J. E., Gibson, D. A., Gillespie, R., and Scott, R. N. Clinical Evaluation of UNB 3-State Myoelectric Control for Arm Prostheses. *Bull. Prosthet. Res., 10-34:* 21–33, 1980.
33. Prior, R. E., Lyman, J., Case, P. A., and Scott, C. M. Supplemental Sensory Feedback for the VA/NU Myoelectric Hand. *Bull. Prosthet. Res., 10-26:* 170–191, 1976.
34. Radcliffe, C. W. The Knud Jansen Lecture. Above-Knee Prosthetics. *Prosthet. Orthot. Int., 1:* 146–160, 1977.
34a. Radcliffe, C. W., and Foort, J. *The Patellar Tendon Bearing Prosthesis.* Biomechanics Laboratory University of California, Berkeley and San Francisco, 1961.
35. Redhead, R. G. Total Surface Bearing Self-Suspending Above-Knee Sockets. *Prosthet. Orthot. Int., 3:* 126–136, 1979.
36. Redhead, R. G., and Snowdon, C. A New Approach to the Management of Wounds of the Extremities. Controlled Environment Treatment and its Derivatives. *Prosthet. Orthot. Int., 2:* 148–156, 1978.
37. Ricci, J., and Gabourie, R. Polypropylene Symes Prosthesis. *Orthotics Prosthet., 2:* 21–22, 1979.
38. Sarmiento, A., May, B. J., Sinclair, W. F., Newton, C. P., McCoulough III, N. C.,

AND WILLIAMS, E. M. Lower-Extremity Amputation—The Impact of Immediate Postsurgical Prosthetic Fitting. *Clin. Orthop. Rela. Res., 68:* 22–31, 1970.

39. SEJRSEN, P. Cutaneous Blood Flow in Man Studied by Freely Diffusible Radioactive Indicators. *Scand. J. Clin. Lab. Inves.,* Suppl. 99, *19:* 52, 1967.
40. SHANNON, G. F., AND AGNEW, P. J. Fitting Below-Elbow Prostheses Which Convey a Sense of Touch. *Med. J. Aust., 1:* 242–244, 1979.
41. SHER, M. H. The Air Splint—An Alternative to the Immediate Postoperative Prosthesis. *Arch. Surg., 108:* 746–747, 1974.
42. SPENCE, V. A., WALKER, W. F., TROUP, I. M., AND MURDOCH, G. Amputation of the Ischemic Limb: Selection of the Optimum Site by Thermography. *Angiology, 32:* 155–169, 1981.
43. STRANDNESS, JR., D. E., RADKE, H. M., AND BELL, J. W. Use of new Simplified Plethysmorgraph in the Clinical Evaluation of Patients with Arteriosclerosis Obliterans. *Surg. Gynecol. Obst., 112:* 751–756, 1961.
44. THOMPSON, R. G., AND CHILDRESS, D. S. *Bull. Prosthet. Res., 10-26:* 285, 1976.
45. THOMPSON, R. G., AND CHILDRESS, D. S. Synergetic Hook and Hand. *Bull. Prosthet. Res., 10-27:* 127–128, 1977.
46. WAGNER, JR., F. W. Orthopedic Rehabilitation of the Dysvascular Lower Limb. *Orthop. Clin. North Am., 9:* 325–350, 1978.
47. WAGNER, JR., F. W. Transcutaneous Doppler Ultrasound in the Prediction of Healing and the Selection of Surgical Level for Dysvascular Lesions of the Toes and Forefoot. *Clin. Orthop. Relat. Res., 142:* 110–114, 1979.
48. WARREN, R. Amputations in the lower limb. *Surg. Annu., 7:* 331–346, 1975.

48a. WEISS, M. Physiologic amputation, immediate prosthesis and early ambulation. *Prosthet. Int. 3:* 38–44, 1969.

49. WILSON, JR., A. B. The Modern History of Amputation Surgery and Artificial Limbs. *Orthop. Clin. North Am., 3:* 267–285, 1972.
50. WILSON, JR., A. B. Ultralight Below-Knee Prosthesis. *Bull. Prosthet. Res. 10-27:* 176–179, 1977.
51. WILSON, D. V. International Prosthetics and the International Society for the Welfare of Cripples. *Prosthet. Int.,* pp. 7–10, (Copenhagen) 1960.

Index